Current Topics in Microbiology 222 and Immunology

Springer-Verlag Berlin Heidelberg GmbH

Reproductive Immunology

Edited by L.B. Olding

With 17 Figures and 10 Tables

Springer

Professor LARS B. OLDING, M.D., Ph.D.

Department of Immunology, Microbiology,
Pathology and Infectious Diseases
Karolinska Institute
Division of Pathology, F42
Huddinge University Hospital
S-141 86 Huddinge
Sweden

Cover illustration: "The human fetus in the uterus". Pencil-drawing by Leonardo Da Vinci around 1510. Royal Library, Windsor Castle.

Cover design: Design & Production GmbH, Heidelberg

ISSN 0070-217X

ISBN 978-3-642-64475-7 ISBN 978-3-642-60614-4 (eBook)
DOI 10.1007/978-3-642-60614-4

Library of Congress Catalog Card Number 15-12910

Typesetting: Scientific Publishing Services (P) Ltd, Madras

SPIN: 10485040 27/3020/SPS – 5 4 3 2 1 0 – Printed on acid-free paper

Foreword

Discrimination of self from nonself is the major function of the immune system and understanding the mechanism(s) involved a main employer of immunologists. Hence, the age-old puzzle of why a fetus that contains a panel of major histocompatibility (MHC) antigens derived from its mother and its father is not rejected (spontaneously aborted) by lymphocytes from its mother who should theoretically recognize foreign MHC molecules from the father has remained of great interest. This dilemma has enticed immunologists and developmental biologists for many years.

This volume was created to present the information currently on hand in this subject to the scientific public. The guest editor, Professor Lars Olding, has a long and distinguished history of contributions in this field, having been one of the main proponents of the argument that lymphocytes from the fetus play an active role in this process by suppressing lymphocytes from the mother from proliferating and thereby acting as killer cells. His work has defined the phenomenon and identified suppressor molecules (factors) involved in the process. In a different but related chapter, Margareta Unander extends such observations to the clinical study of women with repeated "habitual" miscarriages.

But, in addition, there is the topography associated with maternal–fetal lymphoid cell interactions. Knowledge of the structural basis of the human placenta, and the immunobiology of the decidua and of trophoblasts are important issues for solving the puzzle. Information in these areas is supplied by several experts who have contributions in this line of research including Drs. Faulk, Clark, and Redline. To round out this volume, other contributors (Drs. Adinolfi, Chaouat, Menu, Papadogiannakis, Goldman, and Goldblum) discuss trafficking of leukocytes, other issues of T-cell reactivity in the fetus, newborn or mother, and antigen presentation in specialized cells at the maternal–fetal interface.

The lessons to be learned from study of the immunobiology of maternal–fetal interactions are not only important for the area of normal birth and spontaneous miscarriages, but have the potential to provide both understanding and development of pharmacological approaches to enhance successful transplantation and gene therapy.

La Jolla, California MICHAEL B.A. OLDSTONE

Preface

Reproductive immunology encompasses virtually all facets of modern immunobiology; accordingly, a complete review would be encyclopedic. Therefore, this volume includes only selected topics in recent research, older investigations of relevance, and topics which have been to some extent ignored by the international community of scientists in the field.

Recent progress in immunogenetics that sheds light on the major histocompatibility complex (MHC) antigens on trophoblasts, particularly the unique HLA-G antigen on invading "frontier" trophoblasts, is reviewed by Drs. Ober and van der Ven. They also elucidate the old and controversial question of whether parental sharing of one or more HLA antigen compromises gestation, a subject that has been studied in a secluded religious sect. Modern aspects of the human placental structure associated with strictly defined immune cells are then reviewed by Dr. Redline. Next, the decidua and its occupancy by bone-marrow-derived cells with strong immunological potency are thoroughly discussed by Drs. Arck and Clark. Immunomodulation of these cells is crucial for successful implantation of the blastocyst. The important problem of the ontogeny, differentiation, and maturation of fetal immunity is discussed at length by Dr. Adinolfi in terms of both the natural and acquired states. Drs Chaouat and Menu subsequently provide an overview of maternal T-cell reactivity, which is important for the recognition of fetal antigens, as shown in vitro and in animal experiments. The ability of the trophoblast to evade recognition, destruction, and rejection by maternal cytotoxic immune cells is the topic reviewed by Drs. Torrey, McIntyre, and Faulk. They propose that protection might be delivered by "blocking antibody" raised against an antigen common to both trophoblasts and lymphocytes. This observation, although controversial, has attracted great interest. The extent and possible importance of leakage of fetal leukocytes into the maternal circulation within the placenta – and perhaps in the opposite direction as well – is the controversial issue detailed in the chapter by Dr. Papadogiannakis. The importance of nonspecific suppressor-T-cell activity in cord blood, prostaglandins, and alpha-fetoproteins in modulating maternal–fetal immune reactions is the subject of a chapter written by Drs. Olding, Papadogiannakis, Barbieri, and Murgita. New aspects of functional suppressor cells and of the genuine immunomodulatory potency of prostaglandins and alpha-fetoproteins are emphasized.

Despite the mass of new information on reproductive immunobiology during the last three decades, few clinical applications have emerged. The difficulty in extrapolating results from experiments with animals or from in vitro investigations to the conditions of human pregnancy is obvious. Rarely can one study immunological events in vivo at the maternal–fetal interface in the human placenta, and laboratory animals differ too greatly in structure and function from humans for ready application of research outcomes. However, one clinical application is reviewed here by Dr. Unander: the treatment of women who have normal fertility but repeatedly undergo spontaneous (chronic or "habitual") abortions, with leukocyte transfusions that produce the missing blocking antibodies. This kind of treatment is the subject of much controversy, but can apparently be successful. It is a well-known phenomenon that mothers continue to protect their babies after birth by means of antibodies transferred in breast milk. Less well known is that maternal immune cells in this milk might actually penetrate the barrier of the newborn's gut, as reviewed by Drs. Goldman and Goldblume in the chapter that concludes this volume.

I am indebted to the authors for their great efforts in preparing their reviews and to the publishers for their kind cooperation and skill.

Stockholm, April 1997 LARS B. OLDING

List of Contents

List of Contributors

(Their addresses can be found at the beginning of their respective chapters.)

Immunogenetics of Reproduction: An Overview

C. Ober[1] and K. van der Ven[2]

1 Introduction

The survival of allografts in mammals is influenced by genes of the major histocompatibility complex (MHC); in humans incompatibility with respect to HLA genes is associated with rapid rejection of foreign tissues (van Rood and Claas 1990; Ratner et al. 1991). A notable exception is pregnancy, during which allogeneic (fetal) tissues escape rejection. The immunologically privileged nature of the fetal allograft was first noted by Medawar in 1953, and maternal tolerance of an allogeneic fetus is a paradox that remains a central theme in reproductive immunological research today.

Paradigms from transplantation immunology have provided models for investigating the maternal-fetal relationship, both with respect to the influence of maternal-fetal HLA compatibility on pregnancy outcome (reviewed below) and the development of treatments for the prevention of fetal loss (Sollinger et al. 1984; Beer et al. 1981; Taylor and Faulk 1981). However, important differences between fetal allografts and tissue grafts have come to light in recent years, particularly

[1]Department of Obstetrics and Gynecology, MC2050, University of Chicago, 5841 Maryland Avenue, Chicago, IL 60637, USA
[2]University of Bonn, Department of Obstetrics and Gynecology, Sigmund Freud Str. 25, 53105 Bonn-Venusberg, Germany

with discovery of the absence of classical HLA antigens on fetal tissues that are in contact with maternal tissues during pregnancy (Galbraith et al. 1981; Faulk et al. 1982; Johnson and Stern 1986; Sunderland et al. 1981b). Instead, a novel HLA gene, *HLA-G* is expressed at the maternal-fetal interface (Chumbley et al. 1994; Ellis et al. 1990; Kovats et al. 1990; Sunderland et al. 1981a; Yelavarthi et al. 1991). *HLA-G* has many unique properties in addition to its tissue distribution, which may effectively modulate maternal tolerance during pregnancy (Hunt and Orr 1992; Schmidt and Orr 1993; Loke and King 1991; Colbern and Main 1991). However, the function of this unique HLA gene is still largely unknown.

This chapter provides an overview of the genetics of the HLA complex, including a description of the novel gene *HLA-G* and a review of studies evaluating the relationship between maternal-fetal compatibility and pregnancy outcome.

2 The Major Histocompatibility Complex in Humans

The human MHC includes a cluster of genes located on chromosome 6p21 that control cell-cell interactions and regulate immune responses. The MHC is divided into three regions, called the class I, class II, and class III regions (Fig. 1). Although the MHC is one of the most extensively studied regions in the human genome, the exact number and function of many of its genes are still not known.

The class I region is the largest of the three regions, stretching over approximately 2×10^6 bp (Geraghty et al. 1992b; Le Bouteillier 1994). Class I HLA molecules are composed of a transmembrane glycoprotein encoded by MHC genes on chromosome 6 and an associated β_2-microglobulin encoded by a gene on chromosome 15. The class I genes include the classical or class Ia genes, *HLA-A*, *HLA-B,* and *HLA-C*, and the nonclassical or class Ib genes *HLA-E*, *HLA-F*, and *HLA-G*. Class I pseudogenes, such as *HLA-H*, and gene fragments, such as *HLA-J* (Fig. 1) have also been described (Messer et al. 1992; Geraghty et al. 1992a). The class Ia genes have a ubiquitous tissue distribution and are expressed on nearly all nucleated cells. A noteworthy exception are syncytiotrophoblasts and villous cytotrophoblasts, which lack expression of *HLA-A* and *HLA-B* (Galbraith et al. 1981; Faulk et al. 1982; Johnson and Stern 1986; Sunderland et al. 1981b). Recently, expression of *HLA-C* has been demonstrated in extravillous cytotrophoblast (King et al. 1996). The class Ib genes have more limited tissue distributions and unknown functions (Orr 1989; Geraghty 1993; Le Bouteillier 1994). *HLA-E* is expressed in most tissues, including adult and fetal thymus and liver, lymph nodes, spleen, unactivated T and B cells, activated T cells, skin, muscosa colon, eosinophils, placentas, and extravillous membranes. *HLA-F* transcripts have been found in resting T and B cells, activated T cells, peripheral blood lymphocytes, fetal thymus and liver, skin, and lymphoblastoid cell lines. *HLA-G* is expressed in extravillous cytotrophoblasts at the maternal-fetal interface (Chumbley et al. 1994; Ellis et al. 1990; Kovats et al. 1990;

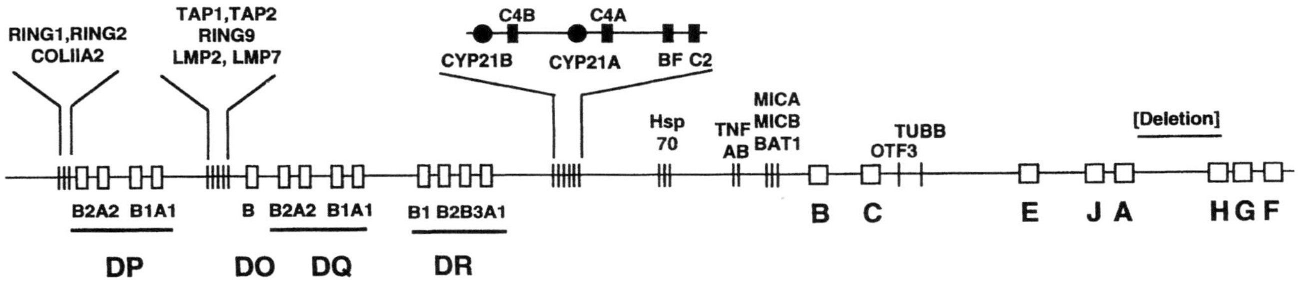

Fig. 1. The major histocompatibility complex on chromosome 6, showing the approximate location of some of the genes in this region. *Above line*, labeling of HLA genes; below line, labeling of non-HLA genes. *Open squares*, class I genes; *open rectangles*, class II genes. Complement component genes: *C2, BF, C4A, C4B;* steroid 21-hydroxylase genes: *CYP21B, CYP21B;* proteosomelike genes: *LMP2, LMP7*; ABC transporter genes: *TAP1, TAP2*; collagen gene: *COLIIA2*; tumor necrosis factor genes: *TNFA, TNFB*; heat shock protein genes: *Hsp70*; transcription factor gene: *OTF3*; tubulin gene: *TUBB*; genes of unknown function: *RING1, RING2, RING9, BAT1*. (Modified from CAMPBELL and TROWSDALE 1993; OBER 1995)

SUNDERLAND et al. 1981a; YELAVARTHI et al. 1991) and in the anterior chamber of the eye and fetal thymus (SHUKLA et al. 1990), first trimester fetal liver (HOULIHAN et al. 1992), and adult peripheral lymphocytes (KIRSZENBAUM et al. 1994). For a detailed review of the class I region genes see GERAGHTY 1993; LE BOUTEILLIER 1994.

Class II molecules consist of two transmembrane glycoproteins (α and β chains), both encoded by MHC genes. Class II gene products have more limited tissue distributions than class I antigens, being restricted primarily to B lymphocytes, macrophages, endothelial cells, and activated T cells. Additional non-HLA class II region genes have been identified by molecular genetic techniques, including genes encoding antigen-processing and transport proteins, such as *TAP1* (formerly *RING4*), *TAP2* (formerly *RING11*), *LMP7* (formerly *RING10*), and *LMP2* (formerly *RING12*; KELLY et al. 1991a,b; GLYNNE et al. 1991; SPIES et al. 1990; TROWSDALE et al. 1990; COLONNA et al. 1992; Fig. 1).

The class III region contains genes encoding complement components (C4A, C4B, C2 and BF), the α and β chains of the tumor necrosis factor, the enzyme cytochrome P450 steroid 21-hydroxylase, and the heat shock protein Hsp70. Additional genes have been mapped to this region but have not yet been characterized (Fig. 1).

2.1 *HLA-G*: Mediator of Maternal Tolerance?

The *HLA-G* gene was cloned in 1987 (GERAGHTY et al. 1987), but it was not discovered that this gene encoded the unusual class I molecule present in extravillous cytotrophoblasts (ELLIS et al. 1986) until 1990 (ELLIS et al. 1990; KOVATS et al. 1990). The unique tissue distribution of *HLA-G* suggests that this molecule plays a key role in the induction of maternal tolerance in pregnancy (reviewed by COLBERN and MAIN 1991; HUNT and ORR 1992; LOKE and KING 1991; SCHMIDT and ORR 1993).

HLA-G, or *HLA-6.0*, as it was provisionally named, is located telomeric to *HLA-A* and shows a high degree of sequence similarity with *HLA-A2* at the nucleotide and amino acid levels (KIRISITS et al. 1991). The *HLA-G* heavy-chain is anchored to the cell membrane in noncovalent association with β_2-microglobulin, similar to the class Ia genes. The structure of the *HLA-G* gene is also similar to the class Ia genes, which includes eight exons encoding a signal peptide (exon 1), the α_1-domain (exon 2), the α_2-domain (exon 3), the α_3-domain (exon 4), the transmembrane domain (exon 5), a cytoplasmic tail (exons 6 and 7), and an untranslated region (exon 8). However, an in-frame termination codon at the second codon of exon 6 of *HLA-G* results in a truncated cytoplasmic tail, which is 19 amino acids shorter than the corresponding regions of *HLA-A, HLA-B,* and *HLA-C* (GERAGHTY et al. 1987). The functional significance of the truncated cytoplasmic tail in *HLA-G* is unknown, but it is similar in this respect to the shortened cytoplasmic tail of the murine Qa antigens (FLAHERTY et al. 1990).

A second feature of *HLA-G* that is also similar to the murine Qa genes (TABACZEWSKI et al. 1994) is that its mRNA undergoes alternative splicing, resulting in at least five different proteins (ISHITANI and GERAGHTY 1992; FUJII et al. 1994). The largest mRNA, HLA-G1, encodes a full length protein that includes the α_1-, α_2-, and α_3-domains, the transmembrane region, and the cytoplasmic tail. A soluble form of this protein, HLA-$G1_{sol}$, includes an additional 21 amino acids following the α_3-domain, which are encoded by nucleotides from intron 4 (FUJII et al. 1994). A smaller message, HLA-G2, lacks the α_2-domain (exon 3 is spliced out), resulting in a protein with the α_1- and α_3-domains joined. A soluble form of this protein, HLA-$G2_{sol}$, also includes an additional 21 amino acids following the α_3-domain (FUJII et al. 1994). HLA-G3, the smallest splice form, has both exons 3 and 4 (corresponding to the α_2- and α_3-domains) removed with the α_1-domain directly connected to the transmembrane region (ISHITANI and GERAGHTY 1992). Because HLA-G3 lacks exon 4 (the α_3-domain), it cannot bind with β_2-microglobulin and may be unstable at the cell surface.

Another characterisitic of *HLA-G* that has received much attention was the apparent low level (or absence) of polmorphism in the *HLA-G* protein. Whereas the class Ia loci, particularly *HLA-A* and *HLA-B*, show high levels of polymorphism at the nucleotide and amino acid levels, *HLA-G* was initially reported to be non-polymorphic (GERAGHTY et al. 1987; KOVATS et al. 1990) or to have very low levels of sequence variation (ELLIS et al. 1990; MCMASTER et al. 1993; MORALES et al. 1993; WARD et al. 1993; CHIANG and MAIN 1993). However, our own molecular genetic studies in healthy African-American individuals revealed extensive nucleotide variation in this gene (VAN DER VEN and OBER 1994). Two sequence variations in exon 2 (α_1-domain) and 24 in exon 3 (α_2-domain) result in amino acid substitutions, i.e., polymorphisms at the level of the protein. Based on these data, we estimated that approximately 67% of African Americans are heterozygous for *HLA-G* proteins, which is fewer than that observed for *HLA-A* and *HLA-B* alleles but is a considerably higher frequency of heterozygotes than that observed for most other human genes. Five *HLA-G* alleles have been detected in an inbred Caucasian population (OBER et al. 1996), suggesting that a greater number of alleles are present in outbred populations.

These data suggest that a single gene, which is uniquely expressed in extravillous cytotrophoblasts, encodes at least five different proteins. The different proteins could simultaneously maintain diverse functions in the placental environment, depending on the molecular structure and the presence or absence of the polymorphic α_2-domain. The membrane-bound and soluble forms of HLA-G1, which include the polymorphic α_2-domain, are potentially capable of presenting a variety of peptides and of eliciting a maternal immune response, similar to the class Ia molecules. The smaller splice forms, HLA-G2 and HLA-G3, which are less variable because they lack the α_2-domain may function as immunologically neutral molecules at the maternal-fetal interface, perhaps playing a role in the induction of maternal tolerance. The timely and quantitative shift of the expression of alternatively spliced forms of *HLA-G* mRNA as observed by ISHITANI and GERAGHTY (1992) may also suggest multiple functions for HLA-G proteins. The smallest mRNA, HLA-G3, was abundant in term placenta, whereas the largest form, HLA-G1, predominated in a cell line from an earlier placental stage (ISHITANI and GER-

AGHTY 1992). Paralleling these findings, expression levels of the peptide transporter genes *TAP1* and *TAP2* were consistently more abundant in early gestation than in late gestational placentas (ROBY et al. 1994), suggesting that an antigen-presentation function of *HLA-G* may be more predominant in placental cell populations in early than in late gestation. Speculations aside, future studies elucidating the function and expression pattern of the *HLA-G* proteins promise to shed light on the mechanisms by which the fetus escapes immunological rejection.

3 The Role of Classical HLA in Pregnancy

Despite the fact that classical HLA genes are not expressed at the maternal-fetal interface, the maternal immune system encounters fetal cells expressing class I and class II HLA as evidenced by the presence of HLA antibodies in multigravidae (PAYNE and ROLFS 1958; VAN ROOD et al. 1958). Although it is likely that sensitization of fetal HLA occurs most commonly around delivery, when fetal blood spills into the maternal circulation, there is evidence to suggest that fetal cells expressing classical HLA are recognized by the maternal immune system *during* pregnancy. The latter hypothesis is supported by a recent study by NELSON et al. (1993), who reported an association between maternal-fetal disparity for class II alleles and remission of rheumatoid arthritis during pregnancy. In this study maternal-fetal disparities for HLA-DRB1, -DQA1, and -DQB1 occurred in 26 of 34 pregnancies (76%) characterized by remission or improvement of RA as compared with 3 of 12 pregnancies (25%) characterized by active rheumatoid arthritis ($p = 0.003$). These data suggest that not only does the maternal immune system recognize fetal class II genes during pregnancy, but that there are different immune responses to class II compatible and incompatible fetuses.

Whether maternal-fetal compatibility for HLA genes is associated with fetal loss remains controversial, although our own prospective studies on HLA and reproduction in a fertile, inbred population continue to provide evidence that HLA sharing between partners influences reproductive outcome (reviewed in OBER 1995). In the following sections we review the retrospective studies of HLA and fertility in outbred couples and summarize the results of prospective studies in an inbred population.

3.1 HLA and Fertility: Retrospective Studies in Outbred Couples

Shortly after the discovery of HLA antibodies in multigravidae (PAYNE and ROLFS 1958; VAN ROOD et al. 1958) it was suggested that maternal recognition of paternally derived HLA may be beneficial (AMOS 1974; BEER and BILLINGHAM 1976). Because sensitization to paternal HLA occurs commonly in pregnancies without any ostensibly deleterious effects but rarely in women with recurrent spontaneous abortion (RSA; BEER et al. 1981), it was proposed that normal pregnancy *requires* maternal recognition of, and response to, paternally derived fetal antigens. Abnormal pregnancy may result from failure of the maternal immune system to recognize or respond to fetal antigens. Inadequate maternal immune recognition and response may be associated with maternal-fetal histocompatibility, i.e., fetuses whose paternally derived HLA do not differ from maternal HLA. Because only couples who share HLA can produce compatible fetuses, increased HLA sharing among couples with poor reproductive outcome (such as RSA) would be consistent with this hypothesis.

3.1.1 HLA Sharing in Recurrent Spontaneous Abortion

Initial data suggesting a role for MHC genes in human pregnancy were derived from retrospective studies of HLA sharing in couples with RSA. These studies tested the hypothesis that maternal-fetal histocompatibility is associated with recurrent abortion by comparing the frequency of HLA sharing among RSA and fertile control couples. Evidence supporting this hypothesis was first reported by Komlos et al. in 1977. They compared the frequency of HLA-A and -B sharing in 18 control couples with at least two or more liveborn children and no history of abortion, to three groups of experimental couples including 13 couples with one abortion only, 23 with repeated abortions, and 25 with hydatidiform moles. The proportion of couples sharing HLA-A or -B antigens was higher in all experimental groups than in control subjects, but the differences reached statistical significance only in recurrent aborters ($p < 0.05$).

Since this initial investigation many studies of HLA sharing and RSA have been reported (Table 1). Overall, about half of studies report higher sharing of HLA in RSA than in control couples. However, even among studies reporting an association there is little agreement with regard to the MHC gene or region associated with spontaneous abortion. For example, some investigators reported associations between RSA and sharing antigens at the class I loci, HLA-A or HLA-B, other reported associations with sharing antigens at the class II loci, HLA-DR or HLA-DQ, and yet others reported increased sharing over all loci (Table 1).

These conflicting data may be due to a variety of factors including chance findings in small samples (28 of the 41 samples described in Table 1 included fewer than 50 couples), differences between centers with regard to tissue typing methodology, the numbers of antigens identified by the laboratory and the numbers of antigens present in a particular population, the choice and numbers of control couples, and the selection and stratification of RSA couples. In addition, genetic heterogeneity could account for some of the discordant results. That is, different MHC genes or regions may have distinct effects on fertility. The latter is supported by results of prospective studies of pregnancy outcome in a fertile population (Ober et al. 1992), discussed below.

In addition to sample heterogeneity and the other potential confounding factors mentioned above, measuring HLA sharing between partners does not provide unambiguous information on the genetic make-up of the fetus because couples

Table 1. HLA-sharing in couples with unexplained recurrent spontaneous abortion (modified from OBER 1992)

Reference	Number of couples	Increased sharing by locus[a]				Increased antigen sharing[a]	Sample[b]
		HLA-A	HLA-B	HLA-DR	HLA-DO		
BEER et al. (1985)	237	+/–	+	+	NA	+	Primary and secondary RSA
BOLIS et al. (1984)	20	+	+/–	NA	NA	+	Primary and secondary RSA
CAUCHI et al. (1988)	46	–	–	+/–	NA	–	Primary RSA
	37	–	–	–	NA	–	Secondary RSA
CAUDLE et al. (1983)	12	–	–	NA	NA	–	Primary and secondary RSA
CHANG et al. (1991)	25	–	+/–	–	NA	–	Primary RSA
	11	+/–	+/–	+/–	NA	+/–	Secondary RSA
CHRISTIANSEN et al. (1989)	39	–	–	–	NA	–	Primary and secondary RSA
COULAM et al. (1987)	32	NA	NA	+	+	+	Primary RSA
	27	NA	NA	+/–	+	+/–	Secondary RSA
GERENCER et al. (1979)	45	–	+	NA	NA	+/–	Primary and secondary RSA
GERENCER and KASTELAN (1983)	105	NA	NA	+	NA	NA	Primary and secondary RSA
EROGLU et al. (1992)	60	NA	NA	–	NA	–	Primary RSA
HO et al. (1990)	91	+	–	+/–	+	+	Primary RSA
	32	+/–	+/–	+/–	+/–	+	Secondary RSA
ITO et al. (1992)	82	NA	NA	–[d]	NA	NA	Primary RSA
	21	NA	NA	–	NA	NA	Secondary RSA
JEANNET et al. (1985)	29	NA	NA	NA	NA	+/–	Primary and secondary RSA[c]
JOHNSON et al. (1988)	80	–	+	–	NA	NA	Primary RSA
	33	+/–	+/–	+/–	NA	NA	Secondary RSA
KILPATRICK and LISTON (1993)	108	+/–	+/–	+/–	NA	+	Primary and secondary RSA
KOMLOS et al. (1977)	23	+	+	NA	NA	+	Primary and secondary RSA
KOYAMA et al. (1991)	56	–	–	+	+	NA	Primary RSA[c]

	20	–	–	–	–	NA	Secondary RSA[c]
Laitinen et al. (1993)	35	NA	NA	–[d]	–	NA	Primary RSA
	15	NA	NA	–	–	NA	Secondary RSA
McIntyre et al. (1986)	35	+	+	+	NA	+	Primary RSA compared to 15 secondary RSA couples
Mowbray et al. (1983)	15	–	–	–	NA	–	Primary and secondary RSA
Ober et al. (1993)	68	NA	NA	NA	+[d]	NA	Primary and secondary RSA
Oksenberg et al. (1984)	60	–	–	–	NA	–	Primary RSA
Purandare et al. (1993)	103	+/–	+/–	+/–	NA	+/–	Primary and secondary RSA[c]
Reznikof-Etievant et al. (1988)	129	–	+	+	NA	NA	Primary and secondary RSA
Sargent et al. (1988)	18	–	–	–	NA	NA	Primary and secondary RSA
Schacter et al. (1984)	16	–	+	–	NA	NA	Primary RSA
	36	+	–	–	NA	NA	Secondary RSA
Smith and Cowchock (1988)	115	NA	NA	NA	NA	–	Primary and secondary RSA compared to couples with "explained" RSA
Takakuwa et al. (1986)	20	–	–	+	NA	NA	Primary RSA
Taylor et al. (1985)	139	NA	NA	NA	NA	+	Primary RSA
Thomas et al. (1985)	21	–	–	–	NA	NA	Primary and secondary RSA[c]
Unander and Olding (1983)	8	+/–	+/–	+/–	NA	+	Primary RSA[c]
Vanoli et al. (1985)	47	+/–	–	+/–	NA	NA	Primary and secondary RSA

+, Increased sharing in RSA (statistically significant); +/–, increased sharing in RSA (not statistically significant); –, no increased sharing in RSA; NA, data not available.
[a] Sharing of serologically defined antigens except where otherwise noted.
[b] RSA compared to fertile control couples unless otherwise noted.
[c] Sharing in RSA compared to theoretically derived expectations based on population frequencies.
[d] Alleles identified by DNA-based typing.

sharing only one antigen at a locus produce compatible and incompatible fetuses at relatively equal (50%) frequencies. In the past, HLA typing of abortus tissues was technically difficult and not practical for large studies. However, with the advent of DNA-based typing methodologies it has become possible to genotype abortus tissue and directly examine the HLA compatibility status of aborted fetuses.

3.1.2 Maternal-Fetal Compatibility in RSA Couples

To directly assess whether RSA couples preferentially abort compatibile fetuses we studied couples with RSA who were undergoing white cell immunization as a treatment for RSA (Ober et al. 1993). Study couples had at least three prior losses, and known causes of miscarriage had been excluded prior to treatment. Couples were selected for treatment without regard to their HLA sharing status. Placental specimens were collected from 106 abortuses over 2.5 years. Fetal tissue was identified in 62 specimens (58.8%), of which 22 were excluded from analysis (fetal chromosomal abnormalities in 7 abortuses; abnormal ultrasound findings prior to the miscarriage in 5; ectopic pregnancies, fetal demise >28 weeks gestation, or elective abortion in 8; the pregnancy was achieved prior to immunotherapy in 1; and the presence of paternal DNA could not be confirmed in the tissue sample in 1). The final sample included 40 abortuses of 37 couples and 31 children born to 31 RSA couples who underwent immunotherapy during the same time period as the 37 couples with abortions. The 31 successful couples also had at least three prior (unexplained) losses. DNA from both partners, abortus tissues, and liveborn children were typed for alleles at the class II locus HLA-DQA1 (Ober et al. 1993; Steck et al. 1995).

Among the 17 abortuses of couples sharing one HLA-DQA1 allele, six were compatible and 11 incompatible with respect to HLA-DQA1 (expected = 8.5 and 8.5, respectively; $p = 0.225$). However, when the liveborn children were included, 7 of 28 "fetuses" were HLA-DQA1 compatible and 21 of 28 were HLA-DQA1 incompatible (expected = 14.0 and 14.0, respectively; $p = 0.0067$; Table 2; Ober et al. 1993). Thus significantly fewer than expected HLA-DQA1 compatible fetuses (abortuses with identifiable fetal tissues plus liveborn) were observed. If the proportions of compatible and incompatible embryos are equal at conception, these data suggest that HLA-DQA1 compatible fetuses are aborted early in pregnancy, either in the peri-implantation period before pregnancy is recognized or early in the

Table 2. Maternal-fetal HLA-DQA1 compatibility in RSA couples; the expected numbers of fetuses based on mendelian expectations (modified from Ober et al. 1993)

Sample	Number fetuses in couples sharing 1 HLA-DQA1 allele	Number observed/expected		p
		Compatible	Incompatible	
Abortuses	17	6/8.5	11/8.5	0.225
Liveborn	11	1/5.5	10/5.5	0.007
Total fetuses	28	7/14.0	21/14.0	0.008

first trimester prior to the time when fetal tissue can be collected. In fact, we were less likely to obtain fetal tissue in the earlier abortuses (mean gestational age = 7.8 weeks among the 44 abortus specimens in which fetal DNA could not be identified and 11.0 weeks among the analyzed samples). Increased over expected proportions of HLA-DQA1 compatible fetuses in the earlier losses could account for the deficit of compatible fetuses in our study (OBER et al. 1993).

Although the results of this study suggest that HLA-DQA1 compatible fetuses are aborted early in gestation, the small sample size requires that these results be replicated in other samples before drawing conclusions regarding the fate of HLA-DQA1 compatible fetuses. However, results of studies in fertile couples (OBER et al. 1992) and in couples with unexplained infertility (JIN et al. 1995) further suggest a role for class II region genes in peri-implantation embryonic losses.

3.1.3 HLA Sharing and Unexplained Infertility

In approximately 10% of couples with primary infertility no cause of infertility can be identified despite thorough diagnostic investigation. Causes of infertility that are currently "unidentifiable" include occult lesions of tubal mucosa and endometrial tissues, temporary endocrinological dysfunctions, sperm dysfunctions, environmental factors, and implantation failures. As a result, couples with unexplained infertility (UI) are etiologically heterogeneous, and a subgroup of patients with UI may experience occult losses of blastocysts during the peri-implantation period. At present technical limitations make it impossible to identify such couples and to estimate the proportion of UI couples experiencing recurrent peri-implantational losses. However, maternal-fetal HLA compatibility may be a contributing factor in some couples with occult peri-implantational pregnancy losses.

Three early studies did not reveal higher sharing of HLA-A, HLA-B or HLA-DR locus antigens in couples with UI than in fertile controls (NORDLANDER et al. 1983; PERSITZ et al. 1985) or compared to theoretically derived expectations of sharing (JEANNET et al. 1985); however, the sample sizes in these studies were small (Table 3). One of these studies did find a marginally significant excess of total antigen sharing ($p < 0.05$), but the small sample size ($n = 16$) and lack of fertile control data limit the interpretation of these results (JEANNET et al. 1985). On the other hand, one larger study of 79 UI subjects reported that couples with primary infertility ($n = 48$) but not secondary infertility ($n = 31$) were less likely to produce HLA-DQ heterozygous offspring (i.e., the couples shared more HLA-DQ antigens) than were fertile controls ($p = 0.014$; COULAM et al. 1987). Differences with respect to sharing antigens at the HLA-A, HLA-B, or HLA-DR loci were not observed in primary or secondary UI couples (COULAM et al. 1987).

More recent studies of HLA sharing in UI have attempted to identify couples who may be experiencing recurrent peri-implantational losses by studying infertile couples who fail to achieve a successful pregnancy with assisted reproductive technology (ART). Following documentation of fertilization in ART, failure to achieve a clinical pregnancy would result from an implantation failure. Associations between HLA sharing and outcome after ART were first reported by

Table 3. HLA-sharing in couples with unexplained infertility (UI)

Reference	Number of couples	Increased sharing by locus[a]				Increased antigen sharing[a]	Sample[b]
		HLA-A	HLA-B	HLA-DR	HLA-DO		
Nordlander et al. (1983)	14	–	–	–	NA	NA	Primary UI
Persitz et al. (1985)[c]	18	–	+/–	+/–	NA	NA	UI[d]
Jeannet et al. (1985)	16	–	–	–	–	+/–	UI[d]
Coulam et al. (1987)	48	–	–	–	+	–	Primary UI
	31	–	–	–	–	–	Secondary UI
Weckstein et al. (1991)	10	+/–	–	+/–	+/–	+	Primary infertile couples who failed ART compared to primary infertile couples with successes after ART[e]
Balasch et al. (1993)	15	+/–	+/–	+/–	NA	+	Primary infertile couples who failed ART compared to primary infertile couples with successes after ART[e]
Ho et al. (1994); Jin et al. (1995)[c]	34	–	–	–	–	–	Primary UI with ART successes
	36	–	–	–	+	+	Primary UI who failed ART

+, Increased sharing in UI (statistically significant); +/–, increased sharing in UI (not statistically significant); –, no increased sharing in UI; NA, data not available.

[a] Sharing of serologically defined antigens.

[b] Couples with unexplained infertility compared to fertile control couples unless otherwise noted.

[c] Sharing in UI compared to theoretically derived expectations based on population frequencies.

[d] Infertile couples with identifiable etiologies included after appropriate treatment.

[e] No information on primary vs. secondary UI.

WECKSTEIN et al. (1991). In this study HLA typing (HLA-A, HLA-B, HLA-DR, HLA-DQ) was performed in ten couples with primary infertility who had not achieved a viable recognizable pregnancy after two or more attempts of in vitro fertilization (IVF) or tubal embryo transfer (TET) and in ten couples with primary infertility who achieved a viable pregnancy after IVF or TET. The subjects in the two study groups were not all unexplained, but the investigators corrected etiological factors prior to the ART cycle (WECKSTEIN et al. 1991). In both groups 30% had tubal factors, 30% had endometriosis, 20% had male factor, and 20% were UI. At least three embryos were transferred in the study cycle. Seven of ten study couples (failures) shared three or more HLA antigens, compared with four of ten control subjects (successes; $p < 0.01$). A second study of infertile couples undergoing ART reported similar results (BALASCH et al. 1993). The proportion of couples sharing HLA-A, -B, and -DR was compared between 15 couples with ART failures (experimental group), 15 couples with ART successes (infertile control group), and 100 fertile couples (fertile control group). In each infertile group seven couples had tubal factors, four had endometriosis as "causes" of the infertility, and four cases were "unexplained." The mean ages, mean duration of infertility, and the number of embryos transferred did not differ between the experimental and infertile control groups. The frequency of antigen sharing was higher in the experimental group than in the infertile controls ($p < 0.005$) and the fertile control group ($p = 0.01$). The frequency of HLA sharing was not lower in the 30 infertile couples than in the fertile control group ($p = 0.10$). The results of these studies (WECKSTEIN et al. 1991; BALASCH et al. 1993) are consistent with the hypothesis that HLA sharing influences peri-implantational losses; however, the small sample sizes preclude drawing any firm conclusions.

A recent study reported similar results in a larger sample of couples with UI (Ho et al. 1994). In this study all known causes of infertility were excluded, and couples were typed for antigens at the HLA-A, HLA-B, HLA-C, HLA-DR, and HLA-DQ loci. Among the 76 couples, 34 had successful pregnancies following IVF or TET, 36 failed to become pregnant, and 6 became pregnant and subsequently aborted. The 34 women with successful pregnancies and the 36 women who failed to become pregnant were similar with respect to age, obstetric histories, duration of infertility, and the number of oocytes retrieved, fertilized, and transferred (Ho et al. 1994). There was significantly more HLA sharing among the women who failed to become pregnant than among women with successful pregnancies: 44.4% of couples with failures and 21.5% of successful couples shared at least three antigens ($p = 0.015$; comparison between couples with failures and fertile controls, $p = 0.021$; comparison between successful couples and normal fertile controls, $p = 0.44$). Among the individual loci there was an excess of sharing at the HLA-DQ locus among the couples with failures, but this difference was not statistically significant after adjusting for multiple comparisons (uncorrected $p = 0.013$; Ho et al. 1994). Subsequently the investigators reanalyzed these data using a shared allele test, which compares the frequencies of shared alleles at a locus to the frequencies expected if there is random mating at this locus (JIN et al. 1995). Empiric p values were determined from computer simulations, which repeatedly sampled a simulated group of couples equal in size to the study groups; genotypes in the simulated population were assigned based on the genotype frequencies in the sampled population (JIN et al. 1995). In the reanalysis of their data there was a significant excess of sharing HLA-DQ antigens among the couples who failed ART (empiric $p = 0.001$) but not among couples with successful pregnancies (empiric $p = 0.949$; JIN et al. 1995). There was no excess of sharing at the HLA-A, HLA-B, or HLA-DR loci in either group.

These data (BALASCH et al. 1993; HO et al. 1994; WECKSTEIN et al. 1991) suggest that a subgroup of couples presenting as "infertile" may in fact be experiencing recurrent implantation failures. Increased HLA sharing among couples who fail ART suggests that incompatibility for HLA genes may enhance the likelihood of implantation. This hypothesis was first suggested by KIRBY in 1970, who demonstrated higher implantation rates in histoincompatible murine zygotes than in histoincompatible murine zygotes. JIN et al. (1995) further demonstrated that sharing antigens at the class II locus HLA-DQ had the single most important effect on success rates after ART in their subjects. These data are consistent with results of prospective studies in the Hutterites, in which couples who share HLA-DR take significantly longer to become pregnant than couples not sharing HLA-DR (OBER et al. 1992). Because alleles at the HLA-DR and HLA-DQ loci are in strong linkage disequilibrium, Hutterite couples who share HLA-DR antigens also share HLA-DQ antigens, and distinguishing the effects of HLA-DR and HLA-DQ loci in this inbred population is not possible using serologically defined antigens. Nonetheless, the combined data from these studies (COULAM et al. 1987; WECKSTEIN et al. 1991; OBER et al. 1992, 1993; HO et al. 1994; JIN et al. 1995) suggest that maternal-fetal histoincompatibility, particularly with respect to class II region genes, enhances implantation and successful pregnancy outcome among both "infertile" outbred couples and "fertile" inbred couples. Additional studies in outbred couples undergoing ART are necessary to determine whether HLA sharing is correlated with success rates after ART in other populations and to determine the magnitude of the HLA-sharing effect on pregnancy success rates.

3.2 HLA Sharing and Pregnancy Outcome: Studies in Hutterite Couples

To elucidate the reproductive effects of parental HLA sharing and to address the methodological limitations inherent in retrospective studies, population-based and prospective studies were initiated in the Hutterites (OBER et al. 1983, 1985, 1988 1992; OBER 1995). Hutterites are well suited as subjects for such studies because their communal lifestyle reduces the effects of nongenetic factors that may influence fertility, and the high level of inbreeding results in many couples sharing HLA. In addition, birth control is prohibited (and used only rarely) and large families are desired (average family size is eight children).

Initial studies of Hutterite couples revealed a trend toward longer birth intervals among couples sharing HLA-A or HLA-B (OBER et al. 1983). The average length of time to produce ten children was 13.73 years among couples sharing no antigens, 14.52 years among couples sharing one antigen, and 19.0 years among couples sharing two or more antigens. While couples sharing antigens showed decreased fertility, it was clear that HLA sharing did not preclude normal fertility. Subsequent studies revealed significantly longer intervals from marriage to each birth among couples sharing HLA-A, -B, or -DR than among couples not sharing antigens (OBER et al. 1985, 1988). For example, the median interval lengths from marriage to fifth birth was 7.63 years, 8.79 years, and 8.69 years among couples sharing no, one, and multiple HLA-A, B, and DR antigens, respectively (two-tailed test, $p = 0.040$). Analyzing the effects of individual loci on interval lengths revealed a significant HLA-DR sharing effect ($p = 0.025$). Median completed family sizes were 6.5 children among couples sharing HLA-DR and 9.0 children among couples not sharing HLA-DR (one-tailed test, $p = 0.041$). Recognized fetal loss rates, calculated retrospectively on the basis of interview data, were not increased among Hutterite couples sharing HLA-A, -B, or -DR antigens (OBER et al. 1988; HAUCK and OBER 1991). These data suggested that longer birth intervals associated with HLA-DR sharing may result in fetal losses occurring very early in gestation before Hutterite women recognize pregnancy.

A prospective study of pregnancy outcome was initiated to clarify the effects of HLA-DR sharing on birth interval lengths, (OBER et al. 1992). Hutterite women who had not yet completed their families were provided with pregnancy test kits and calendar diaries. Study participants tested for pregnancy 1 month after the first day of their last menses and recorded in the diaries the first day of each menses, the results of all pregnancy tests, dates of pregnancy outcomes (spontaneous abortion, ectopic pregnancy, or delivery), and any other factors that might affect pregnancy rates (e.g., nursing, travel away from spouse, illness).

The length of the interval from the resumption of menses following the birth of the most recent offspring to the next positive pregnancy test was significantly longer among Hutterite couples sharing HLA-DR than among couples not sharing HLA-DR ($p = 0.015$; OBER et al. 1992). The median time to a positive test was 2.0 ± 0.4 months among couples not sharing HLA-DR and 5.1 ± 0.5 months among couples sharing HLA-DR. Fetal loss rates after the first missed period were 16.3% (23 losses/141 pregnancies). Loss rates among couples sharing and not sharing antigens

Table 4. Fetal loss rates[a] by HLA sharing in Hutterite couples (modified from OBER et al. 1992)

HLA locus	Number of antigens shared		p^b
	0	≥1	
A	0.15 (9/61)	0.18 (13/72)	0.466
B	0.12 (10/82)	0.23 (10/43)	0.041
DR	0.18 (11/62)	0.15 (10/66)	0.399

[a]Fetal loss rates calculated as: the number of losses/(total number of pregnancies > 20 weeks gestation + number of losses).
[b]Multivariate logistic regression analysis (adjusted for age, gravidity, and kinship), one-tailed test.

at each locus are shown in Table 4. Recognized loss rates were increased in couples sharing HLA-B antigens compared to couples not sharing HLA-B antigens (0.23 vs. 0.12; $p = 0.041$, respectively; Table 4; OBER et al. 1992). Additional data on 31 fetal losses collected since this report have strengthened this association ($p = 0.007$; OBER, unpublished data).

These data suggest that increased birth interval lengths among Hutterite couples sharing HLA are due predominantly to longer intervals to a clinical pregnancy among couples sharing HLA-DR and, to a lesser degree, to increased fetal loss rates among couples sharing HLA-B. Thus in Hutterites more than one MHC region may mediate reproductive processes. Class II region genes may affect pre-or peri-implantational embryonic survival, consistent with the results of studies in outbred couples with unexplained infertility (COULAM et al. 1987; JIN et al. 1995) and in abortuses of outbred couples with RSA (OBER et al. 1993), discussed above. Class I region HLA-B-linked genes may contribute to early fetal loss. The fact that different MHC genes may underlie different reproductive disorders could account for some of the conflicting data regarding the role of HLA sharing in RSA in outbred couples discussed above.

It should be noted that among the more than 400 Hutterite women who have participated in these studies, none meets the definition of RSA (at least three consecutive spontaneous abortions) and all Hutterite couples with at least three spontaneous abortions have had at least two successful pregnancies (OBER 1995). Therefore it is not clear whether the HLA-B-associated mechanism of fetal loss in the Hutterites influences either recurrent or sporadic miscarriages in outbred couples, although associations between HLA-B sharing and RSA have been reported (Table 1). On the other hand, longer intervals to recognized pregnancies among Hutterite couples may result from peri-implantational losses, which may be mediated by mechanisms similar to those in outbred couples with UI or early RSA as discussed above (Table 5).

At the present time it is unknown whether the HLA-sharing effects on fertility in the Hutterites are due to HLA genes per se or to alleles at non- HLA loci that are in

Table 5. Interval lengths to a positive pregnancy test among Hutterite couples who stopped nursing prior to their first menses after their last pregnancy (modified from OBER et al. 1992)

Antigens shared	n	Median (months)	75th percentile (months)	p (two-tailed)
HLA-A				
0	20	2.2 ± 0.3	6.6 ± 0.6	
≥1	18	2.4 ± 0.8	4.5 ± 1.2	0.518
HLA-B				
0	26	2.2 ± 0.2	6.0 ± 1.1	
≥1	8	3.1 ± 1.4	4.5 ± 1.5	0.782
HLA-DR				
0	21	2.0 ± 0.4	2.4 ± 0.8	
≥1	14	5.1 ± 0.5	8.2 ± 1.0	0.015
All couples	40	2.4 ± 0.5	6.0 ± 1.0	

linkage disequilibrium with HLA alleles. The human MHC contains many genes that could potentially affect reproductive outcome (reviewed in KOSTYU 1994; LE BOUTEILLIER 1994). In other mammals the MHCs include genes that control spermatogenesis, embryo cleavage rates, fetal development, and mating preferences (CHAPMAN and WOLGEMUTH 1993; KUNZ et al. 1980; KIRISITS et al. 1994; LYON 1981; POTTS et al. 1991; UEHARA 1991; WARNER et al. 1987; YEOM et al. 1992). Thus MHC genes could influence reproductive outcome in humans through a variety of immunologic, genetic and even behavioral mechanisms, which at present are still unknown.

4 Conclusions

Although the mechanisms by which the fetal allograft escapes immunological rejection are still poorly understood, evidence has accumulated suggesting that maternal-fetal compatibility for HLA region genes influences pregnancy outcome. Compatibility for class II region genes may influence implantation (COULAM et al. 1987; OBER et al. 1992; JIN et al. 1995) as well as the loss of clinically recognized pregnancies (BEER et al. 1985; COULAM et al. 1987; GERENCER and KASTELAN 1983; JIN et al. 1995; KOYOMA et al. 1991; MCINTYRE et al. 1986; OBER et al. 1993; REZNIKOF-ETIEVANT et al. 1988; TAKAKUWA et al. 1986). Compatibility for class I region genes may also influence recognized fetal losses, at least in an inbred population (OBER et al. 1992). However, the many retrospective studies that did not observe increased sharing of HLA antigens among RSA couples (Table 1) suggest that the effects of HLA sharing on pregnancy outcome in outbred couples may be small or may be causative only in a small proportion of RSA couples. In addition, many outbred fertile couples share HLA without any apparently deleterious effects (summarized by EROGLU et al. 1992). Even among the Hutterites, couples sharing HLA-DR have on average 6.5 children (OBER et al. 1988), and many Hutterite couples sharing antigens at two or more loci have more than ten children and report never having had a miscarriage (OBER et al. 1985). In this light it is not surprising that HLA-sharing status is not a significant predictor of pregnancy outcome among untreated RSA couples or RSA couples undergoing leukocyte immunization (CHRISTIANSEN et al. 1994; COWCHOCK and SMITH 1992; COWCHOCK et al. 1990; MOWBRAY et al. 1983; SMITH and COWCHOCK 1988). Therefore HLA typing should not be included as part of the clinical evaluation of RSA couples because it offers little information about the cause of the miscarriages in any particular couple, does not identify a subgroup of couples that would benefit from a particular treatment, and provides no information on the likelihood of another abortion.

The recent reports of associations between HLA sharing and failure to become pregnant after ART (WECKSTEIN et al. 1991; HO et al. 1994) are intriguing. However, additional studies replicating these findings are necessary before HLA studies are considered in infertile couples considering ART. Likewise, any novel treatments that are offered to UI couples based these findings should be offered as research protocols within the context of a controlled trial so that the efficacy and safety of the treatments(s) can be evaluated.

Future studies of *HLA-G* expression patterns and allelic variations in couples with normal and abnormal pregnancies may elucidate additional mechanisms through which HLA genes influence reproduction. Because of the large physical distance between the *HLA-G* and *HLA-B* loci (Fig. 1) it is unlikely that associations between HLA-B sharing and fetal loss are due to linkage disequilibrium between alleles at these loci. On the other hand, many studies have reported associations between HLA haplotypes and RSA in both population studies (Bolis et al. 1984; Cauchi et al. 1988; Gerencer and Kastelan 1983; Jeannet et al. 1985; Johnson et al. 1988; Reznikoff-Etievant et al. 1988; Smith et al. 1989; Takamizawa et al. 1987) and family studies (Christiansen et al. 1989). It will be interesting to see whether these RSA-associated haplotypes carry specific "high-risk" *HLA-G* alleles, a hypothesis that we are currently investigating in our laboratories. Lastly, because of its unique expression pattern in extravillous cytotrophoblast, abberations of *HLA-G* expression or maternal-fetal compatibility for *HLA-G* alleles may be associated with gestational disorders of trophoblast invasion, such as in preeclampsia, or of trophoblast growth, such as in low birth weight – conditions which have previously been reported to be associated with HLA in selected samples (Bolis et al. 1987; Christiansen et al. 1990a,b; Fujisawa 1985; Jenkins et al. 1978; Kilpatrick et al. 1990; Peterson et al. 1994; Schneider et al. 1994).

Immunogenetic studies of normal and abnormal pregnancy have identified specific MHC regions that contain genes affecting a variety of reproductive processes. It is likely that in the near future the functions of *HLA-G* isoforms will be elucidated, additional MHC genes that influence reproduction will be identified, and ultimately the mechanisms of maternal-fetal tolerance will be revealed.

Acknowledgements. C.O. is supported by NIH grants HD21244, HD27686, and HL49596. K.v.d.V. is supported by DFG VE 174/1-1 and VE 174/1-2.

References

Amos DB (1974) HL-A, fertility, and natural selection. In: Diczfalusy E (ed) Karolinska symposium on research methods in reproductive endocrinology, 7th edn. Karolinska Institutet, Stockholm, pp 318–327

Balasch J, Inmaculada J, Martorell J, Gayá A, Vanrell JA (1993) Histocompatibility in in vitro fertilization couples. Fertil Steril 59:456–458

Beer AE, Billingham RE (1976) The immunobiology of reproduction. Prentice-Hall, Englewood cliffs

Beer AE, Quebbeman JF, Ayers JWT, Haines RF (1981) Major histocompatibility complex antigens, maternal and paternal immune responses, and chronic habitual abortions in humans. Am J Obstet Gynecol 141:987–997

Beer AE, Semprini AE, Xiaoyu Z, Quebbeman JF (1985) Pregnancy outcome in human couples with recurrent spontaneous abortions: HLA antigen profiles, female serum MLR block factors, and paternal leukocyte immunization. Exp Clin Immunogenet 2:137–153
Bolis PF, Bianchi MM, Soro V, Belvedere M (1984) HLA typing in couples with repetitive abortion. Biol Res Pregnancy 5:135–137
Bolis PF, Martinetti Bianchi M, Fianza A, Franchi M, Cuccia Belvedere M (1987) Immunogenetic aspects of pre-eclampsia. Biol Res Pregnancy Perinatol 8:42–45
Campbell RD, Trowsdale J (1993) Map of the human MHC. Immunol Today 14:349–352
Cauchi MN, Tait B, Wilshire MI, Koh SH, Mraz G, Kloss M, Pepperell R (1988) Histocompatibility antigens and habitual abortion. Am J Reprod Immunol 18:28–31
Caudle MR, Rote NS, Scott JR, DeWitt C, Barney MD (1983) Histocompatibility in couples with recurrent spontaneous abortion and normal fertility. Fertil Steril 39:793–797
Chang M-Y, Soong Y-K, Huang C-C (1991) Comparison of histocompatibility between couples with idopathic recurrent spontaneous abortion and normal multipara. Formosan Med Assoc 90:153–159
Chapman DL, Wolgemuth DJ (1993) Isolation of the murine cyclin B2 cDNA and characterization of the lineage and temporal specificity of expression of the B1 and B2 cyclins during oogenesis, spermatogenesis, and early embryogenesis. Development 118:229–240
Chiang MH, Main EK (1993) Identification of HLA-G polymorphism using denaturing gradient gel electrophoresis (DGGE) followed by DNA sequence analysis. Serono Symposia on the Immunobiology of Reproduction, 29A
Christiansen OB, Riisom K, Lauritsen JG, Grunnet N (1989) No increased histocompatibility antigen-sharing in couples with idiopathic habitual abortion. Hum Reprod 4:160–162
Christiansen OB, Mathiesen O, Grunnet N, Jersild C, Lauritsen JG (1990a) Is there a common genetic background for pre-eclampsia and recurrent spontaneous abortion? Lancet 335:361–362
Christiansen OB, Mathiesen O, Riisom K, Lauritsen JG, Grunnet N (1990b) HLA or HLA-linked genes reduce birthweight in families affected by idiopathic recurrent abortion. Tissue Antigens 36:156–163
Christiansen OB, Mathiesen O, Husth M, Lauritsen JG, Grunnet N (1994) Placebo-controlled trial of active immunization with third party leukocytes in recurrent miscarriage. Acta Obstet Gynecol Scand 73:261–268
Chumbley G, King A, Gardner L, Lowlett S, Holmes N, Loke YW (1994) Generation of an antibody to HLA-G in transgenic mice and demonstration of the tissue reactivity of this antibody. J Reprod Immunol 27:173–186
Colbern GT, Main EK (1991) Immunology of the maternal-placental interface in normal pregnancy. Semin Perinatol 15:196–205
Colonna M, Bresnahan M, Bahram S, Strominger JL, Spies T (1992) Allelic variants of the human putative peptide transporter involved in antigen processing. Proc Natl Acad Sci USA 89:3932–3936
Coulam CB, Moore SB, O'Fallon WM (1987) Association between major histocompatibility antigen and reproductive performance. Am J Reprod Immunol Microbiol 14:54–58
Cowchock FS, Smith JB (1992) Predictors for livebirth after unexplained spontaneous abortion: correlations between immunologic test results, obstetric histories, and outcome of next pregnancy without treatment. Am J Obstet Gynecol 167:1208–1212
Cowchock FS, Smith JB, David S, Scher J, Batzer F, Corson S (1990) Paternal mononuclear cell immunization therapy for repeated miscarriage: predictive variables for success. Am J Reprod Immunol 22:12–17
Ellis SA, Sargent IL, Redman CWG, McMichael AJ (1986) Evidence for a novel HLA antigen found on human extravillous trophoblast and a choriocarcinoma cell line. J Immunol 59:595–601
Ellis SA, Palmer MS, McMichael AJ (1990) Human trophoblast and the choriocarcinoma cell line BeWo express a truncated HLA class I molecule. J Immunol 144:731–735
Eroglu G, Betz G, Torregano C (1992) Impact of histocompatibility antigens on pregnancy outcome. Am J Obstet Gynecol 166:1364–1369
Faulk WP, Hsi BL, McIntyre JA, Yeh CJG, Mucchielli A (1982) Antigens of the human extra-embryonic membranes. J Reprod Fertil Suppl 31:181–189
Flaherty L, Elliott E, Tine JA, Walsh AC, Waters JB (1990) Immunogenetics of the Q and Tl regions of the mouse. CRC Crit Rev Immunol 10:131–175
Fujii T, Ishitani A, Geraghty DE (1994) A soluble form of HLA-G antigen is encoded by a messenger ribonucleic acid contraining intron 4. J Immunol 153:5516–5524
Fujisawa S (1985) HLA antigens-antibodies system and its association with severe toxemia of pregnancy. Acta Obstet Gynaecol Jpn 37:124–130

Galbraith RM, Werner P, Kantor RR, Galbraith GM (1981) Studies of the interaction between human transferrin and specific receptors on the trophoblast membrane. Placenta Suppl 3:49–59
Geraghty DE (1993) Structure of the HLA class I region and expression of its resident genes. Curr Opin Immunol 5:3–7
Geraghty DE, Koller BH, Orr HT (1987) A human major histocompatibility complex class I gene that encodes a protein with a shortened cytoplasmic segment. Proc Natl Acad Sci USA 84:9145–9149
Geraghty DE, Koller BH, Hansen JA, Orr HT (1992a) The HLA class I gene family includes at least six genes and twelve speudogenes and gene fragments. J Immunol 149:1934–1946
Geraghty DE, Pei J, Lipsky B, Hansen JA, Taillon-Miller P, Bronson SK, Chaplin DD (1992b) Cloning and physical mapping of the HLA class I region spanning the HLA-E-to-HLA-F interval by using yeast artificial chromosomes. Proc Natl Acad Sci USA 89:2669–2673
Gerencer M, Kastelan A (1983) The role of HLA-D region in feto-maternal interactions. Transplant Proc 15:893–895
Gerencer M, Drazancic A, Kuvacic I, Tomaskovic Z, Kastelan A (1979) HLA antigen studies in women with recurrent gestational disorders. Fertil Steril 31:401–404
Glynne R, Powis SH, Beck S, Kelly A, Kerr L-A, Trowsdale J (1991) A proteasome-related gene between the two ABC transporter loci in the class II region of the human MHC. Nature 353:357–360
Hauck WW, Ober C (1991) Statistical analysis of outcomes from repeated pregnancies: effects of HLA sharing on fetal loss. Genet Epidemiol 8:187–197
Ho H-N, Gill TJ, Nsieh R-P, Hsieh H-J, Lee T-Y (1990) Sharing of human leukocyte antigens in primary and secondary recurrent spontaneous abortions. Am J Obstet Gynecol 163:178–188
Ho H–N, Yang Y-S, Hsieh R-P, Lin H-R, Chen S-U, Chen H0F, Huang S0C, Lee T-Y, Gill TJ III (1994) Sharing of human leukocyte antigens in couples with unexplained infertility affects the success of in vitro fertilization and tubal embryo transfer. Am J Obstet Gynecol 170:63–71
Houlihan JM, Biro PA, Fergar-Payne A, Simpson KL, Holmes CH (1992) Evidence for the expression of non HLA-A,-B,-C class I genes in the human fetal liver. J Immunol 149:668–675
Hunt J, Orr HT (1992) HLA and maternal-fetal recognition. FASEB J 6:2344–2348
Ishitani A, Geraghty DE (1992) Alternative splicing of HLA-G transcripts yields proteins with primary structures resembling both class I and class II antigens. Proc Natl Acad Sci USA 89:3947–3951
Ito K, Obata F, Tanaka T, Tsutsumi N, Kashiwagi N (1992) Analysis of HLA-DR types of unexplained recurrent spontaneous aborters in the Japanese population by oligonucleotide-DNA typing. Tissue Antigens 40:204–209
Jeannet M, Bischof P, Bourrit B, Vuagnat P (1985) Sharing of HLA antigens in fertile, subfertile, and infertile couples. Transplant Proc 17:903–904
Jenkins DM, Need JA, Scott JS, Morris H, Pepper M (1978) Human leukocyte antigens and mixed lymphocyte reaction in severe pre-eclampsia. Br Med J 1:542–544
Jin K, Ho H-N, Speed TP, Gill TJ III (1995) Reproductive failure and the major histocompatibility complex. Am J Hum Genet 56:1456–1467
Johnson PM, Stern PL (1986) Antigen expression at human materno-fetal interfaces. Prog Immunol 6:1056–1069
Johnson PM, Chia KV, Risk JM, Barnes RMR, Woodrow JC (1988) Immunological and immunogenetic investigation of recurrent spontaneous abortion. Dis Markers 6:163–171
Kelly AP, Powis SH, Glynne R, Radley E, Beck S, Trowsdale J (1991a) Second proteasome-related gene in the human MHC class II region. Nature 353:667–668
Kelly Ap, Monaco JJ, Cho S, Trowsdale J (1991b) A new human class II-related locus, DM. Nature 353:571–573
Kilpatrick DC, Liston WA (1994) Influence of histocompatibility antigens in recurrent spontaneous abortion and its relevance to leukocyte immunotherapy. Hum Reprod 8:1645–1649
Kilpatrick DC, Gibson F, Livingston J, Liston WA (1990) Pre-eclampsia is associated with HLA-DR4 sharing between mother and fetus. Tissue Antigens 35:178–181
King A, Boocock C, Sharkey AM, Gardner L, Beretta A, Siccardi AG, Loke YW (1996) Evidence for the expression of *HLA-C* class I mRNA and protein by human first trimester trophoblast. J Immunol 156:2068–2076
Kirby DR (1970) The egg and immunology. Proc R Soc Med 63:59–61
Kirisits MJ, Kunz HW, Gill TJ III (1991) Analysis of the sequence similarities of classical and non-classical class I genes. In: Tsuji M, Aizawa M, Sasuzuki T (eds) HLA 1991, vol 1. Oxford University Press, Oxford, pp 1021–1030
Kirisits MJ, Sawai H, Kunz HW, Gill TJ III (1994) Multiple TL-like loci in the grc-G/C region of the rat. Immunogenetics 39:301–315

Kirszenbaum M, Moreau P, Gluckman E, Dausset J, Carosella E (1994) An alternatively spliced form of HLA-G mRNA in human trophoblasts and evidence for the presence of HLA-G transcript in adult lymphocytes. Proc Natl Acad Sci USA 91:4209–4213

Komlos L, Zamir R, Joshua H, Halbrecht I (1977) Common HLA antigens in couples with repeated abortions. Clin Immunol Immunopathol 7:330–335

Kostyu DD (1994) HLA: Fertile territory for developmental genes? Crit Rev Immunol 14:29–59

Koyoma M, Saji F, Takahashi S, Takemura M, Samejima Y, Kameda T, Kimura T, Tanizawa O (1992) Probabilistic assessment of the HLA sharing of recurrent spontaneous abortion couples in the Japanese population. Tissue Antigens 37:211–217

Kovats S, Main EK, Librach C, Stubblebine M, Fisher SJ, Demars R (1990) A class I antigen, HLA-G, expressed in human trophoblasts. Science 248:220–223

Kunz HW, Gill TJ III, Dixon BD, Taylor FH, Greiner DL (1980) The growth and reproduction complex in the rat: genes linked to the major histocompatibility complex which affect development. J Exp Med 152:1506–1508

Laitinen T, Koskimies S, Westman P (1993) Foeto-maternal compatibility in HLA-DR, -DQ, and -DP loci in Finnish couples suffering from recurrent spontaneous abortions. Eur J Immunogenet 20:249–258

Le Bouteiller P (1994) HLA class I chromosomal region, genes, and products: facts and questions. Crit Rev Immunol 14:89–129

Loke YW, King A (1991) Recent developments in the human maternal-fetal immune interaction. Curr Opin Immunol 3:762–766

Lyon MF (1981) The t-complex and the genetical control of development. Symp Zool Soc London 47: 455

McIntyre JA, Faulk WP, Nichols-Johnson VR, Taylor CG (1986) Immunologic testing and immunotherapy in recurrent spontaneous abortion. Obstet Gynecol 67:169–174

McMaster MT, Librach CL, Zhon Y, Lim KH, Janatpour MJ, De Mars R, Kovats S, Damsky C, Fisher SJ (1995) Human placental HLA-G expression is restricted to differentiated cytotrophoblasts, J Immunol 154:3771–3778

Medwar PB (1953) Some immunological and endocrinological problems raised by the evolution of viviparity in vertebrates. Symp Soc Exp Biol 7:320–338

Messer G, Zemmour J, Orr HT, Parham P, Weiss EH, Girdlestone J (1992) HLA-J, a second inactivated class I HLA gene related to HLA-G and HLA-A. Implications for the evolution of the HLA-A-related genes. J Immunol 148:4043–4053

Morales PSJ, Corell A, Martinez-Laso J, Martin-Villa M, Varela M, Paz-Artal E, Allende L, Arnaiz-Villena A (1993) Three new HLA-G alleles and their linkage disequilibria with HLA-A. Immunogenetics 38:323–331

Mowbray JF, Gibbings CR, Sidgwick AS, Ruszkiewicz M, Beard RW (1983) Effects of transfusion in women with recurrent spontaneous abortion. Transplant Proc 15:896–899

Nelson JL, Hughes KA, Smith AG, Nisperos BB, Branchaud AM, Hansen JA (1993) Maternal-fetal disparity in HLA class II alloantigens and the pregnancy-induced amerlioration of rheumatoid arthritis. N Engl J Med 329:466–471

Nordlander C, Fuchs T, Hammarström L, Smith CIE (1983) Human leukocyte anigens group A in couples with unexplained infertility. Fertil Steril 40:60–65

Ober C (1992) The maternal-fetal relationship in human pregnancy: an immunogenetic perspective. Exp Clin Immunogenet 9:1–14

Ober C (1995) HLA and reproduction: lessons from studies in Hutterites. Placenta 16:569–577

Ober C, Martin AO, Simpson JL, Hauck WW, Amos DB, Kostyu DD, Fotino M, Allen FH (1983) Shared HLA antigens and reproductive performance in the Hutterites. Am J Hum Genet 35:990–1004

Ober C, Hauck WW, Kostyu DD, O'Brien E, Elias S, Simpson JL, Martin AO (1985) Adverse effects of HLA-DR sharing on fertility: a cohort study in a human isolate. Fertil Steril 44:227–232

Ober C, Elias S, O'Brien E, Kostyu DD, Hauck WW, Bombard A (1988) HLA sharing and fertility in Hutterite couples: evidence for prenatal selection against compatible fetuses. Am J Reprod Immunol Microbiol 18:111–115

Ober C, Elias S, Kostyu DD, Hauck WW (1992) Decreased fecundability in Hutterite couples sharing HLA-DR. Am J Hum Genet 50:6–14

Ober C, Steck T, van der Ven K, Billstrand C, Messer L, Kwak J, Beaman K, Beer AE (1993) MHC class II compatibility in aborted fetuses and term infants of couples with recurrent spontaneous abortion. J Reprod Immunol 25:195–207

Ober C, Rosinsky B, Grimsley C, van der Ven K, Robertson A, Runge A (1996) Population genetic studies of *HLA-G*: allele frequencies and linkage disequilibrium with *HLA-A*. J Reprod Immunol (in press)

Oksenberg JR, Persitz E, Amar A, Brautbar C (1984) Maternal-paternal histocompatibility: lack of association with habitual abortions. Fertil Steril 42:389–395

Orr HT (1989) Characterization of genes encoding non-HLA-A,B,C proteins. In: Dupont B (ed) Immunobiology of HLA. Springer Berlin, Heidelberg New York, pp 33–40

Payne R, Rolfs MR (1958) Fetomaternal leucocyte incompatibility. J Clin Invest 37:1756–1763

Persitz E, Oksenber JR, Margalioth EH, Hacohen S, Schenker J, Brautbar C (1985) Histoincompatibility in couples with unexplained infertility. Fertil Steril 43:733–738

Peterson RDA, Tuck-Miller CM, Spinnato JA, Peevy K, Giattina K, Hoff C (1994) An HLA haplotype associated with preeclampsia and intrauterine growth retardation. Am J Reprod Immunol 31:177–179

Potts WK, Manning CJ, Wakeland EK (1991) Mating patterns in seminatural populations of mice influenced by MHC genotype. Nature 352:619–621

Purandare AS, Smith DS, Wilson PJ (1993) HLA frequency, HLA sharing, and the management of recurrent miscarriage. Int J Fertil 38:219–224

Ratner LE, Hadley GA, Hanto DW, Mohanakumar T (1991) Immunology of renal allograft rejection. Arch Pathol Lab Med 115:283–287

Reznikoff-Etievant MF, Durieux I, Huchet J, Salmon C, Netter A (1988) Human MHC antigens and paternal leucocyte injections in recurrent spontaneous abortions. In: Beard RW, Sharp F (eds) Early pregnancy loss: mechanisms and treatments. Peacock, Ashton-under-Lyne, pp 375–384

Roby KF, Fei K, Yang Y, Hunt JS (1994) Expression of HLA class II-associated peptide transporter and proteasome genes in human placentas and trophoblast cell lines. Immunology 83:444–448

Sargent IL, Wilkins T, Redman CWG (1988) Maternal immune responses to the fetus in early pregnancy and recurrent miscarriage. Lancet 2:1099–1104

Schacter B, Weitkamp LR, Johnson WE (1984) Parental HLA compatibility in parents of offspring with neural-tube defects: evidence for a T/t-like locus in humans. Am J Hum Genet 36:1082–1091

Schmidt CM, Orr Ht(1993) Maternal/fetal interactions: the role of the MHC class I molecule HLA-G. Crit Rev. Immunol 13:207–224

Schneider K, Knutson, Tamsen L, Sjöberg O (1994) HLA antigen sharing in preeclampsia. Gynecol Obstet Invest 37:87–90

Shukla H, Swaroop A, Srivastava R, Weissman SM (1990) The mRNA of a human class I gene HLA G/ HLA 6.0 exhibits a restricted pattern of expression. Nucleic Acids Res 18:2189

Smith JB, Cowchock FS (1988) Immunological studies in recurrent spontaneous abortion: effects of immunization of women with paternal mononuclear cells on lymphocytotoxic and mixed lymphocyte reaction blocking antibodies and correlation with sharing of HLA and pregnancy outcome. J Reprod Immunol 14:99–113

Smith JB, Cowchock FS, Hankinson B, Iftekhar A (1989) Association of HLA-DR5 with recurrent spontaneous abortion in women treated with paternal leukocytes. Arthritis Rheum 32:1572–1576

Sollinger Hw, Burlingham WJ, Sparks EM, Glass NR, Belzer FO (1984) Donor-specific transfusions in unrelated and related HLA-mismatched donor-recipient combinations. Transplantation 38:612–615

Spies T, Bresnaham M, Bahram S, Arnold D, Blanck G, Mellins E, Pious D, DeMars R (1990) A gene in the human major histocompatibility complex class II region controlling the class I antigen presentation pathway. Nature 348:744–747

Steck T, van der Ven K, Kwak J, Beer AE, Ober C (1995) HLA-DQA1 and HLA-DQB1 haplotypes in aborted fetuses and couples with recurrent spontaneous abortion. J Reprod Immunol 29:95–104

Sunderland CA, Naiem M, Mason DY, Redman CWG, Stirrat GM (1981a) The expression of major histocompatibility antigens by human chorionic villi. J Reprod Immunol 3:323–331

Sunderland CA, Redman VWG, Stirrat GM (1981b) HLA-A, -B, -C antigens are expressed on nonvillous trophoblasts of the early human placenta. J Immunol 127:2614–2615

Tabaczewski P, Shirwan H, Lewis K, Stroynowski I (1994) Alternative splicing of class Ib major histocompatibility complex transcripts in vivo leads to the expression of soluble Qa-2 molecules in murine blood. Proc Natl Acad Sci USA 91:1883–1887

Takakuwa K, Kanazawa K, Takeuchi S (1986) Production of blocking antibodies by vaccination with husband's lymphocytes in unexplained recurrent aborters: the role of successful pregnancy. Am J Reprod Immunol Microbiol 10:1–9

Takamizawa M, Juji T, Tsuneyoshi H, Neida M, Fujii T, Kawana T, Mizuno M (1987) Recurrent spontaneous abortion and human leucocyte antigen DRw8. Am J Obstet Gynecol 157:514–515

Taylor CG, Faulk WP (1981) Prevention of recurrent abortions with leucocyte transfusions. Lancet 2:68–69
Taylor CG, Faulk WP, McIntyre JA (1985) Prevention of recurrent spontaneous abortions by leukocyte tranfusions. J R Soc Med 78:623–627
Thomas ML, Harger JH, Wagener DK, Rabin BS, Gill TJ III (1985) HLA sharing and spontaneous abortion in humans. Am J Obstet Gynecol 151:1053–1058
Trowsdale J, Hanson I, Mockridge I, Beck S, Townsend A, Kelly A (1990) Sequences encoded in the MHC related to the 'ABC' superfamily of transporters. Nature 348:741–743
Uehara H (1991) Mouse *Oct-3* maps between the tcl^{12} embryonic lethal gene and the *Qa* gene in the H-2 complex. Immunogenetics 34:266–269
Unander AM, Olding LB (1983) Parental sharing of HLA antigens, absence of maternal blocking antibody, and suppression of maternal lymphocytes. Am J Reprod Immunol 4:171–178
Van der Ven K, Ober C (1994) HLA-G polymorphisms in African Americans. J Immunol 153:5628–5633
Van Rood JJ, Claas FHJ (1990) The influence of allogeneic cells on the human T and B cell repertoire. Science 248:1388–1393
Van Rood JJ, van Leeuwen A, Eernisse JG (1958) Leucocyte antibodies in sera from pregnant women. Nature 181:1735–1736
Vanoli M, Fabio G, Bonara P, Eisera N, Pardi G, Acaia B, Scorza Smeraldi R (1985) Histocompatibility in Italian couples with recurrent spontaneous abortions of unknown origin and with normal fertility. Tissue Antigens 26:227–233
Ward K, Edwin SS, Nelson L, Byrne JLB, Branch DW (1993) Analysis of parental human leukocyte antigen -G(HLA-G) in recurrent pregnancy loss. Soc Gynec Invest 129A
Warner CM, Gollnick SO, Flaherty L, Goldbard SB (1987) Analysis of Qa-2 antigen expression by preimplantation mouse embryos: possible relationship to the preimplantation-embryo-development (PED) gene product. Biol Reprod 36:611–616
Weckstein LN, Patrizio P, Balmaceda JP, Asch RH, Branch DW (1991) Human leukocyte antigen compatibility and failure to achieve a viable pregnancy with assisted reproductive technology. Acta Eur Fertil 22:103–107
Yelavarthi K, Fishback JI, Hunt JA (1991) Analysis of HLA-G mRNA in human placental and extraplacental membrane cells by in situ hybridization. J Immunol 146:2847–2854
Yeom YI, Abe K, Bennett D, Artzt K (1992) Testis-/embryo-expressed genes are clustered in the mouse H-2K region. Proc Natl Acad Sci USA 89:773–777

The Structural Basis of Maternal-Fetal Immune Interactions in the Human Placenta

R.W. REDLINE

1 Introduction

More than 40 years ago Sir PETER MEDAWAR (1955) proposed a set of immunological mechanisms to explain how a semiallogeneic fetus can survive in the maternal host. Since that time a variety of investigators have sought to explain reproductive loss using this framework. Despite validation of many of the mechanisms, significant questions remain regarding the existence and nature of immunologically mediated reproductive failure. Much of the past work has been performed in rodents. Although the hemochorial placentas of primates and rodents have significant homology, it is difficult to overcome two major differences between these two mammalian orders: mass of gestational tissue and duration of pregnancy. The human placenta is several hundred times larger than the rodent placenta and persists in the mother for an average of 280 versus 21 days for the mouse. These different parameters are likely to have exerted divergent evolutionary pressures in the two orders, leading to significant differences in function. The limitation of rodent models is exemplified by the fact that two major causes of perinatal mortality in humans, preterm labor and preeclampsia, do not occur in rodents. For these reasons it is likely that future progress in reproductive immunology will require the increased use of nonhuman primates and the development of better techniques to study immunopathology in human placentas.

Interpretation of experimental and clinical data pertaining to maternal fetal interactions in human pregnancy depends on an understanding of placental

Institute of Pathology, Case Western Reserve University, Cleveland, OH 44106, USA structure. This review considers the anatomic relationships between maternal and fetal tissues at three critical interfaces: the implantation site, the interhemal membrane, and the amniochorion. Simple cataloguing of anatomic relationships, however, provides an incomplete picture of the dynamic interactions that determine placental structure. Among the other topics considered are changes in the antigenic profile of differentiating trophoblast at each interface, the frequency and phenotype of local bone marrow derived leukocytes, and potential sites for normal and abnormal antigen presentation.

Before discussing placental structure it is useful to consider what human obstetrical conditions might be explained by understanding abnormal immune reactivity. While a considerable literature has accumulated implicating aberrant immune regulation in recurrent spontaneous abortion, this is an uncommon and multifactorial syndrome (Stirrat 1990a,b). This review summarizes evidence supporting the following three arguments: (a) that aberrant interactions between trophoblast and uterine cells at the implantation site are involved in preeclampsia and other maternal vasculopathies of pregnancy, (b) that violation of the interhemal membrane by maternal T-cells causes villitis of unknown etiology, a major cause of intrauterine growth retardation in nonhypertensive pregnancies, and (c) that inappropriate activation of fetal and/or maternal macrophages in the placental membranes can upset delicate balance of regulatory factors which prevents premature labor and delivery.

2 Development

Very early stages of pregnancy involving transport of the fertilized zygote through the fallopian tube, adhesion of the blastocyst to the endometrial epithelium, and translocation to the uterine stroma may have relevance to later immunologic reactivity but are not considered here. All later placental development represents elaboration on the same basic structural unit; the early postimplantation blastocyst consisting of the developing trilaminar embryo surrounded by a shell of trophectoderm (days 7.5–10; Hertig 1968; Benirschke and Kaufmann 1995). Invasive syncytial trophoblast differentiates from mononuclear trophectoderm at the periphery of the blastocyst following implantation and invades endometrial capillaries allowing maternal serum and blood products to flow into an intrasyncytial meshwork of lacunar spaces, the future intervillous space (days 10–12.5). The mononuclear trophectoderm (cytotrophoblast) underlying the outer syncytium remains undifferentiated and represents the stem cell lineage for all subsequent trophoblastic growth and differentiation. Fibrous connective tissue, possibly derived from mesenchyme associated with the primary yolk sac, adheres to the inner surface of this layer of cytotrophoblast forming the fibrous chorion (Bianchi et al. 1993). Invaginations of connective tissue project out from the fibrous chorion into the trophoblastic shell. These invaginations interdigitate with the enlarging syn-

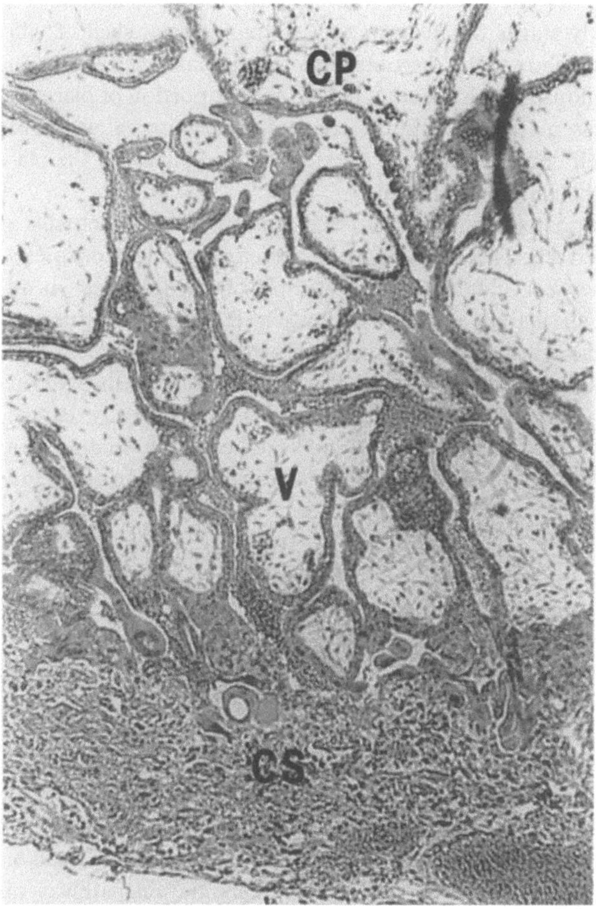

Fig. 1. Basic structure of the early developing placenta. Fibrous connective tissue of the chorionic plate (*CP*) sends projections into the trophoblast forming pillarlike villi (*V*). Cytotrophoblast at the distal tips of the villi punctures the syncytial trophoblast forming a circumferential cytotrophoblast shell (*CS*) around the conceptus

cytial lacunae to form pillar like anchoring villi that serve as struts supporting the intervillous space (days 13–15; Fig. 1).

The distal tips of the anchoring villi become the niduses for proliferative and invasive trophoblast which remodels the uterus and uterine vessels as the placenta grows (see below). Within the anchoring villi fetal connective tissue and lining trophoblast proliferate and undergo branching morphogenesis filling the intervillous space with free-floating villous trees. Villi become vascularized in three stages. First, capillary blood vessels with associated hematopoietic elements develop in situ in the fetal villous mesenchyme adjacent to cytotrophoblast (days 18–21). Second, larger vessels (two arteries and a vein) form along the allantoic duct in the body stalk (later umbilical cord). Finally, the two elements of the placental circulation anastomose and become functional following cardiogenesis at 6 week's gestation. During these early stages the placenta is a circumferential shell of villi connecting the inner fibrous chorion to the outer cytotrophoblast shell. Later in pregnancy (10–12 weeks) villous growth becomes limited to that portion of placenta directly facing the uterine vasculature (the implantation site). The intervillous space in the remainder of the shell collapses, leaving a tough water-tight layer, the placental membranes, facing the endometrial cavity.

From the above it is apparent that the maternal fetal interface is actually a maternal trophoblastic interface. Trophoblast, or its secretory product oncofetal fibronectin, is interposed between maternal and nontrophoblastic fetal cells at all locations of the placenta (Feinberg et al. 1991). Among the features distinguishing trophoblast from other fetal cell lineages are the expression of novel genes (e.g., *HCG, HPL, HLA-G*) (Kurman et al. 1984; Kovats et al. 1990), different patterns of chromosomal imprinting (e.g., preferential inactivation of the paternally derived X chromosome; De Groot and Hochberg 1993), and the occasional finding of a completely different karyotype (confined placental mosaicism) (Kalousek and Dill 1983).

3 Implantation Site/Basal Plate

As described above, the early implanting blastocyst consists of an inner mononuclear and an outer syncytial layer of trophoblast. Proliferative mononuclear trophoblast at the tips of the anchoring villi (cytotrophoblast columns) punctures the syncytium and spreads around the periphery of the blastocyst to form a shell of mononuclear trophoblast (cytotrophoblast shell). The differentiation pathway of shell trophoblast is described in the next paragraph, but the end result is two additional types of trophoblast: intermediate trophoblast, which invades the uterine stroma, and endovascular trophoblast, which migrates centrifugally within the lumina of the uterine arteries. Early in gestation endovascular trophoblast forms nearly occlusive intra-arterial plugs which prevent maternal blood from entering the intervillous space (Hustin and Schaaps 1987). Later (10–12 weeks) trophoblast in these plugs invades the arterial muscle wall, disrupting the continuity of the circumferential smooth muscle layers and thereby transforming the normally contractile arteries into dilated funnel-shaped conduits which allow maternal blood to flow into the intervillous space at low pressure (Ramsay and Donner 1980). As gestation progresses, expansion of the chorionic sac and uterine invasion deplete the cytotrophoblast shell, leaving a layer of extracellular matrix and scattered trophoblast (basal plate). Shortly thereafter (14–22 weeks) the anchoring villi become the focal points for a second wave of trophoblast invasion which extends the implantation site into myometrium and the larger myometrial arteries (Pijnenborg et al. 1981).

The process of uterine invasion and placental remodeling depends on two interacting components, trophoblast and the uterine environment. Considering trophoblast first, a number of different phenotypes can be distinguished as one moves outward from the trophoblast lining the anchoring villus to that which deeply invades the myometrium (Fig. 2). The first cell type is cytotrophoblast, in direct contact with the anchoring villus basement membrane. This cell expresses few specific proteins other than the α_6 β_4 integrin chains which anchor it to the basement membrane (DAMSKY et al. 1992). Later these cells are believed to contribute to a thickening of the anchoring villous basement membrane by elaborating a meshwork of 10-nm fibrils (KING and BLANKENSHIP 1994a). This protective layer

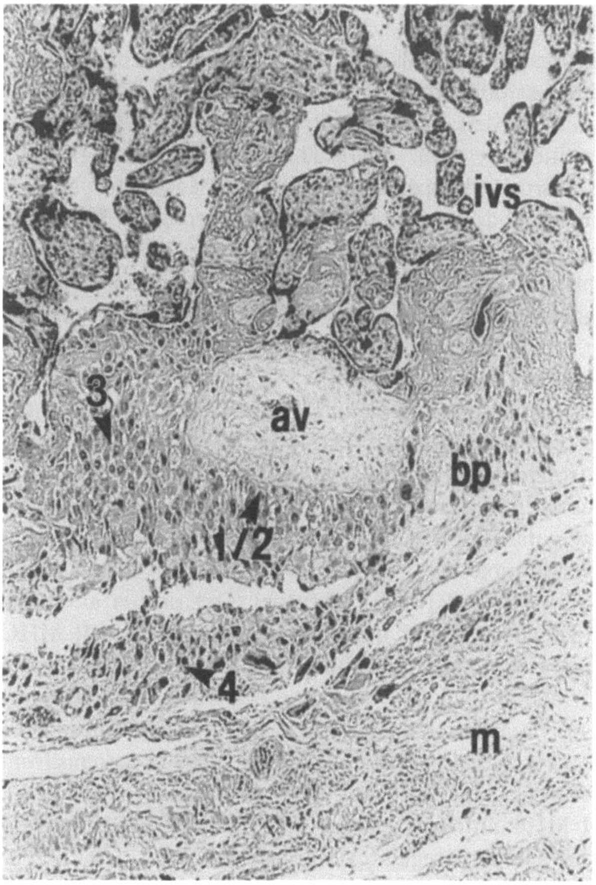

Fig. 2. Implantation site/basal plate. Anchoring villi (*av*) embedded in the basal plate (*bp*) give rise to invasive intermediate trophoblast. *1/2*, Types 1 and 2 (see text) are adjacent to the villous basement membrane; *3*, type 3 forms loosely cohesive aggregates of nonmotile cells surrounded by a prominent extracellular matrix of fibronectin; *4*, type 4 are discohesive invasive cells permeating the endometrium and myometrium (*m*). Note the intervillous space (*ivs*) overlying the basal plate

could be of some importance in view of the relatively common finding of lymphoplasmacytic deciduitis and basal villitis in pathologic pregnancies.

The second cell type is proliferative cytotrophoblast, characterized by clear cytoplasm, high nuclear cytoplasmic ratio, and abundant mitotic figures. These cells maintain cell-cell contact with one another and express a variety of growth-related antigens such as c-*myc*, platelet-derived growth factor-β and its receptor, insulin-like growth factor IGF II, and IGF binding protein 3, proliferating-cell nuclear antigen, and Ki67 (Pfeiffer-Ohlsson et al. 1984; Goustin et al. 1985; Glaser et al. 1992; Blankenship and King 1994a). The first two cell types lack MHC antigens.

The third cell type is a nonmotile discohesive population of trophoblast characterized by abundant fibronectin secretion and the expression of fibronectin binding receptors (α_5/β_1 integrins; Damsky et al. 1992). These cells also synthesize human placental lactogen and express class I MHC antigens. The major class I MHC antigen expressed by these cells is HLA-G, a class Ib MHC molecule with limited but potentially significant polymorphism (van der Ven and Ober 1994). Recently it was reported that conventional HLA-B/C antigens may also be expressed in this third layer (Shorter et al. 1993). This intriguing finding awaits further confirmation. The fourth cell type is invasive intermediate trophoblast which expresses the polyfunctional decidual matrix binding receptor α_1 β_1 integrin (Damsky et al. 1992), several different degradative proteases (72- and 92-kDa collagenases, urokinase plasminogen activator; Blankenship and King 1994b; Polette et al. 1994; Multhaupt et al. 1994), and a number of potential regulators of invasion [transforming growth factor-β (TGF-β), plasminogen-activator inhibitor 1; Selick et al. 1994; Feinberg et al. 1989].

The fifth and final cell type is the endovascular trophoblast, described in the previous paragraph. While the first four cell types represent a continuum of differentiation, endovascular trophoblast diverges at an earlier stage, possibly corresponding to type 1 or 2. The phenotype of endovascular trophoblast overlaps with types 3 and 4 but has a few notable differences, including the expression of polysialyated neuronal-cell adhesion molecule (NCAM), the E-selectin binding ligand sialyl Le-X (Burrows et al. 1994) and IGF-II receptors (Ohlsson et al. 1989). Recently it was reported that endovascular trophoblast expresses class II MHC antigens in pathologic pregnancies (Labarrere and Faulk 1995a). This intriguing finding awaits further confirmation. Type 3, type 4, and endovascular trophoblast all express HLA-G, but not conventional HLA-A/B antigens. In addition to membrane-bound HLA-G, these cells also synthesize soluble HLA-G proteins from alternatively spliced transcripts lacking the transmembrane domain (Fujii et al. 1994). Such soluble class I MHC antigens released into the maternal circulation could be immunogenic or have immunoregulatory properties.

The second component of the basal plate is the uterine environment. One prominent feature of this environment is the presence of decidualized endometrial stromal cells. Decidualization is a hormonally mediated process which converts the normally loose fibroblastic endometrial stroma into a basement membrane-rich epithelioid layer (Finn 1971). Individual decidual cells become encapsulated by a thick basement membrane layer of laminin and types IV and V collagen. The interstitium between cells is filled by types I and III collagen fibrils and fibronectin, which are merocrine secretions of the decidual cells themselves (KISALUS et al. 1987). Undoubtedly the milieu is considerably more complex, including stromal modulators such as Secreted Protein, Acidic, Rich in Cysteine (SPARC), tissue inhibitor of metalloprotease (TIMP-1), IGF binding protein 1, and TGF-β, and agonists such as TGF-α, relaxin, and prolactin (WEWER et al. 1988; RODGERS et al. 1994; RUTANEN et al. 1991; LYSIAK et al. 1995; HOROWITZ et al. 1993; BOGIC et al. 1995; SHAW et al. 1989; ROSENBERG et al. 1980). Decidualized endometrium is widely believed to modulate trophoblast invasiveness, in part because of its absence in invasive conditions such as placenta acreta and ectopic pregnancy. Decidua may also play an immunomodulatory role by regulating allospecific effector cells (BEER and BILLINGHAM 1976) and certain aspects of macrophage function (REDLINE et al. 1988, 1990). The latter activity appears to reside in the matrix rather than the cells themselves (MCKAY et al. 1992).

In addition to decidualized stromal cells, the pregnant human endometrium contains a prominent maternal leukocyte population known as endometrial granulocytes. Endometrial granulocytes include natural killer cells, T-cells bearing the γ/δ T-cell receptor, and cells with features of both natural killer and T-cells (MINCHEVA-NILSSON et al. 1992, 1994). These cells are only weakly cytolytic (FERRY et al. 1990) but secrete cytokines that could play a role in immunoregulation, host defense, placental growth, and/or endometrial remodeling. These include colony-stimulating factor 1, tumor necrosis factor-α (TNF-α), interferon-γ. TGF-β, leukocyte inhibition factor, and granulocyte-macrophage colony-stimulating factor (GM-CSF; JOKHI et al. 1994). Endometrial granulocytes express high-affinity interleukin IL 2 receptors but do not themselves secrete IL-2 (FERRY et al. 1990). While some evidence suggests a specificity for trophoblast (HEYBORNE et al. 1994), these cells cluster much more commonly around the basement membranes of endometrial glands and vessels. The finding of positivity for HSP-60, a common ligand for γ/δ T-cell receptors, at the base of endometrial glands lends support to the hypothesis that these cells are concerned primarily with uterine remodeling (MINCHEVA-NILSSON et al. 1994). In addition to endometrial granulocytes, pregnant endometrium also contains numerous macrophages which seem to encircle but not damage basal plate trophoblast (BULMER et al. 1988). T-cells expressing α/β receptors are infrequent, and B-cells are essentially absent except in pathologic conditions such as preeclampsia, infections, and idiopathic chronic inflammatory conditions (REDLINE 1995).

Additional important components of the uterine environment are the vascular and lymphatic circulations. Interestingly, arteries in the basal plate, but not in the membrane decidua, express L-selectin, the receptor for sialyl Le-X, which is selectively expressed on endovascular trophoblast (BURROWS et al. 1994).

Large veins near the basal plate are occasionally invaded by trophoblast, but from the outside in rather than vice versa as for arteries (BLANKENSHIP et al. 1993). Some evidence in rodents suggests that decidua has a paucity of draining lymphatics, which could limit primary immune responses (HEAD and BILLINGHAM

1986). Evidence for this latter feature, however, is indirect and requires further study. Clearly trophoblast cells, membrane fragments, and various oncofetal antigens have ample access to the maternal circulation from whence they can lodge in either the pulmonary or splenic circulatory beds, depending on their size. The nature of the immune response they elicit in these locations is beyond the scope of this review but could have implications for conditions such as preeclampsia and recurrent spontaneous abortion.

It is a well-known feature of preeclampsia and other maternal vascular disorders that uterine implantation is inappropriately superficial (Brosens et al. 1972). While it is beyond the scope of this review to consider this evidence in detail, three major leads as to the underlying etiology of preeclampsia are being considered at this time. The first relates to the observation that integrin adhesion receptors are not expressed appropriately on intermediate trophoblast in preeclampsia (Zhou et al. 1993), although this has recently been challenged by a second group (Divers et al. 1995). The second involves data linking a particular HLA-G allele to an increased risk of preeclampsia (Main et al. 1994). The third implicates aberrant regulation of vascular tone in preeclampsia which might interact with vascular remodelling in the implantation site. Specifically, particular angiotensinogen alleles (Ward et al. 1993) and acquired defects in calcium homeostasis have been reported in preeclamptic mothers (Zemel et al. 1990; Belizan et al. 1991). Major progress in elucidating the underlying biology is anticipated in the next few years.

4 Interhemal Membrane/Terminal Villi

As described above, the combination of lacunae in the primitive syncytium and invaginated vascularized fetal connective tissue forms an interhemal membrane between the maternal and fetal circulations. Branching morphogenesis of the vascularized fetal connective tissue generates different subtypes of villi, a description of which is beyond the scope of this review (Benirschke and Kaufmann 1995). The important point is that only the most distal branches, known as terminal villi, are normally involved in gas and nutrient exchange. The remainder of the villous tree provides structural support, conducts fetal blood in and out of terminal villi, and generates new terminal villi as the placenta enlarges. Leukocytes and soluble mediators of maternal origin circulate through the intervillous space while leukocytes and mediators of fetal origin flow through the terminal villous capillary bed. Separating the two circulations and constituting the interhemal membrane are syncytiotrophoblast and its basement membrane, villous fibroblasts and their associated extracellular matrix, and fetal capillary endothelium with its basement membrane. The latter basement membrane is a continuous layer in humans (as opposed to the fenestrated type seen in some rodent placentas) but does not become fully established until the third trimester of pregnancy (Demir et al. 1989). Another prominent population in terminal villi are fetal tissue mac-

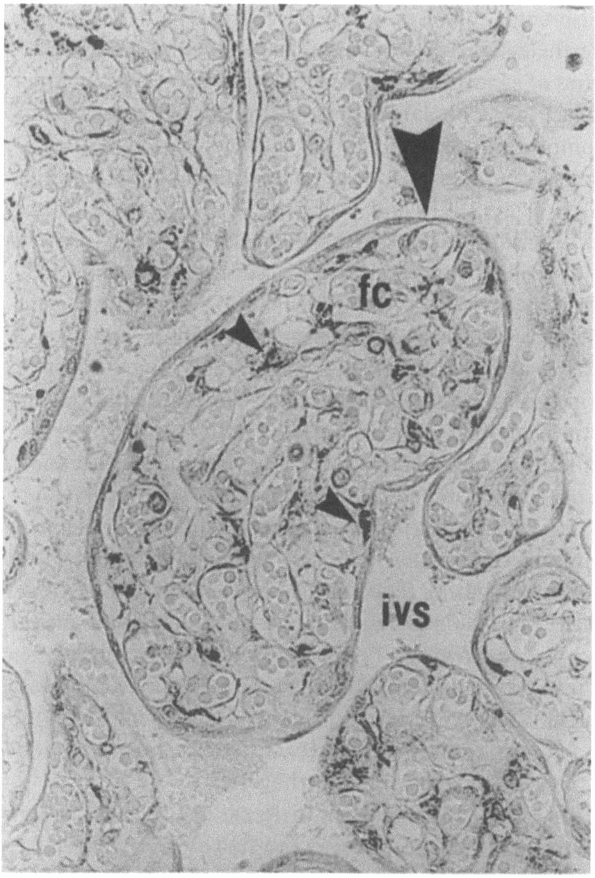

Fig. 3. Interhemal membrane/terminal villi. The interhemal membrane (*large arrow*) separates maternal blood in the intervillous space (*ivs*) from fetal blood in fetal capillaries (*fc*). Moving from the intervillous space inward its layers are syncytiotrophoblast, trophoblastic basement membrane, villous stromal fibroblasts and associated extracellular matrix, and endothelial basement membrane. Note the prominent villous macrophages, also known as Hofbauer cells, indicated by small arrows. Section is immunostained for CD68, a specific macrophage marker

rophages (Hofbauer cells), which are interspersed throughout the fetal connective tissue (Fig. 3).

A detailed consideration of the presence or absence of systemic immunosuppression during pregnancy is beyond the scope of this review. Most evidence suggests that, despite some hormonally mediated immunomodulation, pregnant women retain full capacity to initiate and execute humoral and cell-mediated immune responses (STIRRAT 1994). This capacity is manifest clinically at the interhemal membrane by the pronounced perivillitis and intervillositis observed in *Listeria* infections and in some women with recurrent reproductive failure (DRISCOLL et al. 1962; VALDERRAMA 1992). Furthermore, it is known that a subset of women have complement-fixing antibodies which are reactive with trophoblast (McCrae et al. 1993). Nevertheless, direct attack on the interhemal membrane is uncommon. Specific properties of syncytiotrophoblast may protect it from immune attack. First, unlike trophoblast in the implantation site, syncytiotrophoblast lacks major histocompatibility complex antigens on its cell surface (Galbraith et al. 1981). Second, it fails to express a number of adhesion molecules (e.g., intracellular adhesion molecule 1; Salafia et al. 1991) and procoagulant (e.g., tissue factor; Drake et al. 1989) molecules. Third, it expresses complement regulatory proteins which prevent complement-dependent cell lysis (decay-accelerating factor, CD59, membrane cofactor protein Holmes et al. 1990). Finally, damaged syncytiotrophoblastic cells are constantly shed into the maternal circulation (Chua et al. 1991). This shedding leaves the underlying basement membrane intact and is repaired by a sequence of fibrin deposition, cytotrophoblast stem cell migration, and reepithelialization by syncytiotrophoblast (Nelson et al. 1990).

An indirect mechanism for immune reactivity at the interhemal membrane is through inadvertent mixing of the two circulations. Evidence exists for both fetal to maternal and maternal to fetal trafficking of blood-borne leukocytes. Fetal to maternal traffic involves rupture of terminal villi and probably happens in all pregnancies based on studies of circulating fetal cells in the maternal bloodstream (Medearis et al. 1984). When transfusion is massive, fetuses can die, with anemia and hypovolemia (de Almeida and Bowman 1994). Pathologic pregnancies often have increased fetal-maternal traffic, as evidenced by their frequent association with elevated maternal α-fetoprotein, a large fetal serum protein (Waller et al. 1991). It is likely that the frequent finding of anti-fetal HLA antibodies in multiparous women results from these small fetal-maternal hemorrhages.

Traffic in the opposite direction, from mother to fetus, also occurs, as evidenced by the spread of maternal viral infections to the fetus via passenger leukocytes (Lin et al. 1987). Experiments in rodents suggest that transplacental passage of maternal cells to the fetus can elicit a host versus graft reaction resulting in fetal death (Beer and Billingham 1973). Anecdotal evidence suggests that a similar scenario may occur in some human infants with severe intrauterine growth retardation (Seemayer 1980). An important pathologic lesion, villitis of unknown etiology (VUE) has been shown by two independent methods, chromosome-specific in situ hybridization in male fetuses (Redline and Patterson 1993) and HLA immunostaining in HLA-disparate pregnancies (Labarrere and Faulk 1995b), to be associated with infiltration of fetal villous connective tissue by CD4-positive maternal T-cells (Labarrere et al. 1990). One hypothesis is that VUE represents an in vivo mixed leukocyte reaction since it is known that fetal villous stromal macrophages express class II HLA antigens. Villous inflammation in VUE might even be a mechanism preventing entry of maternal lymphocytes into the fetus itself. A particularly interesting group of patients are those with recurrent VUE and reproductive loss in multiple pregnancies (Redline and Abramowsky 1985). These cases might represent enhanced reactivity of maternal T-cells for fetal antigen or a facilitated pathway for T-cells to enter the villous stroma and/or fetal circulation.

In contrast to barriers blocking maternal cell transfer, maternal immunoglobulin transport to the fetus is actually facilitated by receptor-mediated endocytosis via trophoblast Fc γ receptors and vesicular transport across the fetal endothelium. It is generally felt that maternal immunoglobulin plays a critical opsonic function protecting the fetus from various perinatal pathogens. The receptors involved in facilitated immunoglobulin transport have been extensively studied and recently reviewed (SAJI et al. 1994). Lying between the trophoblast and the endothelium are macrophages which bear fetal target antigens and express Fc γ receptors of several subclasses. One school of thought is that macrophages act as either an antigen-specific or -nonspecific sink regulating the passage of potentially pathogenic antibodies across the fetomaternal barrier (WOOD 1983). Clearly any such mechanism is overwhelmed in cases of hemolytic disease due to maternal blood group antibodies.

Finally, although the ontogeny of the fetal immune system is beyond the scope of this review, we should briefly consider the potential reactivity of fetal leukocytes at the interhemal membrane. Fetal macrophages in mice have a deficit in the upregulation of class II MHC antigens and accessory molecules necessary for antigen presentation (LU and UNANUE 1982). Some evidence suggests that this macrophage defect is due to unique fetal lipid constituents carried by the fetal serum protein, α-fetoprotein (LU et al. 1984; KHAIR-EL-DIN et al. 1995). Prior to term, only long-standing bacterial infections lead to significant fetal neutrophil responses. Lymphoid follicles and plasma cells are seen only in severe congenital infections such as toxoplasmosis or syphilis (KYRIAZIS and ESTERLY 1971). Most fetal T-cells have a naive phenotype bearing only the CD45RA antigen or, in some cases, lacking both CD45RA and CD45RO T-cells (BOFILL et al. 1994). An increased CD45RO-positive population (memory phenotype) in cord blood has recently been touted as a diagnostic test for congenital infections (MICHIE and HARVEY 1994). Finally, an interesting population of fetal γ/δ receptor positive T-cells has been described which lyse maternal T-cells in an allospecific class I MHC dependent manner (MIYAGAWA et al. 1992). Whether these cells provide an additional layer of defense against potential maternal host versus graft reactions remains speculative.

5 Placental Membranes/Decidua and Amniochorion

The final maternal fetal interface to be considered is that formed between decidua and amniochorion in the placental membranes. Endometrium overlying the implanting blastocyst (decidua capsularis) bulges outward toward the uterine lumen as the gestational sac enlarges until it fuses with the lining of the remainder of the uterus (decidua parietalis) to form the membranous decidua. Placental tissue under the decidua capsularis becomes attenuated through atrophy, collapse of the intervillous space, and deposition of a tough extracellular matrix to form the membranous chorion (chorion laevae). Trophoblast in the chorion laevae is a mixture of vacuolated villous-type trophoblast expressing alkaline phosphatase and α_6/β_4 integrins and eosinophilic intermediate-type trophoblast expressing human placental lactogen and α_1/β_1 integrins (YEH et al. 1989; MALAK and BELL 1994). The former cells predominate on the inside near the fibrous chorion, and the latter cells predominate on the outside near the fused decidual layers. Lining the inner surface of the chorion laevae is the amnion, a circumferential sac of ectodermally derived epithelial cells which is continuous with and antigenically similar to fetal skin (ROBINSON et al. 1984). Separating amnionic epithelium from fibrous chorion are

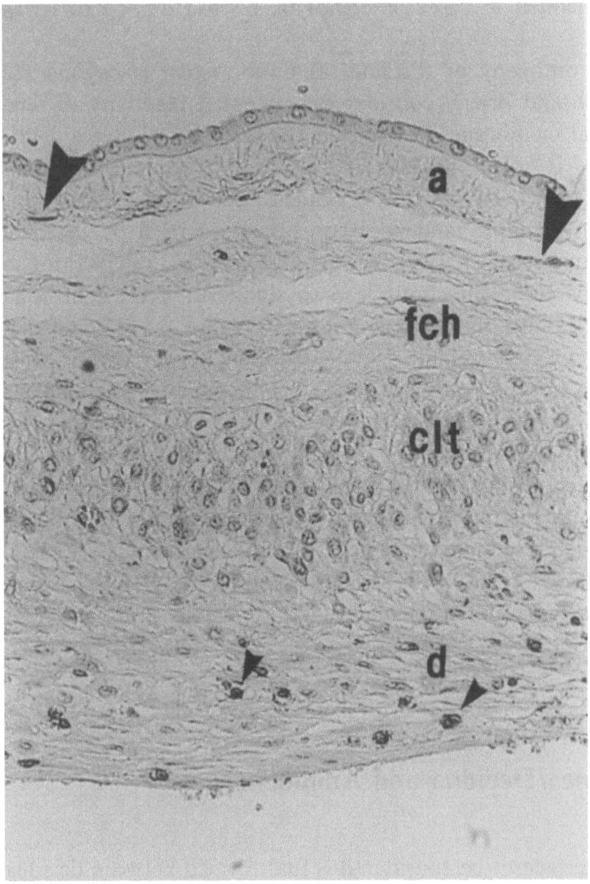

Fig. 4. Placental membranes/decidua and amniochorion. Maternally derived decidua (*d*) represents endometrial stroma separating fetal amniochorion from contractile maternal smooth muscle. Fibrous chorion (*fch*) and chorion laevae trophoblast (*clt*) represent the collapsed shell of the early circumferential placenta. Amnion (*a*) consists of an epithelial layer, basement membrane, and several layers of fibrous connective tissue. Section is immunostained for CD68, a specific macrophage marker by *Large arrows*, fetal macrophages in amniochorionic connective tissue; small arrows, maternal macrophages in the decidua

several layers of connective tissue and a basement membrane (BOURNE 1960; VAN HERENDAEL et al. 1978). Amnion and chorion are only loosely attached to one another while chorion and decidua are tightly adherent (Fig. 4). A final component of the membrane environment in utero is the junction between decidua and myometrium. Considered from this perspective, the decidua is strategically placed between fetal amniochorion and myometrium where it can act as a regulator of signals controlling the timing of labor and delivery.

Fetal and maternal cells can potentially interact at two separate locations in the membranes. The first is the decidual-chorion laevae interface where inflammatory cells exiting from decidual postcapillary venules encounter chorion laevae trophoblast, and the second is the amnion-amniotic fluid interface where maternal inflammatory cells from the cervix and vagina encounter fetal amnionic epithelial cells. Interestingly, both of these fetal cell types, chorion laevae trophoblast and amnionic epithelium, express HLA-G molecules (YELAVARTHI et al. 1991; HOULIHAN et al. 1995). In addition to parenchymal cells, fetal and maternal leukocytes (predominantly macrophages) share the membrane environment. Unlike the situation described above for VUE, there is no direct evidence that mixing of fetal and maternal cells in the membranes leads to alloreactivity.

It is likely that inappropriate activation of inflammatory cells in the membrane environment contributes to the pathogenesis of preterm labor. To understand the potential impact of immune mediators on premature delivery it is necessary to digress briefly on the normal mechanism of labor. The control of parturition is incompletely understood and undoubtedly involves multiple regulatory systems. The final events in the labor cascade are believed to be the formation of gap junctions between myometrial cells allowing for coordination of uterine contractions, effective stimulus-contraction coupling for the induction of contractions (HUSZAR and NAFTOLIN 1984), and protease activation allowing for the dissolution of the tensile strength imparted by membrane connective tissue (VADILLO-ORTEGA et al. 1995). The exact order in which these events occur is unclear and may not always be the same. Among the literally hundreds of mediators studied several are considered key by virtue of changes in their concentration or activity at the time of labor. Decreased myometrial nitric oxide synthetase activity enhances the formation of myometrial gap junctions (RADETSKY 1994). Release of decidual prostaglandin $PGF_{2\alpha}$ is believed to be the final inducer of contractions (MITCHELL 1984). $PGF_{2\alpha}$ release may depend on signaling mediated through oxytocin receptors (TAKEMURA et al. 1994) and, possibly, priming by cortiocotropin-releasing hormone released by the adjacent chorion laevae (PERKINS and LINTON 1995). The major membrane protease elevated at the time of labor is mmp-9 (BRYANT-GREENWOOD and YAMAMOTA 1995). Inhibition of labor, on the other hand, is thought to involve mediators released by fully differentiated decidual stromal cells including relaxin, prolactin, IGF binding protein 1, and antiproteases such as TIMP-1 and plasminogen-activator inhibitor 1 (BRYANT-GREENWOOD et al. 1993; BRYANT-GREENWOOD and YAMAMOTA 1995; LOCKWOOD 1994). Initiation of labor is thought to be signaled by the mature fetus itself via mediators released into the amniotic fluid from urine or lung fluid (CASEY et al. 1983a,b; BILLAH and JOHNSTON

1983). These signals are believed to act on amnionic epithelial cells, possibly by eliciting synthesis of amnionic PGE_2, and transduced across chorion laevae and decidua to myometrium through a series of poorly characterized steps (Mitchell 1984).

It has been hypothesized that fetal and maternal macrophages are pivotal regulatory cells in the membrane environment (Hunt 1989). Noxious stimuli such as bacterial infection, ischemia, and the products of activated maternal lymphocytes at the maternal fetal interface are all potential activators of these cells. These stimuli are poorly dealt with in the immunologically privileged and sequestered fetal environment. There may have been considerable evolutionary pressures to develop mechanisms to short-circuit the normal labor pathway in these situations to deliver the nearly mature fetus rapidly before the well-being of both mother and offspring is jeopardized. Several points are germane. First, fetal and maternal macrophages are strategically placed in amniochorion and decidua, respectively (Fig. 4; Bulmer and Johnson 1985). Second, recent data suggest that decidua is an environment dominated by cytokines generally associated with type 2 T-helper cell immune responses such as IL-10, which is synthesized by decidual cells in mice (Lin et al. 1993; IL-4, which is synthesized by human amniocytes (Jones et al. 1995), a and a variety of other cytokines such as IL-3, GM-CSF, and TGF-beta which are products of decidual natural killer cells and/or trophoblast (Jokhi et al. 1994; Dudley et al. 1993). This type 2 T-helper cell environment may be disrupted by activated macrophages which can produce IL-1, TNF-α, IL-6, IL-8, PGE_2, platelet-activating factor and other proinflammatory mediators (reviewed in Hunt 1989). These cytokines could act in a variety of ways. IL-1 and TNF-α are known to inhibit decidual stromal cell differentiation and function (Frank et al. 1995; Inoue et al. 1994; Jikihara and Handwerger 1994; Jikihara et al. 1995) and induce 72- and 92-kDa metalloproteinases (reviewed in Woessner 1991). IL-1 by itself elicits preterm labor in rhesus monkeys (Witkin et al. 1994) and IL-1 induced labor is blocked in mice by injecting IL-1RA, a specific IL-1 antagonist (Romero and Tartakovsky 1992). IL-6 and IL-8 are attractants for and activators of neutrophils which secrete additional inflammatory mediators and proteases. PGE_2 is a potent inducer of uterine contractions, and platelet-activating factor is a potent potentiator of smooth muscle contraction and PG synthesis (reviewed in Lockwood 1994).

6 Conclusion

The picture that has emerged over the past decade is one in which direct immunologic attack on the placenta is subverted at multiple levels by structural barriers, lack of target and accessory molecules, and immunoregulatory factors released by maternal, placental, and fetal cells. Nevertheless, in contrast to rodent gestation, inflammatory lesions are not infrequent in the human placenta. Placental pathologists commonly encounter processes such as chronic villitis, massive intervillositis, lymphoplasmacytic deciduitis, decidual perivasculitis, and chronic chorionitis in association with reproductive failure (REDLINE 1995). Among the underlying causes under investigation at this time are antigen-specific maternal responses to placental implantation, inadvertent mixing of maternal and fetal leukocytes, and inappropriate activation of placental macrophages. Future progress will depend on the contributions of geneticists, immunologists, and perinatal pathologists to identify genetic and epigenetic factors contributing to the distinctive phenotypes observed in these patients.

References

Beer AE, Billingham RE (1973) Maternally acquired runt disease: immune lymphocytes from the maternal blood can traverse the placenta and cause runt disease in the progeny Science 179:240–243

Beer AE, Billingham RE (1976) The immunobiology of mammalian reproduction. Prentice-Hall, Englewood Cliffs, pp 23–40

Belizan JM, Villar J, Gonzalez L, Campodonico L, Bergel E (1991) Calcium supplementation to prevent hypertensive disorders of pregnancy N Engl J Med 325:1399–1405

Benirschke K, Kaufmann (1995) Pathology of the human placenta. 3rd edn. Springer Berlin Heidelberg, New York

Bianchi DW, Wilkins-Huag LE, Enders AC, Hay ED (1993) Origin of extraembryonic mesoderm in experimental animals: relevance to chorionic mosaicism in humans. Am J Med Gen 46:542–550

Billah MM, Johnston JM (1983) Identification of phospholipid platelet-activating factor (1-O-alkyl-2-acetyl-sn-glycero-3-phosphocholine) in human amniotic fluid and urine. Biochem Biophys Res Commun 113:51–58

Blankenship TN, King BF (1994a) Developmental expression of Ki-676 antigen and proliferating cell nuclear antigen in macaque placentas Dev Dyn 201:324–333

Blankenship TN, King BF (1994b) Identification of 72-Kilodalton type IV collagenase at sites of trophoblastic invasion of macaque spiral arteries Placenta 15:177–187

Blankenship TN, Enders AC, King BF (1993) Trophoblastic invasion and modification of uterine veins during placental development in macaques Cell Tissue Res 274:135–144

Bofill M, Akbar AN, Salmon M, Robinson M, Burford G, Janossy G (1994) Immature CD45RA^{low}-RO^{low} T cells in the human cord blood. I. Antecedents of CD45RA^{+} unprimed T cells. J Immunol 152:5613–5623

Bogic LV, Mandel M, Bryant Greenwood GD (1995) Relaxin gene expression in human reproductive tissues by in situ hybridization. J Clin Endocrinol Metab 80:130–137

Bourne GL (1960) The microscopic anatomy of the human amnion and chorion. Am J Obstet Gynecol 79:1070–1073

Brosens IA, Robertson WB, Dixon HG (1972) The role of the spiral arteries in the pathogenesis of preeclampsia. In: Wynn R (ed) (Contributions to Obstetetrics and Gynecology) Annual Appleton Century Crofts, New York, pp 177–191

Bryant-Greenwood GD, Yamamoto SY (1995) Control of peripartum collagenolysis in the human chorion-decidua. Am J Obstet Gynecol 172:63–70

Bryant-Greenwood GD, Rutanen EM, Partanen S, Coelho TK, Yamamoto SY (1993) Sequential appearance of relaxin, prolactin and IGFBP-1 during growth and differentiation of the human endometrium, Mol Cell Endocrinol 95:23–29

Bulmer JN, Johnson PM (1985) Identification of leucocytes within the human chorion laeve. J Reprod Immunol 7:89–92

Bulmer JN, Smith J, Morrison L, Wells M (1988) Maternal and fetal cellular relationships in the human placental basal plate. Placenta 9:237–246

Burrows TD, King A, Loke YW (1994) Expression of adhesion molecules by endovascular trophoblast and decidual endothelial cells: implications for vascular invasion during implantation. Placenta 15:21–33

Casey ML, MacDonald PC, Mitchell MD (1983a) Stimulation of prostaglandin E2 production in amnion cells in culture by a substance(s) in human fetal and adult urine. Biochem Biophys Res Commun 114:1056–1063

Casey ML, Cutrer SI, Mitchell MD (1983b) Origin of prostanoids in human amniotic fluid: the fetal kidney as a source of amniotic fluid prostanoids. Am J Obstet Gynecol 147:547–551

Chua S, Wilkins T, Sargent I, Redman C (1991) Trophoblast deportation in pre-eclamptic pregnancy, Br J Obstet Gynaecol 98:10

Damsky CH, Fitzgerald ML, Fisher SJ (1992) Distribution patterns of extracellular matrix components and adhesion receptors are intricately modulated during first trimester cytotrophoblast differentiation along the invasive pathway, in vivo. J Clin Invest 89:210–222

De Almeida V, Bowman JM (1994) Massive fetomaternal hemorrhage: Manitoba experience. Obstet Gynecol 83:323–328

De Groot N, Hochberg A (1993) Gene imprinting during placental and embyronic development. Mol Reprod Dev 36:390–406

Demir R, Kaufmann P, Castellucci M, Erbengi T, Kotowski A (1989) Fetal vasculogenesis and angiogenesis in human placental villi. Acta Anat (Basel) 136:190–203

Divers MJ, Bulmer JN, Miller D, Lilford RJ (1995) Beta 1 integrins in third trimester human placentae: no differential expression in pathological pregnancy. Placenta 16:245–260

Drake TA, Morrissey JH, Edgington TS (1989) Selective cellular expression of tissue factor in human tissues. Am J Pathol 134:1087–1097

Driscoll SG, Gorbach A, Feldman D (1962) Congenital listeriosis: diagnosis from placental studies. Obstet Gynecol 20:216–220

Dudley DJ, Chen C-L, Mitchell MD, Daynes RA, Araneo BA (1993) Adaptive immune responses during murine pregnancy: pregnancy-induced regulation of lymphokine production by activated T lymphocytes. Am J Obstet Gynecol 168:1155–1163

Feinberg RF, Kao L-C, Haimowitz JE, Queenan JT Jr, Wun T-C, Strauss JF III, Kliman HJ (1989) Plasminogen activator inhibitor types 1 and 2 in human trophoblasts: PAI-1 is an immunocytochemical marker of invading trophoblasts. Lab Invest 61:20–26

Feinberg RF, Kliman HJ, Lockwood CJ (1991) Is oncofetal fibronectin a trophoblast glue for human implantation? Am J Pathol 138:537–543

Ferry BL, Starkey PM, Sargent IL, Watt GMO, Jackson M, Redman CWG (1990) Cell populations in the human early pregnancy decidua: natural killer activity and response to interleukin-2 of CD56-positive large granular lymphocytes. Immunology 70:446–452

Finn CA (1971) The biology of decidual cells. Adv Reprod Physiol 5:1–26

Frank GR, Brar AK, Jikihara H, Cedars MI, Handwerger S (1995) Interleukin-1 beta and the endometrium: an inhibitor of stromal cell differentiation and possible autoregulator of decidualization in humans. Biol Reprod 52:184–191

Fujii T, Ishitani A, Geraghty DE (1994) A soluble form of the HLA-G antigen is encoded by a messenger ribonucleic acid containing Intron 4. J Immunol 153:5516–5524

Galbraith RM, Kantor RRS, Ferrara GB, Ades EW, Galbraith GMP (1981) Differential anatomical expression of transplantation antigens within the normal human placental chorionic villus. Am J Reprod Immunol 1:331–335

Glaser A, Luthman H, Stern I, Ohlsson R (1992) Spatial distribution of active genes implicated in the regulation of insulin-like growth factor stimulatory loops in human decidual and placental tissue of first-trimester pregnancy. Mol Reprod Dev 33:7–15

Goustin AS, Betsholtz C, Pfeifer-Ohlsson S, Persson H, Rydnert J, Bywater M, Holmgren G, Heldin C-H, Westermark B, Ohlsson R (1985) Coexpression of the sis and myc proto oncogenes in developing human placenta suggests autocrine control of trophoblast growth. Cell 41:301–312

Head JR, Billingham RE (1986) Concerning the immunology of the uterus. Am J Reprod Immunol Microbiol 10:76–81

Hertig AT (1968) Human trophoblast. Thomas, Springfield

Heyborne K, Fu Y-X, Nelson A, Farr A, O'Brien R, Born W (1994) Recognition of trophoblasts by $\gamma\delta$ T cells. J Immunol 153:2918–2926

Holmes CH, Simpson KL, Wainwright SD, Tate CG, Houlihan JM, Sawyer IH, Rogers IP, Spring FA, Anstee DJ, Tanner MJ (1990) Preferential expression of the complement regulatory protein decay accelerating factor at the fetomaternal interface during human pregnancy. J Immunol 144:3099–3105

Horowitz GM, Scott RT, Drews MR, Navot D, Hofmann GE (1993) Immunohistochemical localization of transforming growth factor-alpha in human endometrium, decidua, and trophoblast. J Clin Endocrinol Metab 76:786–792

Houlihan JM, Biro PA, Harper HM, Jenkinson HJ, Holmes CH (1995) The human amnion is a site of MHC class 1b expression: evidence for the expression of HLA-E and HLA-G. J Immunol 154:5665–5674

Hunt JS (1989) Cytokine networks in the uteroplacental unit: macrophages as pivotal regulatory cells. J Reprod Immunol 16:1–17

Hustin J, Schaaps JP (1987) Echographic and anatomic studies of the maternotrophoblastic border during the first trimester of pregnancy. Am J Obstet Gynecol 157:162–168

Huszar G, Naftolin F (1984) The myometrium and uterine cervix in normal and preterm labor. N Engl J Med 311:571–581

Inoue T, Kanzaki H, Iwai M, Imai K, Narukawa S, Higuchi T, Katsuragawa H, Mori T (1994) Tumour necrosis factor alpha inhibits in vitro decidualization of human endometrial stromal cells. Hum Reprod 9:2411–2417

Jikihara H, Handwerger S (1994) Tumour necrosis factor-alpha inhibits the synthesis and release of human decidual prolactin. Endocrinology 134:353–357

Jikihara H, Poisner AM, Handwerger S (1995) Tumor necrosis factor-alpha and interleukin-1 beta inhibit the synthesis and release of renin from human decidual cells. J Clin Endocrinol Metab 80:195–199

Jokhi PP, King A, Sharkey AM, Smith SK, Loke YW (1994) Screening for cytokine messenger ribonucleic acids in purified human decidual lymphocyte populations by the reverse-transcriptase polymerase chain reaction. J Immunol 153:4427–4435

Jones CA, Williams KA, Finlay Jones JJ, Hart PH (1995) Interleukin 4 production by human amnion epithelial cells and regulation of its activity by glycosaminoglycan binding. Biol Reprod 52:839–847

Kalousek DK, Dill F (1983) Chromosomal mosaicism confined to the placenta in human conceptions. Science 221:665–667

Khair-El-Din TA, Sicher SC, Vazquez MA, Wright WJ, Lu CY (1995) Docosahexaenoic acid, a major constituent of fetal serum and fish oil diets, inhibits IFN γ-induced Ia-expression by murine macrophages in vitro. J Immunol 154:1296–1306

King BF, Blankenship TN (1994) Ultrastructure and development of a thick basement membrane-like layer in the anchoring villi of macaque placentas. Anat Rec 238:498–506

Kisalus LL, Herr JC, Little CD (1987) Immunolocalization of extracellular matrix proteins and collagen synthesis in firsttrimester human decidua. Anat Rec 218:402–415

Kovats S, Main EK, Librach C, Stubblebine M, Fisher SJ, DeMars R (1990) A class I antigen, HLA-G, expressed in human trophoblasts. Science 248:220–223

Kurman RJ, Young RH, Norris HJ, Main CS, Lawrence WD, Scully RE (1984) Immunocytochemical localization of placental lactogen and chorionic gonadotropin in the normal placenta and trophoblastic tumors, with emphasis on intermediate trophoblast and the placental site trophoblastic tumor. Int J Gynecol Pathol 3:101–121

Kyriazis AA, Esterly JR (1971) Fetal and neonatal development of lymphoid tissues. Arch Pathol 91:444–451

Labarrere CA, Faulk WP (1995a) Intercellular adhesion molecule-1 (ICAM-1) and HLA-DR antigens are expressed on endovascular cytotrophoblasts in abnormal pregnancies. Am J Reprod Immunol 33:47–53

Labarrere CA, Faulk WP (1995b) Maternal cells in chorionic villi from placentae of normal and abnormal human pregnancies. Am J Reprod Immunol 33:54–59

Labarrere CA, McIntyre JA, Faulk WP (1990) Immunohistologic evidence that villitis in human normal term placentas is an immunologic lesion. Am J Obstet Gynecol 162:515–522

Lin HH, Lee TY, Chen DS (1987) Transplacental leakage of HBeAg-positive maternal blood as the most likely route in causing intrauterine infection with hepatitis B virus. J Pediatr 111:877–881

Lin H, Mosmann TR, Guilbert L, Tuntipopipat S, Wegmann TG (1993) Synthesis of T helper 2-type cytokines at the maternal-fetal interface. J Immunol 151:4562-4573

Lockwood CJ (1994) Recent advances in elucidating the pathogenesis of preterm delivery, the detection of patients at risk, and preventative therapies. Curr Opin Obstet Gynecol 6:7–18

Lu CY, Unanue ER (1982) Ontogeny of murine macrophages: functions related to antigen presentation. Infect Immun 36:169–175

Lu CY, Changelian PS, Unanue ER (1984) α-Fetoprotein inhibits macrophage expression of Ia antigens. J Immunol 132:1722–1727

Lysiak JJ, Hunt J, Pringle GA, Lala PK (1995) Localization of transforming growth factor β and its natural inhibitor decorin in the human placenta and decidua throughout gestation. Placenta 16:221–231
Main E, Chiang M, Colbern G (1994) Nulliparous preeclampsia (PE) is associated with placental expression of a variant allele of the new histocompatibility gene: HLA-G. Am J Obstet Gynecol 170:289
Malak TM, Bell SC (1994) Differential expression of the integrin subunits in human fetal membranes. J Reprod Fertil 102:269–276
McCrae KR, DeMichele AM, Pandhi P, Balsai MJ, Samuels P, Graham C, Lala PK, Cines DB (1993) Detection of antitrophoblast antibodies in the sera of patients with anticardiolipin antibodies and fetal loss. Blood 82:2730–2741
McKay DB, Vasquez MA, Redline RW, Lu CY (1992) Macrophage functions are regulated by murine decidual and tumor extracellular matrices, J Clin Invest 89:134–142
Medawar PB (1953) Some immunological and endocrinological problems raised by the evolution of viviparity in vertebrates. Symp Soc Exp Biol 7:320–338
Medearis AL, Hensleigh PA, Parks DR, Herzenberg LA (1984) Detection of fetal erythrocytes in maternal blood post partum with the fluorescence-activated cell sorter. Am J Obstet Gynecol 148:290
Michie C, Harvey D (1994) Can expression of CD45RO, a T-Cell surface molecule, be used to detect congenital infection? Lancet 343:1259–1260
Mincheva-Nilsson L, Hammarstrom S, Hammarstrom M-L (1992) Human decidual leukocytes from early pregnancy contain high numbers of $\gamma\ \delta^+$ cells and show selective down-regulation of alloreactivity. J Immunol 149:2203–2211
Mincheva-Nilsson L, Baranov V, Yeung MM-W, Hammarstrom S, Hammarstrom M-L (1994) Immunomorphologic studies of human decidua-associated lymphoid cells in normal early pregnancy. J Immunol 152:2020–2032
Mitchell MD (1984) The mechanism(s) of human parturition. J Dev Physiol 6:107–118
Miyagawa Y, Matsuoka T, Baba A, Nakamura T, Tsuno T, Tamura A, Agematsu K, Yabuhara A, Uehara Y, Kawai H, Miyasaka K (1992) Fetal liver T cell receptor γ / δ^+ T cells as cytotoxic T lymphocytes specific for maternal alloantigens. J Exp Med 176:1–7
Multhaupt HAB, Mazar A, Cines DB, Warhol MJ, McCrae KR (1994) Expression of urokinase receptors by human trophoblast: a histochemical and ultrastructural analysis. Lab Invest 71:392–400
Nelson DM, Crouch EC, Curran EM, Farmer DR (1990) Trophoblast interaction with fibrin matrix: epithelialization of perivillous fibrin deposits as a mechanism for villous repair in the human placenta. Am J Pathol 136:855–865
Ohlsson R, Holmgren L, Glaser A, Szpecht A, Pfeifer-Ohlsson S (1989) Insulin-like growth factor 2 and short-range stimulatory loops in control of human placental growth. EMBO J 8:1993-1999
Perkins AV, Linton EA (1995) Identification an isolation of corticotrophin-releasing hormone-positive cells from the human placenta. Placenta 16:233–243
Pfeifer-Ohlsson S, Goustin AS, Rydnert J, Wahlstrom T, Bjersing L, Stehelin D, Ohlsson R (1984) Spatial and temporal pattern of cellular myc oncogene expression in developing human placenta: implications from embryonic cell proliferation. Cell 38:585–596
Pijnenborg R, Bland JM, Robertson WB, Dixon G, Brosens I (1981) The pattern of interstitial trophoblastic invasion of the myometrium in early human pregnancy. Placenta 2:303–316
Polette M, Nawrocki B, Pintiaux A, Massenat C, Maquoi E, Volders L, Schaaps JP, Birembaut P, Foidart JM (1994) Expression of gelatinases A and B and their tissue inhibitors by cells of early and term human placenta and gestational endometrium. Lab Invest 71:838–846
Radetsky P (1994) Stopping premature births before it's too late. Science 266:1486–1488
Ramsay EM, Donner MW (1980) Placental vasculature and circulation. Saunders, Philadelphia, pp 26–30
Redline RW (1995) Placenta and adnexa in late pregnancy. In: Reed GB, Claireaux AE, Cockburn F (eds) Disease of the fetus and newborn, 2nd edn. Chapman and Hall, London, pp 319–338
Redline RW, Abramowsky CR (1985) Clinical and pathologic aspects of recurrent placental villitis. Hum Pathol 16:727–731
Redline RW, Patterson P (1983) Villitis of unknown etiology is associated with major infiltration of fetal tissue by maternal inflammatory cells. Am J Pathol 143:473–479
Redline RW, Shea CM, Papaioannou VE, Lu CY (1988) Defective anti-listerial responses in deciduoma of pseudopregnant mice. Am J Pathol 133:485–497
Redline RW, McKay DB, Vasquez MA, Papaioannou VE, Lu Cy (1990) Macrophage functions are regulated by the substratum of murine decidual stromal cells. J Clin Invest 85:1951–1958
Robinson HN, Anhalt GJ, Patel HP, Takahashi Y, Labib RS, Diaz LA (1984) Pemphigus and pemphigoid antigens are expressed in human amnion epithelium. J Invest Dermatol 83:234–237

Rodgers WH, Matrisian LM, Giudice LC, Dsupin B, Canon P, Svitek C, Gorstein F, Osteen KG (1994) Patterns of matrix metalloproteinase expression in cycling endometrium imply differential functions and regulation by steroid hormones. J Clin Invest 94:946–953
Romero R, Tartakovsky B (1992) The natural interleukin-1 receptor antagonist prevents interleukin-1-induced preterm delivery in mice. Am J Obstet Gynecol 167:1041–1045
Rosenberg SM, Maslar IA, Riddick DH (1980) Decidual production of prolactin in late gestation: further evidence for a decidual source of amniotic fluid prolactin. Am J Obstet Gynecol 138:681–685
Rutanen E-M, Partanen S, Pekonen F (1991) Decidual transformation of human extrauterine mesenchymal cells is associated with the appearance of insulin-like growth factor-binding protein-1. J Clin Endocrinol Metab 72:27–31
Saji F, Koyama M, Matsuzaki N (1994) Current topic: human placental Fc receptors. Placenta 15:453–466
Salafia CM, Haynes N, Merluzzi VJ, Rothlein R (1991) Distribution of ICAM-1 within decidua and placenta and its gestational age-associated changes. Pediatr Pathol 11:381–388
Seemayer TA (1980) The graft-versus-host reaction: a pathogenetic mechanism of experimental and human disease. In: Rosenberg HS, Bolande RP (eds) Perspectives in pediatric pathology, vol 5. Masson, New York, pp 93–135
Selick CE, Horowitz GM, Gratch M, Scott RT Jr, Navot D, Hofmann GE (1994) Immunohistochemical localization of transforming growth factor-β in human implantation sites. J Clin Endocrinol Metab 78:592–596
Shaw KJ, Do YS, Kjos S, Anderson PW, Shinagawa T, Dubeau L, Hsueh WA (1989) Human decidua is a major source of renin. J Clin Invest 83:2085–2092
Shorter SC, Starkey PM, Ferry BL, Clover LM, Sargent IL, Redman CWG (1993) Antigenic heterogeneity of human cytotrophoblast and evidence for the transient expression of MHC Class I antigens distinct from HLA-G. Placenta 14:571–582
Stirrat GM (1990a) Recurrent miscarriage. I. Definition and epidemiology. Lancet 336:673–675
Stirrat GM (1990b) Recurrent miscarriage. II. Clinical associations, causes, and management. Lancet 336:728–733
Stirrat GM (1994) Pregnancy and immunity. BMJ 308:1385–1386
Takemura M, Kimura T, Nomura S, Makino Y, Inoue T, Kikuchi T, Kubota Y, Tokugawa Y, Nobunaga T, Kamiura S, Onoue H, Azuma C, Saji F, Kitamura Y, Tanizawa O (1994) Expression and localization of human oxytocin receptor mRNA and its protein in chorion and decidua during parturition. J Clin Invest 93:2319–2323
Vadillo-Ortega F, Gonzalezavila G, Furth EE, Lei HQ, Muschel RJ, Stetlerstevenson WG, Strauss JF (1995) 92 kd type IV collagenase (matrix metalloproteinase-9) activity in human amniochorion increases with labor. Am J Pathol 146:148–156
Valderrama E (1992) Massive chronic intervillositis. Report of three cases. Lab Invest 66:10
Van der ven K, Ober C (1994) HLA-G polymorphisms in African Americans. J Immunol 153:5628–5633
Van Herendael BJ, Oberti C, Brosens I (1978) Microanatomy of the human amniotic membranes: a light microscopic, transmission, and scanning electron microscopic study. Am J Obstet Gynecol 131:872–880
Waller DK, Lustig LS, Cunningham GC, Golbus MS, Hook EB (1991) Second-trimester maternal serum alpha-fetoprotein levels and the risk of subsequent fetal death. N Engl J Med 325:6–10
Ward J, Hata A, Jeunemaitre X, Helin C, Nelson L, Namikawa C, Farrington PF, Ogasawara M, Suzumori K, Toomoda S, Berrebi S, Sasaki M, Crovol P, Lifton RP, Lalouel J-M (1993) A molecular variant of angiotensinogen associated with preeclampsia. Nature [Genet] 4:59–61
Wewer UM, Albrechtsen R, Fisher LW, Young MF, Termine JD (1988) Osteonectin/SPARC/BM-40 in human decidua and carcinoma, tissues characterized by De Novo formation of basement membrane. Am J Pathol 132:345–355
Witkin SS, Gravett MG, Haluska GJ, Novy MJ (1994) Induction of interleukin-1 receptor antagonist in rhesus monkeys after intraamniotic infection with group B streptococci or interleukin-1 infusion. Am J Obstet Gynecol 171:1668–1672
Woessner JF Jr (1991) Matrix metalloproteinase and their inhibitors in connective tissue remodeling. FASEB J 5:2145–2154
Wood GW (1983) Role of macrophages in the elimination of anti-fetal antibody during its transport through the human placenta. Surv Synth Pathol Res 1:196–207
Yeh I-T, O'Connor DM, Kurman RJ (1989) Vacuolated cytotrophoblast: a subpopulation of trophoblast in the chorion laeve. Placenta 10:429–438

Yelavarthi KK, Fishback JL, Hunt JS (1991) Analysis HLA-G mRNA in human placental and extraplacental membrane cells by in situ hybridization. J Immunol 146:2847–2854
Zemel MB, Zemel PC, Berry S, Norman G, Kowalczyk C, Sokol RJ, Standley PR, Walsh MF, Sowers JR (1990) Altered platelet calcium metabolism as an early predictor of increased peripheral vascular resistance and preeclampsia in urban black women. N Engl J Med 323:434–438
Zhou Y, Damsky CH, Chiu K, Roberts JM, Fisher SJ (1993) Preeclampsia is associated with abnormal expression of adhesion molecules by invasive cytotrophoblasts. J Clin Invest 91:950–960

Immunobiology of the Decidua

P.C. Arck and D.A. Clark

McMaster University, Departments of Medicine, Pathology, Obstetrics and Gynecology, Molecular Virology-Immunology Program, 1200 Main Street West, Hamilton L8N 3Z5, Canada

1 Introduction

In mammalian reproduction the fertilized oocyte develops into an embryo which attaches to the uterine tissue from which it obtains nutrition sufficient to develop to maturity, at which point it is born alive (Bell 1983). In different species the details of the embryo-uterine lining interactions differ. In primates and rodents trophoblast cells which form the outer layer of the preimplanting blastocyst attach to the uterine epithelium, invade or destroy the epithelial barrier, and ultimately establish direct contact with maternal blood and maternal uterine lining stromal cells (Enders 1991). The latter rapidly differentiate into large glycogen-filled cells called decidual cells (Bell 1983). In other species, such as the horse, the trophoblast interdigitates with epithelium, and part of the trophoblasts invade and form "cups" in stroma, but decidualization does not occur (Allen et al. 1986). The lifespan of the "cup" trophoblast is brief, and the fundamental relationship sustaining nourishment of the growing fetus is a maternal epithelium-fetal trophoblast (epitheliochorial) interface. It follows then that decidual transformation plays an important role where trophoblast interfaces with maternal blood and stroma, and where this relationship must survive for the full duration of pregnancy.

Because the embryo usually arises by mating of histoincompatible individuals, the embryo has been viewed as a foreign graft (Billingham 1964). Indeed, in humans, rodents, and horses a maternal antibody response to antigens on the "graft" is not uncommon, and yet the embryo is not rejected or compromised (Bell and Billington 1986). Enders (1991) has proposed that decidualization represents a key element in creating a relationship that minimizes chances of rejection. As is seen below, rejection, when it occurs spontaneously in the form of abortion, is more akin to rejection of a tumor (a collection of primitive neoplastic cells) by natural effector cells. In the process of rejection by natural effector cells, the decidua may facilitate or inhibit, and classical immune responses, where they occur, may enhance protection against rejection rather than promote it.

Decidualized endometrium is more complex than a mere collection of enlarged glycogen-filled stromal cells. There are arteries and veins, lymphatics, and maternal lymphomyeloid cells that must be considered. The epithelium of the endometrium contains intraepithelial lymphocytes, and in the stroma, T cells, B cells, natural killer (NK) cells, and lymphatics are present (Bulmer et al. 1988; Starkey et al. 1988; Clark et al. 1994a; King and Loke 1991; Hunt 1994). There are changes in the composition of decidual tissue as pregnancy progresses, differences between species, and differences depending on the nature of the stimulus initiating decidualization (Pace et al. 1991; Bulmer 1992; Chernyshov et al. 1993; Clark 1995). The endometrium may be exposed to pathogens, and thus must be able to mount both natural and antigen-specific immune responses (Bell and Billington 1986; Clark 1991; Enders 1991). The success of pregnancy, however, requires avoiding rejection of the embryo. The latter is due in large measure to fetal trophoblast cells, which are resistant to killing by antigen-specific and natural effector cells of the type present in the decidua (Drake and Head 1989a; Head 1989; Ljunggren and

KÄRRE 1990; LOKE 1990; KING and LOKE 1991). However, pregnancy rejection does occur, and decidua-associated cells play an important role.

This review focuses on two species, the mouse and the human, and two types of decidual stimuli:

- Murine species:
  Direct contact with trophoblast
  Epithelial trauma (causing deciduoma) (in pseudopregnant or hormone primed mice)
- Human species:
  Direct contact with trophoblast
  Remote, as in ectopic pregnancy

The role of decidua in pregnancy failure is also discussed. We first discuss rodent pregnancy since more direct experimental data are available. Based on information obtained from investigations in mouse models, successful and aborting human pregnancies have been studied with similar findings (CLARK 1990).

2 Murine Pregnancy Decidua

2.1 Description of Implantation and Decidualization

The trophoblast of the blastocyst contacts and attaches to endometrial epithelium on the antimesometrial side of the uterus and induces the local formation of decidua, called the primary decidua. As the embryo grows, its ectoplacental cone (EPC) trophoblast grows across the lumen of the uterus and attaches to the mesometrial endometrium. This results in the formation of the mesometrial decidua, called secondary decidua (BELL 1983).

2.2 Secondary Versus Primary Decidua

The primary decidua zone excludes macrophages and lymphatic tissue, but in the mesometrial decidua there are granulated lymphatic cells present at the time of EPC invasion (LYSIAK and LALA 1992). Both antimesometrial and mesometrial decidua cells are considered to arise by in situ differentiation of local stromal fibroblast-type cells (CLARKE et al. 1994). As pregnancy progresses, trophoblast invasion and proliferation are altered in favour of differentiation into a placenta. Initially there are three layers: an outer layer of giant trophoblast cells, which degenerate by the middle of pregnancy, leading to decidual contact with the spongiotrophoblast, the middle layer, and an inner layer of labyrinthine trophoblast (REDLINE and LU 1989). Spongiotrophoblast cells act as precursors for other trophoblastic tissue; cell marker studies suggest about 40% of the cells in the spongy zone are maternal and not fetal (REDLINE and LU 1989; ROSSANT et al. 1983).

Concerning the inner layer of labyrinthine trophoblast, the labyrinth consists of fetal vessels and stroma separated from maternal blood by a trilaminar trophoblast. In the mouse spongiotrophoblast cells express paternal class I major histocompatibility complex (MHC) whereas giant cells and labyrinthine trophoblast do not (HEDLEY et al. 1989; VAN Kaer et al. 1991).

2.3 Local and Systemic Host Responses to Placenta

A systemic maternal immunresponse to the placenta, the fetal "graft", may lead to generation of IgG antibody and to cytotoxic T cells (RAGHUPATHY et al. 1981; BELL and BILLINGTON 1986; SMITH et al. 1978). Fetectomy studies have shown that the placenta alone is sufficient to induce an antibody response (BELL and BILLINGTON 1986). Further, there is enlargement of regional lymph nodes that is greater in allogenic than in syngeneic pregnancy, suggesting an immune response, but no cytotoxic T lymphocytes (CTL) are present (CLARK and MCDERMOTT 1978). There is little evidence of either antigen-specific or non-specific systemic immunosuppression (by α_2-macroglobulin or blocking antibody or suppressor cells) of sufficient magnitude to prevent graft rejection in a pregnant host (NAGARKATTI and CLARK 1983).

Spongiotrophoblast cells which express paternal class I MHC alloantigens are in direct contact with the uterine decidua from days 13.5 until 21.5 of pregnancy in the mouse (BILLINGTON and BURROWS 1989; HEDLEY et al. 1989; CLARK 1990). While trophoblast cells express class I MHC, they are not immunogenic when transferred to another host, and the nature of the immune stimulus for antibody formation by the placenta is therefore uncertain. CTL may also be generated in spleen by pregnancy (SMITH et al. 1978; MANJUNATH et al. 1985). It is notable that primed effector cells can also be generated in the spleens of pregnant rodents by immunization, but this does not lead to rejection (WEGMANN et al. 1979). Antibody to MHC can bind to placenta, and putative CTL generated in vitro in opti-MEM CTL medium may kill trophoblast (DRAKE and HEAD 1989b). Nevertheless, one does not find accumulation of effector cells (CTL or antibody-dependent cellular cytotoxicity effectors) at the fetomaternal interface where antigen is expressed. What may prevent such accumulation? NK and natural cytotoxic cells are present at the interface in small numbers; what is their significance (CLARK et al. 1994a)?

2.4 Local Immunological Mechanisms in Decidua

2.4.1 Granulated Material Gland Cells

During placentation some of the granulated cells differentiate by enlarging and forming 15–20 μm diameter granulated metrial gland (GMG) cells (CROY et al. 1988, 1991; WOOD et al. 1988; CLARKE et al. 1994). The accumulation of these cells in the mesometrial area outside the uterus suggested a "gland", and here the cells were called GMG or metrial gland (MG) cells. GMG cells do not express mature T cell markers and are present in SCID and *nu/nu* mice; therefore they are not an endproduct of T cell differentiation (KINSKY et al. 1990; LINNEMEYER and POLLACK 1991; CLARK et al. 1994b). Studies by a number of investigators indicate a haemopoietic origin of GMG cells (KEARNS and LALA 1983; LYSIAK and LALA 1992). The best evidence that precursors of GMG cells migrate from the bone marrow to the uterus is derived from rat bone marrow reconstituted in mice (PEEL and STEWART 1989). In the pregnant murine decidua GMG cells share numerous surface markers with NK cells and may exhibit NK-like cytotoxic activity in YAC target cells when deliberately activated by interleukin (IL) 2 (CROY and KASSOUF 1989; CROY et al. 1991; LINNEMEYER and POLLACK 1991). Interestingly, NK cells found in spleen that kill YAC without IL-2 cannot kill trophoblast or most types of freshly isolated malignant tumor cells, but when activated by IL-2 into lymphokine activated killer (LAK) cells, they efficiently kill both. By contrast, GMG cell can kill some trophoblast cells without IL-2 activation (STEWART and MUKHTARD 1994).

As mentioned above, GMG share numerous surface markers with NK cells and exhibit cytotoxic activity in the presence of IL-2, and their granules contain cytolytic molecules such as perforin and serine esterase (PARR et al. 1987; CROY et al. 1991; LINNEMEYER and POLLACK 1991). The role of GMG cells in murine pregnancy remains unknown; one function may be to prevent trophoblast from invading through the full thickness of the uterine wall. However, this idea is difficult to test since there are no published data on GMG knockout pregnant mice available, and anti-asialo-GM1 antibody treatment does not significantly deplete GMG cell numbers in decidua (PARR et al. 1987). GMG cells produce a variety of cytokines, including IL-2, and embryotoxic factor, but not tumor necrosis Factor-α (TNF-α; CROY et al. 1991). Metrial gland tissue did appear to release immunosuppressive activity and also had growth factor activity. Supernatants of isolated GMG cells (kindly provided by Dr. B.A. Croy) were not immunosuppressive in assays performed in our laboratory (unpublished data). Recently TNF-α has been detected in situ and may promote trophoblast differentiation via production of TNF-α (HUNT 1994). However, studies using a highly sensitive TNF-α reporter gene transgenic system has failed to detect TNF-α gene expression in decidua where GMG cells occur (GIROIR et al. 1992); rather, it is the placenta that expresses the gene in the mouse (GIROIR et al. 1992).

2.4.2 Macrophages

Macrophages derived from explanted murine decidua or blood and cultured in vitro synthesize high levels of prostaglandin (PG) E_2, which inhibits NK cell proliferation into LAK cells in response to IL-2 synthesis (HUNT and POLLARD 1992). However, in the decidua at the fetomaternal interface, macrophages are absent due to their failure to migrate from perivascular areas (REDLINE et al. 1990). Also, uterine macrophages show significant impairment in their ability to deal with intracellular pathogens such as Listeria as their function is inhibited by decidual stroma (REDLINE et al. 1990). Although uterine macrophages may present antigens in vitro, it is unclear whether they possess this ability in situ (DULCOS et al. 1994). Therefore, the in situ functional activities of macrophages in decidua are uncertain.

2.4.3 T Cells

Immunohistochemicl studies have shown significant numbers of T cells in murine decidual tissue. The number of cells increases as pregnancy progresses, and is greater in allogenic than in syngeneic pregnancy (Kearns and Lala 1983). The location of the T cells in the uterus is uncertain, but certainly there should be some within maternal blood in vascular spaces. Large $CD8^+$ cells with immunosuppressive activity develop in the endometrium immediately after mating and persist through the time of implantation until day 8.5 when the placenta begins to form (Bierley and Clark 1987; Clark et al. 1989). In early pregnancy $CD8^+$ cells in peripheral blood and spleen are induced to express progesterone receptors and secrete in response to progresterone a 34-kDa molecule that inhibits cytotoxic cells such as NK and LAK cells. Alloactivation seems to be an important stimulus increasing expression of progesterone receptors (Szekeres-Bartho et al. 1990). However, depletion of CD8-positive cells in vivo has little effect on pregnancy success in *most* strains of mice or rats, but in CBA/J females that have a high abortion rate when mated to DBA/2J males, anti-CD8 antibody treatment greatly increases the abortion rate. Indeed, anti-CD8 causes a significant increase in the abortion rate in CBA/J females mated to BALB/c, where the abortion rate is usually very low (Clark et al. 1994a); a pregnancy by BALB/c or immunization with BALB/c spleen cells lowers the abortion rates of DBA/2J-mated CBA/J females (Chaouat and Lankar 1988). These data show $CD8^+$ cells to be crucial in immune reactions that prevent abortion in susceptible strains of females. The physiological importance of $CD8^+$ T cells remain uncertain for most types of pregnancy, but in abortion-prone mice they may play a role. Cloned $CD8^+$ T cells secrete a TH_1 pattern of proinflammatory cytokines [i.e. γ-interferon (γ-INF), TNF-α and IL-2], *but* some $CD8^+$ T cells become $CD4^- 8^-$ T cells and secrete a TH_2 pattern of cytokines (i.e. IL-10, IL-4 and IL-5; Erard et al. 1993). IL-4 production at the fetomaternal interface could activate the switch from TH_1 to TH_2 differentiation pathways (Delassus et al. 1994).

2.4.4 Non-T Non-B Immunosuppressor Cells

A small granulated suppressor cell has been identified in the murine decidua and where GMG cells occur, which has previously been described as a non-B/non-T suppressor cell that releases a suppressor effect resembling that of, transforming growth factor-β_2 (TGF-β_2) which appears to be secreted in situ (Clark et al. 1991a, 1993b, 1995; Lea et al. 1992). Recent observations suggest that CD3 is present on these cells, and hence the suppressor cell may have a T cell lineage (unpublished data, manuscript in preparation). However, TGF-β_2 producing suppressor cells are present in the decidua of pregnant *nu/nu* and SCID mice (Clark et al. 1994b). $CD3^+$ bone marrow derived natural suppressor cells have been found in the spleen of pregnant mice and have been shown to secrete TGF-β_1 in vitro; these cells carry αβ T cell receptors and react with the monoclonal antibodies 2C1.1 and 1E5B5.1

(Brooks-Kaiser and Hoskin 1993). Decidual natural suppressor cells that produce TGF-β_2-like factor react with 1E5B5.1 but not 2C1.1 (Merali et al. 1995).

The TGF-β_2-like molecule has a number of effects potentially relevant to pregnancy. NK cell activation and LAK cell generation are inhibited, as is macrophage activation, by cytokines; adherence of neutrophils to endothelial cells and endothelial cell damage by granulocytes may be prevented (Clark et al. 1985, 1990b; Gordon and Galli 1990; Clark 1993). The TGF-β_2-like factor has a novel molecular weight and appears deficient in certain properties of conventional TGF-β such as stimulation of collagen synthesis (Clark et al. 1995). Monoclonal anti-TGF-β_2 increases abortion rates even in low-aborting strains such as C3H/HeJ as well as in CBA/J. Thus the TGF-β_2-like factor could prevent accumulation and activation of a number of different types of potentially abortogenic effector cells at the fetomaternal interface.

TJ6 is another novel suppressor T cell related protein found in the uterus during murine pregnancy and particularly on placenta (Nichols et al. 1994; Mandal and Beaman 1995). TJ6 was originally detected using a monoclonal antibody against a CD4 T cell derived factor that induces CD8$^+$ suppressor T cell activity (Lee et al. 1990). Mice treated with anti-TJ6 monoclonal antibody prior to the time of implantation manifest implantation failure, whereas mice treated during later stages of pregnancy showed no effect on the pregnancy (Nichols et al. 1994). Therefore TJ6 may be important in early pregnancy at the time of implantation when CD8$^+$ suppressor cells are present in the decidua. Downregulation of NK activity may be important at the time of implantation (Povea-Pacci and Roberts 1995).

IL-10 is another potently immunosuppressive T cell product that may be present in the decidua (Clark 1993; Lin et al. 1993; Wegmann et al. 1993). While IL-10 usually comes from the TH_2 subset of CD4$^+$ cells, as mentioned above CD8$^+$ cells may be induced to produce TH_2-type cytokines, and IL-10 is present in supernatants of cultured decidua taken on days 6.5 and 12.5 of pregnancy (Erard et al. 1993; Lin et al. 1993). By polymerase chain reaction analysis, however, IL-10 should be present in situ only at the earlier time point (Delassus et al. 1994). Therefore generation of IL-10 may be induced by culturing. In situ hybridization data suggest a uterine stromal cell origin of IL-10 (Lin et al. 1993). However, a major source of IL-10 in supernatants of cultured pregnancy tissue appears to be in the placenta (Chaouat et al. 1995); with immunization, which prevents abortion, it is placental IL-10 production that is boosted. IL-10 is known selectively to suppress TH_1-mediated cellular immunity, and IL-10 strongly inhibits the production of inflammatory cytokines such as γ-INF, TNF-α and IL-2 during early pregnancy (Mosmann and Moore 1991; Lin et al. 1993). Interestingly, TNF-α is produced mostly by the placenta in vitro (Raghupathy et al. 1981). Anti-IL-10 antibody causes abortion, but primarily in CBA/J mated DBA/2J; there is little effect in matings that normally have a low abortion rate. Hence IL-10 may be one of the cytokines involved in countering rejection when proinflammatory cytokine production is upregulated in placenta, but IL-10 may play little role in the success of pregnancy in low abortion rate mating combinants. The role of IL-10 in early pregnancy is uncertain, and the TGF-β_2-like factor represents the main contribution made by *decidua* to ensure continued viability and resistance to trophoblast damage by NK cells.

Another source of suppression are cytokines such as granulocyte macrophage-colony stimulating factor (GM-CSF) and IL-3 (CLARK 1993). GM-CSF may be produced by T cells and uterine stromal cells; its role in the control of placental cell proliferation has been proposed as part of the immunotropism theory (WEGMANN 1988). In murine pregnancy GM-CSF is produced by endometrial cells from mice of the genotype *nu/nu* and *scid/scid* which lack functional T cells, and T cell depletion does not affect GM-CSF production (BANCROFT et al. 1989; ROBERTSON et al. 1991). GM-CSF does not appear to have any direct effect on embryo or trophoblast, as tested in vitro (LEA and CLARK 1993); however, it may influence maternal tubal and endometrial cells. Recombinant GM-CSF reduces the activity of a subset of spontaneously activated NK-lineage cells in the spleens of injected mice that are capable of killing trophoblast target cells, and $CD8^+$ T cells are required for this effect (CLARK et al. 1994a). GM-CSF may also be produced by murine trophoblast, based on the presence of mRNA detection in northern blots (CRAINIE et al. 1990), and GM-CSF protective effects also occur early (day 6.5–7.5) during pregnancy (CLARK 1993).

2.4.5 Roles of Cytokines in the Decidua

Cytokines produced by T cells and macrophages may be important for normal trophoblast development, and bidirectional interactions in the maternal-fetal relationship have been proposed (WEGMANN 1988; CLARK et al. 1991b; CLARK 1993; WEGMANN et al. 1993). Some cytokines are abortogenic and are discussed below.

2.5 Placental Barrier Model and the Role of the Decidua

Resistance of trophoblast to killing by CTL and conventional NK cells led to a concept of a shield interposed between the fetal allograft and the mother. This barrier was thought to prevent contact between maternal effector cells and the fetus which can be killed by CTL. Labelled maternal lymphocytic cells enter only a small percentage of fetuses and in small numbers (HUNZIKER et al. 1984). However, labelled cells do not circulate/recirculate normally, and we now know that significant numbers of maternal lymphocytes enter the fetus and induce tolerance to the maternal MHC haplotype (ZHANG and MILLER 1993). The way in which the fetus avoids a fatal graft-versus-host reaction is not discussed here. Suffice it to say, the fetus has its own suppressor mechanisms. Nevertheless, any cells entering the placental maternal blood pool may be exposed to factors produced by decidua (CLARK et al. 1993a) and by trophoblast (see CHAOUAT and MENU, this volume). Evidence for in situ suppression in decidua was provided by experiments of SIO (1985), where skin allografts at the choriodecidual junction of rats were partially protected from strong transplantation immunity; grafts on decidua remote from the implants were not. It is of interest that the development of small-sized non-T non-B suppressor cells in the decidua requires local signals from the trophoblast (SLAPSYS et al. 1988). These observations indicate the presence of an unique immunosuppressive environment in the decidua associated with trophoblast.

2.6 Pregnancy Failure in Murine Animal Models

2.6.1 Spontaneous Abortions

Studies with the abortion-prone mouse model CBA/J × DBA/2J show that by contrast to nonabortive pregnancies there is a cellular infiltration at the resorption/abortion site which contains NK cells, and CTL treatment with anti-T-cell antibodies or an anti-IL-2 receptor antibody that is effective in vivo does not prevent abortion (CHAOUAT 1994), but injection with antibody to asialo-GM1, which depletes NK cells, *is* able to prevent abortion (CLARK 1991). The primary importance of natural effector cells in rejection has been supported by the observation that freshly isolated trophoblast is resistant to lysis by CTL and antibody-dependent cell-mediated killing mechanisms (DRAKE and HEAD 1989a), but NK cells can be activated into LAK cells by IL-2, and LAK kill trophoblast. TNF-α also boosts the activity of NK-lineage cells in spleen that kill a murine trophoblast cell line in vitro (CLARK et al. 1993a).

Most studies of determinants of normal and aborting pregnancies have used the CBA/J × DBA/2J model system (CHAOUAT et al. 1990; CLARK et al. 1990a). As mentioned above, prevention of abortion in CBA/J mice mated to DBA/2J can be induced by immunization using BALB/c-strain lymphoid cells, which carry the same MHC antigens as DBA/2J but are more immunogenic (CHAOUAT and LANKAR 1988). Pregnancy by BALB/c male is also protective (CHAOUAT et al. 1988). The mechanism of protection requires $CD8^+$ T cells (see CHAOUAT and MENU, this volume), IL-10 production by placenta is increased by immunization, and TGF-β_2 producing suppressor cell activity in decidua is boosted (CHAOUAT et al. 1995; CLARK et al. 1990a). From this data it is postulated that DBA/2J antigens fail to activate $CD8^+$ maternal T cells required for adequate protection. Abortion in CBA/J mice can also be prevented by the use of clean cage housing, and it is thought exposure to the endotoxin of normal flora activates abortogenic mechanisms in these mice (CLARK et al. 1993). Not all strains of mice are affected, and hence $CD8^+$ T cell dependent suppressor cell function is not always crucial for successful pregnancy (CLARK et al. 1994a).

2.6.2 Induced Murine Pregnancy Failure

Murine pregnancy failure can be induced in a variety of ways. Injection of lipopolysaccharide stimulates macrophages to release TNF-α; LPS abortion can be abrogated by treatment with pentoxifylline which inhibits TNF-α production or by alloimmunization (CHAOUAT 1994; CLARK 1990). Poly I:C is also abortogenic and appears to act via asialo-$GM1^+$ NK cells (KINSKY et al. 1990).

Additional information about mechanisms of abortion and its prevention has recently been obtained by exposing the females to a brief period of stress during early gestation (CLARK et al. 1993c). Stress is known to increase the abortion rate in several strains of mice, and stress-triggered abortions in CBA/J mice pregnant by DBA/2J can be corrected by preimmunization with BALB/c lymphocytes or by injection of antibody to the asialo-GM1 determinant of NK cells (ARCK et al. 1995a). It is logical to suspect that stress can cause abortion by altering the endocrine system, but lowered levels of progesterone do not occur as a result of stress, and there is little change in cortisol or prolactin (ARCK et al. 1995b). In stressed mice increased levels of the abortogenic cytokine TNF-α have been found in decidua in early pregnancy, and this is associated with decreased levels of pregnancy-protective TGF-β_2 related suppressive activity in uterine decidua later in pregnancy. In the alloimmunized animals, where stress fails to boost the abortion rate, these effects are abrogated. It is unclear how stress increases TNF-α production. The neurotransmitter substance P (SP) is known to be able to increase the production of TNF-α by both mast cells and macrophages (STEAD and BIENENSTOCK 1990); both cells may be present in the decidua, and SP-positive afferent nerve fibers are also present (ARCK et al. 1995b). Neural stimulation is known to promote SP release in tissues (STANISZ 1994). TNF-α is known to cause abortion when injected into mice and rats, and appears to act on the placental vasculature resulting in haemorrhage and necrosis (CHAOUAT et al. 1995; CLARK 1993). TNF-α has also been demonstrated to inhibit DNA synthesis and proliferation in trophoblast cells and may also be involved in the activation of NK cells into LAK-type cells, able to damage fetal trophoblast cells (CLARK et al. 1993a).

Functional receptors for SP have also been detected lymphocytes and neutrophils (STANISZ et al. 1987). SP modulates a variety of host responses, including T cell proliferation, immunoglobulin synthesis, lymphocyte traffic, macrophage activation, mast cell degranulation, and release of histamine, as well as mast cell dependent granulocyte infiltration (WAGNER et al. 1987; STEAD and BIENENSTOCK 1990; BOST and PASCUAL 1992). Also, SP may induce the production of IL-1, IL-6 and γ-IFN by certain cell types (WAGNER et al. 1987); IL-1 and γ-IFN have been reported to cause abortion in rodents similar to TNF-α (CLARK 1993). In our model, blocking SP prevented abortion as effectively it did immunization, and blocking SP also prevented the cytokine changes induced by stress (ARCK et al. 1995b). It is therefore necessary to consider neurotransmitters and neurone cells as well as mast cells as important players in the immunobiology of decidual tissue.

3 Deciduoma

A variety of artificial stimuli, such as oil droplets, and physical trauma are capable of inducing decidualization in rodents; the resulting mass of tissue is referred to as a deciduoma (BELL 1985). Deciduoma tissue closely mimics the decidua of true pregnancy; however, major differences in the tissue which arises after induction with either natural or artificial stimuli have been identified. Cellular components of decidua and deciduoma differ. In the deciduoma no GMG cells have been identified, and there are no small lymphocyte suppressor cells (SLAPSYS et al. 1986). BADET (1984) described secretion of a 60-kDa suppressor factor by deciduoma tissue, but further characterization has not been produced. Macrophage functions are paralysed as in regular pregnancy decidua (REDLINE et al. 1990; CHOUDHURI and WOOD 1992).

4 Human Pregnancy Decidua

At the time of implantation a single-celled outer layer of the blastocyst, the trophectoderm, and its cellular descendant, the cytotrophoblast, invade the uterine epithelium and come into direct and increasingly intimate contact with maternal decidua and blood. Where there is contact with blood, cytotrophoblast cells fuse to form a nonproliferating syncytium. At other sites cytotrophoblast invades into decidua and forms anchoring columns and penetrates the decidua as extravillous trophoblast (BELL 1983).

4.1 Decidua-Associated Cells

4.1.1 Granulated Lymphocytes

Maternal lymphomyeloid cells are present in human decidua in significant numbers (DAYA et al. 1985). Some 75%–80% of leucocytes in the human decidua in the early pregnancy are large granulated lymphocytes (LGL), which decrease in number during pregnancy and are scant at term (BULMER et al. 1988; BULMER 1992; MARUYAMA et al. 1992; HALLER et al. 1995). LGL may represent the human analogue of rodent GMG cells but are much smaller (BELL 1983). These LGL have been called *Körnchenzellen* or endometrial granulated lymphocytes and bear an atypical antigenic phenotype. They are intensely positive for CD56, a surface antigen which is expressed by NK cells, do not express T cell antigens such as CD3, CD4 and CD8, and lack the peripheral blood NK cell antigens CD16 and CD57 (CHRISTMAS et al. 1990; KING et al. 1991, 1993; LOKE et al. 1993; DENIZ et al. 1994; COULAM et al. 1995). NK cells of this phenotype are largely uterus specific, but are present in 1% of blood NK cells (KING et al. 1991).

The role of LGL in normal pregnancy is unclear. Since LGL are scarce during the proliferative phase of the menstrual cycle but accumulate in increasing number at the luteal phase and remain in significant numbers throughout the first trimester of pregnancy, they may regulate the extent of trophoblast invasion (LOKE 1990; BULMER 1992). The mechanisms by which they control trophoblast invasion are not clear. Invading cytotrophoblast cells are allogenic fetal cells but lack classical class I and II MHC antigens (HEDLEY et al. 1989; KOVATS et al. 1990). However, extravillous cytotrophoblast expresses a nonclassical MHC class I protein, HLA-G, which may reduce susceptibility to maternal NK and LAK cells (CHUMBLEY et al. 1994b). The interaction of HLA-G and NK cells may play an important role during trophoblast invasion since the expression of HLA-G could be a strategy adapted by the trophoblasts to escape destruction by NK cells (CHUMBLEY et al. 1994a). LGL in peripheral blood mediate NK cell activity, and LGL purified from first trimester decidua have been shown to lyse NK target cells, although they are poor effectors compared with peripheral blood lymphocytes (KING et al. 1989; MANASEKI and SEARLE 1989; BULMER et al. 1991; FERRY et al. 1991). Cultured human trophoblast can be lysed by LAK cells, but fresh trophoblast cells are resistant (KING and LOKE 1990; FERRY et al. 1991). Taken together, these data suggest decidual LGL would not likely inhibit human trophoblast by a cytolytic mechanism. However, cytokines released by decidual LGL could be crucial in the regulation of trophoblast invasion by altering differentiation and expression of adhesion receptors. CD $56^{+}16^{-}$ decidual LGL release novel TGF-β_2 related factors and GM-CSF and may make other cytokines based on mRNA analysis (CLARK 1994a; CLARK et al. 1994a; JOKHI et al. 1994).

4.1.2 Macrophages

Macrophages have been observed in the areas proximate to the implantation site and express the tissue macrophage antigens $CD14^{+}$ and $CD68^{+}$; most are MHC class II antigen positive cells (TACHI et al. 1981; OKSENBERG et al. 1986; HUNT and POLLARD 1992; MIZUNO et al. 1994). Decidual macrophages when removed from the uterus may present antigens to maternal T lymphocytes, but, as in rodents, in situ function is uncertain. It has been suggested human decidual macrophages have important regulating functions for the maintenance of pregnancy (HILL 1990). First trimester human decidual macrophages suppress T lymphocyte alloreactivity in vitro by secreting PGE_2, which blocks activation of NK cells (PARHAR et al. 1989). Decidualized stromal cells have also been shown to mediate immunosuppression in vitro by secretion of PGE_2. However, the in vivo importance of PGE_2 suppressor mechanisms in human pregnancy has not been demonstrated. PG production is likely inhibited in situ as PGs may be abortogenic (CLARK 1985). Interestingly, decidual macrophages from spontaneous aborters produced higher levels of IL-1 in vitro than macrophages from normal pregnant women, possibly providing a cytokine mechanism for abortion (MIZUNO et al. 1994). Decidual macrophages also possess lysosomal enzyme activity, including acid phosphatase, nonspecific esterase, α_1-antitrypsin and α_1-antichymotrypsin. Therefore one function of decidual macrophages may be the phagocytosis of tissue debris resulting from trophoblast invasion of uterine tissue (EARL et al. 1989). This phagocytic function of macrophages is also suppressed in normal pregnancy, and enhanced phagocytosis has been described in decidua from spontaneous aborters (HILL 1990). Macrophages are present in the human decidua and in close contact with trophoblast. Indeed, one might suspect human macrophages to have some of the functions of GMG cells that are present in the decidua in the mouse. Characterization of the maternal cell compartment in the spongiotrophoblast of the mouse placenta may provide more useful information concerning cells in human decidua that are in close contact with the trophoblast.

4.1.3 T Cells

T lymphocytes are scattered throughout human decidua, and 60%–75% are $CD8^+$ T cells (PACE et al. 1991). However, decidual T cells differ from T cells elsewhere. $CD3^+$ T cells are present, but expression of the $\alpha\beta$ and $\gamma\delta$ heterodimer of the T cell receptor is reduced (DIETL et al. 1992; HALLER et al. 1995). MINCHEVA-NILSSON et al. (1994) have claimed that T cells expressing the $\gamma\delta$ heterodimer are particularly abundant in the decidua, but the expression of the $\alpha\beta$ heterodimer on a majority of T cells in the human decidua has also been reported; some of the cells may arise from blood contamination (CHERNYSHOV et al. 1993).

The function of T cell in the human decidua has not been fully investigated. $\gamma\delta$ T cells may be able to react with antigens expressed by trophoblasts (PORCELLI et al. 1989; VAN KAER et al. 1991; HEYBORNE et al. 1994); in vitro this reaction leads to the production of cytokines such as IL-2 or IL-4 by T cells. These could be TH_0 cells that differentiate into either TH_1 or TH_2 (FONG and MOSMANN 1990). IL-2, known to be abortogenic in rodent pregnancies, may activate NK cells into LAK cells, which can kill trophoblast target cells in vitro (ARONSON et al. 1988; KING et al. 1989; KING and LOKE 1990; STARKEY 1991); interestingly, trophoblast cells may also produce IL-2 (BOEHM et al. 1989). The importance of having antagonists to IL-2 effects is obvious, and these data may direct subsequent fate of $CD8^+$ cells. On the other hand, IL-4 would have different effects and enhance antibody formation (WEGMANN et al. 1993). One interesting possibility is that trophoblast growth may be controlled by IL-2 producing $\gamma\delta$ T cells; it is uncertain whether trophoblast in situ can be killed by LAKs, and effects of cytokine products of $\gamma\delta$ T cells on trophoblast differentiation have not been evaluated.

4.2 Human Pregnancy Pathology

4.2.1 Spontaneous Abortion

Recurrent pregnancy loss affects 1%–3% of couples, and a number of potential causes have been proposed (STRAY and STRAY-PEDERSEN 1984). However, more than 60% of cases are unexplained by conventional genetic, anatomical, infectious and endocrinological criteria (STRAY and STRAY-PEDERSEN 1984). Immunological theories have been proposed to account for these otherwise unexplained reproductive losses since embryo and trophoblast are semiallogenic and potential targets for rejection. Based on studies in mice and evidence of resistance of human trophoblast to maternal effector cells, suppressor cell activity and NK cells have been studied (CLARK et al. 1994a). These studies led to the detection of decidual suppressor cell deficiency in biopsies from women with malimplantation following in vitro fertilization and embryo transfer and in the decidua of recurrently aborting women suffering from incipient abortion using in situ hybridization specific for TGF-β_2 producing suppressor cells (Daya et al. 1985; Lea et al. 1995). Macrophage activation and function, normally suppressed in human pregnancy, appears to be enhanced in the decidua from women with spontaneous abortion (Hill 1990). Macrophages and NK cells are known to interact in the mouse system, and this interaction may lead to abortion (Clark 1991). In cases of human recurrent spontaneous abortion (RSA) 40%–50% of the abortion tissue is chromosomally abnormal, and these women have normal blood NK cells. In the 40%–50% of aborting patients with normal karyotyped embryos NK levels are significantly elevated (Coulam and Beaman 1995). In normal pregnancy $CD8^+$ T cells upregulate their progesterone receptors, but in RSA patients this upregulation fails to occur (Clark et al. 1991a; Szekeres-Bartho et al. 1990). Generation of TGF-β_2 related suppressor activity in decidua may also be defective in about 50% of women with RSA (Lea et al. 1995). There are significant parallels in many women between abortion of normal embryo tissue in mice via NK-mediated rejection of suppressor cell failure and unexplained miscarriages of chromosomally normal embryo.

4.2.2 Therapies

Immunization can prevent abortion in mice, and data have also been reported which suggest that immunization using paternal leucocytes, third-party leucocytes, or infusion of gammaglobulin prevents abortion in human couples with partner-specific recurrent losses with an efficacy of 70% (Mueller-Eckhardt et al. 1989; Clark and Daya 1991; Coulam et al. 1994). The underlying mechanisms of protection via immunotherapy remain unclear. Protection against abortion in patients receiving psychotherapy rather than immunization is now more readily understood (Stray-Pedersen and Stray-Pedersen 1988). Women with recurrent pregnancy loss experience considerable stress, and offering putatively effective treatment may reduce stress, resulting in decreased levels of TNF-α. From studies in mice one would expect immunization to protect as effectively against stress-triggered loss as would psychotherapy.

Recently a maternal alloantibody bound to a unique 80-kDa trophoblast antigen (R80K) has been identified in term placenta of successfully pregnant women, and this antibody is absent in the serum of many females suffering from recurrent miscarriages (Clark and Blair 1991; Jalali et al. 1995). This antigen is resistant to trypsin digestion on intact placental microvesicles; after acid elution of the IgG bound to it trypsin released a soluble 50-kDa fragment which reacted with the eluted antibody. The antigen appears to be determined by the father's and by his father's genes, is expressed on the father's and on his father's lymphocytes, and immunization of women lacking this antibody with their partner lymphocytes generates it (Jalali et al. 1995). However, it is not known whether the R80K antigen is present on first trimester trophoblast. One interesting possibility is that antibodies to the 80-kDa antigen enhance the ability of trophoblast to induce a local immunosuppressive environment in the decidua. Indeed, luteal-phase lymphocytes incubated with trophoblast membrane vesicles release suppressor factors in vitro; vesicles from which IgG have been stripped by acid treatment fail to induce suppression (DAYA et al. 1989). These data imply that trophoblast has antigens that do induce immune response when antibody is bound to them, and these responses trigger suppressor cell function in luteal-phase lymphocytes. Detergent-treated vesicles, by contrast, are able to activate suppression in the absence of surface IgG (DAYA et al. 1989). These vesicles may have lost R80K (J. Mowbray, personal communication).

4.2.3 Preeclampsia

Between 7% and 10% of pregnancies are affected by preeclampsia, with increasing blood pressure, renal dysfunction with proteinuria, and oedema developing in the third trimester (ZHOU et al. 1993). Preeclampsia is accompanied by increased perinatal mortality and intrauterine growth retardation. The decidua is of central importance in the pathogenesis of preeclampsia. Trophoblast invasion is retarded, and invasion of spiral arteries is subnormal (ROBERTSON et al. 1986; KHONG et al. 1987; BRANCH et al. 1989; REDMAN 1991). This invasion is thought to be necessary for reduced arterial resistance and a high blood flow in late pregnancy (KHONG et al. 1987). In normal pregnancies trophoblast invasion through the decidua is downregulated by the integrins α_6/β_4, which bind to laminin (SONNENBERG et al. 1988; BURROWS et al. 1993). In normal pregnancy the β_4 is switched to β_1, which binds collagen and fibronectin and stimulates trophoblast invasion. In preeclamptic patients the $\alpha_6\beta_4$ subunit continues to be strongly expressed, and $\alpha_5\beta_1$ is either not upregulated or is weakly expressed on the cytotrophoblast (ZHOU et al. 1993). This leads to the hypothesis that in preeclampsia invading cytotrophoblasts retain cell adhesion molecules that are usually found only on anchoring villus stem cells and fail to upregulate the expression of the $\alpha_5\beta_1$ receptor (ZHOU et al. 1993). Immune responses appear to prevent preeclampsia (CLARK 1994b), and such protection may occur by changing trophoblast differentiation via cytokines.

No differences in the type or quantity of decidual leucocytes from the placental bed decidua of normal and preeclamptic pregnancies at term have been described (KHONG et al. 1987). However, granulated lymphocytes in the decidua parietalis are increased in numbers in mild and severe preeclampsia compared with normal pregnancy (KHONG et al. 1987). The phenotype of these cells is unknown, and the lymphomyeloid cells associated with preeclampsia have not yet been functionally characterized.

5 Ectopic Pregnancy Decidua

As mentioned above, first-timester human pregnancy decidua contains small lymphocytic suppressor cells which release 22-and 43-kDa soluble suppressor factors blocking the action of IL-2. By contrast, luteal-phase endometrium contains large suppressor cells which are similar to the large $CD8^+$ hormone-induced suppressor cells in murine preimplantation endometrium and do not release immunosuppressive factors. Incubation of luteal-phase endometrial lymphocytes from later than 24 days of the menstrual cycle with detergent-treated syncytiotrophoblast membrane demonstrated the release of suppressor factors with 22 and 43 kDa molecular weight (Daya et al. 1989). When uterine decidua was obtained from women with tubal ectopic pregnancy (early first trimester), however, the uterine decidua spontaneously released soluble immunosuppressive factor with 100–135 kDa molecular weight and the suppressor cells were larger (Daya et al. 1989). The data indicate that suppressor cells in ectopic pregnancy decidua remote from trophoblast differ from hormonally induced suppressor cells and from small sized ($CD56^+$) suppressor cells occurring during normal pregnancy. There are similarities between ectopic pregnancy decidua and murine deciduoma tissue.

6 Conclusions

Important advances have been made in elucidating the identity and functions of cells in the decidua in normal and pathological pregnancy. Decidua is more than merely decidualized stromal cells, and decidualization generates an immunologically active immunregulatory tissue that plays a key role in pregnancy outcome. Both trophoblast-dependent and trophoblast-independent changes occur. Several pregnancy disorders, including abortions and preeclampsia, may be related to disturbances in the decidua.

Acknowledgements. This research was supported by the Deutsche Forschungsgemeinschaft and the MRC Canada.

References

Allen WR, Kydd JH, Antczak DF (1986) Successful application of immunotherapy to a model of pregnancy failure in equids. In: Clark DA, Croy BA (eds) Reproductive immunology. Elsevier, Amsterdam

Arck PC, Merali FS, Manuel J, Chaouat G, Clark DA (1995a) Stress-triggered abortion: inhibition of protective suppression and promotion of tumor necrosis factor-α (TNF-α) release as a mechanism triggering resorptions in mice. Am J Reprod Immunol 33:74–80

Arck PC, Merali F, Stanisz A, Stead R, Chaouat G, Manuel J, Clark DA (1995b) Stress-induced murine abortion associated with substance P-dependent alteration in cytokines in maternal uterine decidua. Biol Reprod 53:814–819

Aronson FR, Libby P, Brandon EP, Janicka MW, Mier JW (1988) IL-2 rapidly induces natural killer cell adhesion to human endothelium cells. J Immunol 141:158–163

Badet MT (1984) Specific and non-specific immunosuppressive factors in salamander pregnancy serum. J Reprod Immunol 6:299–311

Bancroft GJ, Sheehan KCF, Schreiber RD, Unanue ER (1989) Tumour necrosis factor is involved in the T cell-independent pathway of macrophage activation in *scid* mice. J Immunol 143:127–130

Bell SC (1983) Decidualization: regional differentiation and associated function. Oxf Rev Reprod Biol 5:220–271

Bell SC, Billington WD (1986) Humoral immune response in murine pregnancy. V. Relationship to the differential immunogenicity of placental and fetal tissues. J Reprod Imunol 9:289–295

Bierley J, Clark DA (1987) Characterization of hormone-dependent suppressor cells in the uterus of mated and pseudopregnant mice. J Reprod Immunol 10:201–217

Billingham RE (1964) Transplantation immunity and the maternal-fetal relation. N Engl J Med. 270:667–672

Billington WD, Burrows FJ (1989) Class I MHC antigens on rat placental trophoblast and yolk sac fetal membrane. Transplant Proc 21:555–556

Boehm KD, Kelley MF, Ilan J, Ilan J (1989) The interleukin-2 gene is expressed in the syncytiotrophoblast of thr human placenta. Proc Natl Acad Sci 86:656–660

Bost KL, Pascual DW (1992) Sunstance P: a late-acting B lymphocyte differentiation factor. Am J Physiol 262:C537

Branch DW, Andres R, Digre KB, Rote NS, Scott JR (1989) The association of antiphospholipid antibodies with severe preeclampsia. Obstot Gynecol 73:541–545

Brooks-Kaiser JC, Hoskin DW (1993) Inhibition of DNA synthesis and IL-2 bioreactivity in MLR by splenic pregnancy-associated natural suppressor cells involves the production of a TGF-β1-like molecule and a second distinct inhibitory factor. J Reprod Immunol 25:31–49

Bulmer JN (1992) Immune aspects of pathology of the placental bed contributing to pregnancy pathology. Baillieres Clin Obstet Gynaecol 6:461–488

Bulmer JN, Pace D, Ritson A (1988) Immunoregulatory cells in human decidua: morphology, immunohistochemistry and function. Reprod Nutr Dev 28:1599–1613

Bulmer JN, Longfellow M, Ritson A (1991) Leukocytes and resident blood cells in endometrium. Ann N Y Acad Sci 622:57–68

Burrows TD, King A, Loke YW (1993) Expression of integrins by human trophoblast and differential adhesion to laminin or fibronectin. Hum Reprod 8:475–484

Chaouat G (1994) Synergy of lipopolysaccharide and inflammatory cytokines in murine pregnancy. Alloimmunization prevents abortion but does not affect the induction of preterm delivery. Cell Immunol 157:328–340

Chaouat G, Lankar D (1988) Vaccination against spontaneous abortion in mice by preimmunization with an anti-idiotypic antibody. Am J Reprod Immunol Microbiol 16:146–150

Chaouat G, Clark DA, Wegmann TG, (1988) Genetic aspects of the CBA × DBA/2 and B10 × B10. A models of murine pregnancy failure and its prevention by lymphocyte immunisation. In: Beard RW, Sharp F (eds) Early pregnancy loss: mechanisms and treatment. Peacock, Ashton-under-Lyne, pp 89–102

Chaouat G, Menu E, Clark DA, Minkowsky M, Dy M, Wegmann TG (1990) Control of fetal survival in CBA × DBA/2 mice by lymphokine therapy. J Reprod Fertil 89:447–458

Chaouat G, Meliani AA, Martal J, Raghupathy R, Elliot J, Mosmann T, Wegmann TG (1995) IL-10 prevents naturally occuring fetal loss in the CBA × DBA/2 mating combination, and local defect in IL-10 production in this abortion-prone combination is corrected by in vivo injection of IFN-τ. JImmunol 154:4261–4268

Cherynyshov VP, Slukvin II, Bondarenko GI (1993) Phenotypic characterization of CD7+, CD3+, and CD8+ lymphocytes from first trimester human decidua using two-color flow cytometry. Am J Reprod Immunol 29:5–16

Choudhuri R, Wood GW (1992) Leukocyte distribution in the pseudopregnant mouse uterus. Am J Reprod Immunol 227:69–76

Christmas SE, Bulmer JN, Meager A, Johnson PM (1990) Phenotypic and functional analysis of human CD3-decidual leukocyte clones. Immunology 71:182–189

Chumbley G, King A, Gardner L, Howlett S, Holmes N, Loke YW (1994a) Generation of an antibody to HLA-G transgenic mice and demonstration of the tissue reactivity to this anitbody. J Reprod Immunol 27:173–186
Chumbley G, King A, Robertson K, Holmes N, Loke YW (1994b) Resistance of HLA-G and HLA-A2 transfectants to lysis by decidual NK cells. Cell Immunol 155:312–322
Clark DA (1985) Prostaglandins and immunogens during pregnancy. Am J Reprod Immunol Microbiol 9:111–112
Clark DA (1990) Animal models of normal and aborting pregnancies. In: Andreani D, Bompiani GD, Di Mario U, Faulk WP, Galluzzo A (eds) Immunobiology of normal and diabetic pregnancy. Wiley, Chichester, pp 23–37
Clark DA (1991) Controversies in reproductive immunology. Crit Rev Immunol 11:215–247
Clark DA (1993) Cytokines, decidua and early pregnancy. Oxf Rev Reprod Biol 15:83–111
Clark DA (1994a) Histocompatibility studies in recurrent spontaneous abortion. Hum Reprod 9:1196–1197
Clark DA (1994b) Does immunological intercourse prevent pre-eclampsia? Lancet 334:973–975
Clark DA (1995) Immunological characterization of the trophoblast-decidual interface in human pregnancy. In: Kurpisz M, Fernandez N (eds) Immunology of human reproduction. Bios Oxford, pp 1–11
Clark DA, Blair C (1991) NICHD Conference on Materno/feto placental interactions. J Reprod Fertil 92:231–244
Clark DA, Daya S (1991) Trials and tribulation in the treatment of recurrent spontaneous abortion. Am J Reprod Immunol 25:18–24
Clark DA, McDermott M (1978) Impairment of host versus graft reaction in pregnant mice. I. Suppression of T cell generation in lymph nodes draining the uterus. J Immunol 121:1389–1395
Clark DA, Chaput A, Walker C, Rosental K (1985) Active suppression of host-versus-graft reaction in pregnant mice. VI. Soluble suppressor activity obtained from decidua of allopregnant mice blocks the response of IL-2. J Immunol 134:1659–1664
Clark DA, Bierley J, Banwatt D, Chaouat G (1989) Hormone-induced preimplantation LYT 2+ murine uterine suppressor cells reduce the spontaneous abortion rate in CBA/J mice. Cell Immunol 123:334–343
Clark DA, Drake B, Head JR, Stedronska-Clark J, Banwatt D (1990a) Decidual-associated suppressor activity and viability of individual implantation sites of allopregnant C3H mice. J Reprod Immunol 17:253–264
Clark DA, Flanders KC, Banwatt D, Millar-Book W, Manuel J, Stedronska-Clark J, Rowley B (1990b) Murine pregnancy decidua produces a unique immunosuppressive molecule related to transforming growth factor β2. J Immunol 144:3008–3014
Clark DA, Lea RG, Rowley B, Denburg J, Banwatt D, Manuel J, Damji N, Underwood J, Michel M, Mowbray J, Daya S, Chaouat G (1991a) Transforming growth factor-β related suppressor factor in mammalian pregnancy decidua: homologies between the mouse and human in successful pregnancy and in recurrent unexplained abortion. In: Chaouat G, Mowbray F (eds) Cellular and molecular biology of the maternofetal relationship. Libbey, Paris pp 171–179 (Proceedings INSERM colloquium, vol 212)
Clark DA, Lea RG, Podor T, Daya S, Banwatt D, Harley C (1991b) Cytokines determining the success of failure of pregnancy. Ann N Y Acad Sci 626:524–536
Clark DA, Lea RG Flanders K, Banwatt D, Chaouat G (1993b) Role of unique species of TGF-β in preventing rejection of the conceptus during pregnancy. In: Gergely J (ed) Progress in immunology vol 8. Springer, Berlin Heidelberg New York, pp 841–847
Clark DA, Lea RG, Flanders KC, Banwatt D, Chaouat G (1993a) Role of a unique species of TGF-β in preventing rejection of the conceptus during pregnancy. In: Gergely J (ed) Progress in immunology, vol 8. Springer Berlin Heidelberg New York, pp 841–847
Clark DA, Banwatt D, Chaouat G (1993c) Stress-triggered abortion in mice prevented by alloimmunization. Am J Reprod Immunol 29:141–147
Clark DA, Chaouat G, Mogil R, Wegmann TG (1994a) Prevention of sponatneous abortion in DBA/2-mated CBA/J mice by GM-CSF involves CD8+ T cell-dependent suppression of natural effector cells. Cell Immunol 154:143–152
Clark DA, Quarrington C, Banwatt D, Manuel J, Fulop G (1994b) Spontaneous abortion in immunodeficient SCID mice. Am J Reprod Immunol 32:15–25
Clark DA, Flanders KC, Hirte H, Dasch JR, Coker R, McAnulty RJ, Laurent GJ (1995) Characterization of murine pregnancy decidual transforming growth factor β1. transforming growth factor β2-like molecules of unusual molecular size released in bioactive form. Biol Reprod 52:1380–1388

Clarke GR, Roberts TK, Smart YS (1994) Natural killer and natural cytotoxic cells are present at the maternal-fetal interface during murine gestation. Immunol Cell Biol 72:153–160
Coulam C, Beaman K (1995) Reciprocal alterations in circulating TJ6+CD19+ and TJ6+ leukocytes in early pregnancy predicts success of miscarriage. Am J Reprod Immunol (in press)
Coulam C, Clark DA, Coulam JA, Scott JS, Schesselmann J, the Recurrent Miscarriage Trialists Group (1994) Worldwide collaborative observational study and metaanalysis on allogenic leukocyte immunotherapy for recurrent spontaneous abortion. Am J Reprod Immunol 32:55–72
Coulam CB, Goodmann C, Roussev RG, Thomason EJ, Beaman KD (1995) Systemic CD56+ cells can predict pregnancy outcome. Am J Reprod Immunol 34:40–46
Crainie M, Guilbert LJ, Wegmann TG (1990) Expression of a novel cytokine transcripts in the murine placenta. Biol Reprod 43:999–1005
Croy BA, Kassouf SA (1989) Evaluation of the murine metrial gland for immunological function. J Reprod Immunol 15:51–70
Croy BA, Waterfield A, Wood W, King GJ (1988) Normal murine and porcine embryos recruit NK cells to the uterus. Cell Immunol 115:471–480
Croy BA, Reed N, Malashenko BA, Kim K, Kwon BS (1991) Demonstration of YAC target cell lysis by murine granulated metrial gland cells. Cell Immunol 133:116–126
Daya S, Clark DA, Devlin C, Jarrell J, Chaput A (1985) Suppressor cells in human decidua. Am J Obstet Gynecol 151:267–270
Daya S, Johnson P, Clark DA (1989) Trophoblast induction of suppressor-type cell activity in human endometrial tissue. Am J Reprod Immunol 19:65–72
Delassus S, Coutinho GC, Saucier C, Darche S, Kourilsky P (1994) Differential cytokine expression in maternal blood and placenta during murine gestation. J Immunol 152:2411–2420
Deniz G, Christmas SE, Brew R, Johnson PM (1994) Phenotypic and functional cellular differences between human $CD3^-$ decidual and peripheral blood leukocytes. J Immunol 152:4255–4261
Dietl J, Ruck P, Horny HP, Handgretinger R, Marzusch K, Ruck M, Kaiserling E, Griesser H, Kabelitz D (1992) The decidua of early human pregnancy: immunohistochemistry and function of immunocompetent cells. Gynecol Obstet Invest 33:197–204
Drake BL, Head JR (1989a) Murine trophoblast can be killed by lymphokine-activated killer cells. JImmunol 143:9–14
Drake BL, Head JR (1989b) Murine trophoblast can be killed by allospecific cytotoxic T lymphocytes generated in GIBCO Opti-MEM medium. J Reprod Immunol 15:71–78
Dulcos AJ, Pomerantz DK, Baines MG (1994) Relationship between decidual leukocyte infiltration and spontaneous abortion in a murine model of early fetal resorption. Cell Immunol 159:184–193
Earl U, Morrison L, Gray C, Bulmer JN (1989) Proteinase and proteinase inhibitor localization in the human placenta. Int J Gynecol Pathol 8:114–124
Enders AC (1991) Current topic: structural responses of the primate endometrium to implantation. Placenta 12:309–325
Erard F, Wild MT, Garcia-Sanz JA, Le Gros G (1993) Switch of CD8 T cells to noncytolytic $CD8^-$ $CD4^-$ cells that make TH_2 cytokines and help B cells. Science 260:1802–1805
Ferry BL, Sargent IL, Starkey PM, Redman CWG (1991) Cytotoxic activity against trophoblast and choriocarcinoma cells of large granular lymphocytes from human early pregnancy decidua. Cell Immunol 132:140–149
Fong TA, Mosmann TR (1990) Alloreactive $CD8^+$ T cell clones secrete the Th_1 pattern of cytokines. J Immunol 144:1744–1752
Giroir BP, Peppel K, Silva M, Beutler B (1992) The biosynthesis of tumor necrosis factor during pregnancy: studies with a CAT reporter transgene and TNF inhibitor. Eur Cyto Network 3:533–538
Gordon JR, Galli SJ (1990) Mast cells as a source of both preformed and immunologically inducible TNF-α. Nature 346:274–276
Haller H, Tedesco F, Rukavina, Radillo O, Gudelj L, Beer AE (1995) Decidual-trophoblast interactions: decidual lymphoid cell populations in basal and parietal dicidua. J Reprod Immunol 28:165–171
Head JR (1989) Can trophoblast be killed by cytotoxic cells? In vitro evidence and invivo possibilities. Am J Reprod Immunol 20:100–105
Hedley ML, Drake BL, Head JR, Tucker PW, Forman J (1989) Differential expression of class I MHC genes in the embryo and placenta during midgestational development in the mouse. J Immunol 142:4046–4053
Heyborne K, Fu YX, Nelson A, Farr A, O'Brien R, Born W (1994) Recognition of trophoblast by $\gamma\delta$ T cells. J Immunol 153:2918–2926

Hill JA (1990) Immunological mechanisms of pregnancy maintenance and failure: a critique of theories and therapy. Am J Reprod Immunol 22:33–42

Hunt JS (1989) Cytokine networks in the uteroplacental unit: macrophages as pivotal regulatory cells. JReprod Immunol 16:1–17

Hunt JS (1994) Immunologically relevant cells in the uterus. Biol Reprod 50:461–466

Hunt JS, Pollard JW (1992) Macrophages in the uterus and placenta. Curr Top Microbiol Immunol 181:39–63

Hunziker RD, Gambel P, Wegmann TG (1984) Placenta as an elective barrier to cellulat traffic. JImmunol 133:667–671

Jalali GR, Rezai A, Underwood JL, Mowbray JF, Allen WR, Surridge S, Matthias S (1995) An 80 kDa syncytiotrophoblast alloantigen bound to maternal alloantibody in term placenta. Am J Reprod Immunol 33:213–220

Jokhi PP, King A, Sharkey AM, Smith SK, Loke YW (1994) Screening for cytokine messenger ribonucleic acids in purified human decidual lymphocyte populations by the reverse-transcriptase polymerase chain reaction. J Immunol 22:4427–4435

Kearns M, Lala PK (1983) Life and history of decidual cells: a review. Am J Reprod Immunol 3:78–82

Khong TY, Lidell HS, Robertson WB (1987) Defective haemochorial placentation as a cause of miscarriage: a preliminary study. Br J Obstet Gynaecol 94:649–655

King A, Loke YW (1990) Human trophoblast and JEG choriocarcinoma cells are sensitive to lysis by IL2-stimulated decidual NK cells. Cell Immunol 129:435–448

King A, Loke YW (1991) On the nature and function of human uterine granular lymphocytes. Immunol Today 12:432–435

King A, Birkby C, Loke YW (1989) Early human decidual cells exhibit NK activity against the K562 cell line but not against first trimester trophoblast. Cell Immunol 118:337–344

King A, Balendran N, Wooding P, Loke YW (1991) CD3 leukocytes present in the human uterus during early placentation: phenotypic and morphologic characterization of the $CD56^{++}$ population. Dev Immunol 1:169–190

King A, Wooding P, Gardner L, Loke YW (1993) Expression of perforin, granzym A, and TIA-1 by human uterine $CD56^{+}$ NK cells implies they are capable of effector functions. Hum Reprod 12:2061–2067

Kinsky R, Delage G, Rosin N, Thang MN, Hoffmann M, Chaouat G (1990) A murine model of NK cell mediated resorption. Am J Reprod Immunol 23:73–77

Kovats S, Main EK, Librach C, Stubbelbine M, Fisher SJ, Demars R (1990) A class I antigen, HLA-G, is expressed on human trophoblast. Science 2248:220–223

Lea RG, Clark DA (1993) Effect of decidual cell supernatants and lymphokines on murine trophoblast growth in vitro. Biol Reprod 48:930–935

Lea RG, Flanders K, Harley CB, Manuel J, Banwatt D, Clark DA (1992) Release of a transforming growth factor (TGF)-β2-related suppressor factor from postimplantation murine decidual tissue can be correlated with the detection of a subpopulation of cells containing RNA for TGF-β2. J Immunol 148:778–787

Lea RG, Underwood J, Flanders KC, Hirte H, Banwatt D, Michel M, Daya S, Harley C, Mowbray JF, Clark DA (1995) A subset of patients with recurrent spontaneous abortion is deficient in transforming growth factor β-2-producing "suppressor cells" in decidua at the placental attachment site. Am J Reprod Immunol 33 (in press)

Lee CK, Chosal K, Beaman KD (1990) Cloning of cDNA for a T-cell produced molecule with a punitative immune regulatory role. Mol Immunol 27:1137–1144

Lin H, Mosmann TR, Guilbert L, Tuntipopitat S, Wegmann TG (1993) Synthesis of T helper 2-type cytokines at the maternal-fetal interface. J Immunol 151:4562–4573

Linnemeyer PA, Pollack SB (1991) Murine granulated metrial gland cells at uterine implantation sites are natural killer lineage cells. J Immunol 147:2530–2535

Ljunggren HG, Kärre K (1990) In search of the "missing self": MHC molecules and NK cell recognition. Immunol Today 11:237–244

Loke YW (1990) Experimenting with human extravillous trophoblast: a personal view. Am J Reprod Immunol 24:22–28

Loke YW, King A, Drake BL (1993) Leucocytic organisation in the endometrium and fallopian tube. WHO Symposium on Local Immunity in Reproductive Tract Tissues, New Delhi, pp 187–204

Lysiak JJ, Lala PK (1992) In situ localization and characterization of bone marrow-derived cells in the decidua of normal murine pregnancy. Biol Reprod 47:603–613

Manaseki S, Searle RF (1989) Natural killer (NK) cell activity of first trimester human decidua. Cell Immunol 121:166–173

Mandal M, Beaman KD (1995) Purification and characterization of a pregnancy associated protein TJ6s. Am J Reprod Immunol 33:60–67

Manjunath R, Ozato K, Mukherjee AB (1985) Stimulation of alloreactive cytotoxic T Cells by paternal major histocompatibility antigens during murine pregnancy. Biol Reprod 33:668–678

Maruyama T, Makimo T, Sugi T, Matsubayshi H, Ozawa N, Nozawa S (1992) Flow-cytometric analysis of immune cell populations in human decidua from various types of first-trimester pregnancy. Hum Immunol 34:212–218

Merali F, Arck P, Flanders K, Manuel J, Hoskin D, Murgita RA, Clark DA (1995) TGF-β2-related decidual suppressor factor (DSF): secreted or synthesized by bone marrow suppressor cells? Abstracts 9th Int Congress San Francisco Immunology, July 23–29, 1995, American Assoc Immunologists, P 186 (Abstr)

Mincheva-Nilsson L, Baranow V, Mo-Wai Yeung M, Hammatström S, Hammarström ML (1994) Immunomorphologic studies of human decidua-associated lymphoid cells in normal early pregnancy. J Immunol 152:2021–2032

Mizuno M, Aoki K, Kimbara T (1994) Functions of macrophages in human decidual tissue in early pregnancy. Am J Reprod Immunol 31:180–188

Mosmann TR, Moore KW (1991) The role of IL-10 in crossregulating of TH_1 and TH_2 responses. Immunol Today 12:A49

Mueller-Eckhardt G, Heine O, Neppert J, Künzel W, Mueller-Eckhardt C (1989) Prevention of recurrent spontaneous abortion by intravenous immunoglobulin. Vox Sang 56:151–155

Nagarkatti PS, Clark DA (1983) In vitro activity and in vivo correlates of alloantigen-specific murine suppressor T cells induced by allogeneic pregnancy. J Immunol 131:638–643

Nichols TC, Kang J, Anckachatchok J, Beer AE, Beaman KD (1994) Expression of a membrane form of the pregnancy-associated protein TJ6 on lymphocytes. Cell Immunol 155:219–229

Oksenberg JR, Mor-Yosef S, Persitzz E, Schenker Y, Mozes E, Brautbar C (1986) Antigen-presenting cells in human decidual tissue. Am J Reprod Immunol 11:82–88

Pace DP, Longfellow M, Bulmer JN (1991) Intraepithelial lymphocytes in human endometrium. Reprod Fertil 91:165–174

Parhar RS, Yagel S, Lala PK (1989) PGE_2-mediated immunosuppression by first trimester human decidual cells blocks activation of maternal leukocytes with potential antitrophoblast activity. Cell Immunol 120:61–74

Parr EL, Parr MB, Young JD (1987) Localization of a pore-forming protein (perforin) in granulated metrial gland cells. Biol Reprod 37:1327–1335

Peel S, Stewart I (1989) Rat granulated metrial gland cells differentiate in pregnant mice and may be cytotoxic for mouse trophoblast. Cell Diff Dev 28:55–61

Porcelli S, Brenner MB, Greenstein JL, Balk SP, Terhorst C, Bleicher PA (1989) Recognition of cluster of differentiation 1 antigens by human $CD4^-$ $CD8^-$ cytolytic T lymphocytes. Nature 341:447–450

Povea-Pacci H, Roberts T (1995) Does murine embryo implantation require a NK cells inhibition window period? Am J Reprod Immunol (in press)

Raghupathy R, Singh B, Leigh JB, Wegmann TG (1981) The ontogeny and turnover kinetics of paternal $H2^k$ antigenic determinants on the allogeneic murine placenta. J Immunol 127:2074–2080

Redline RW, Lu CY (1989) Localization of fetal major histocampatibility complex antigens and maternal leukocytes in murine placenta. Lab Invest 61:27–34

Redline RW, McKay DB, Vasquez MA, Papaioannou VE, Lu CY (1990) Macrophage functions are regulated by the substratum of murine stromal cells. J Clin Invest 85:1951–1958

Redman CWG (1991) Current topic: pre-eclampsia and the placenta. Placenta 12:301–308

Robertson WB, Khong TY, Brosens (1986) The placental bed biopsy: a review from three European centers. Am J Obstet Gynecol 155:401–412

Robertson SA, Seamark RF (1991) Uterine granulocyte-macrophage colony stimulating factor in early pregnancy: cellular origin and potential regulators. In: Chaouat G, Mowbray J (eds) Cellular and molecular biology of the materno-fetal relationship. Libby, Paris, pp 89–102 (Colloque INSERM, vol 212)

Rossant J, Croy BA, Clark DA, Chapman VM (1983) Interspecific hybrids and chimeras in mice. J Exp Zool 228:223–230

Sio JO (1985) Allograft reactivity and progesterone involvement at the choriodecidual junction. PhD thesis, University of Texas, Dallas

Slapsys RM, Younglai E, Clark DA (1988) A novel suppressor cell is recruited to decidua by fetal trophoblast-type cells. Reg Immunol 1:182–189

Smith G (1982) Differential ability of murine trophoblast and embryonic cells to induce cytotoxic lymphocytes in vitro. Transplantation 36:68–74

Smith JA, Burton RC, Barg M, Mitchell GF (1978) Maternal alloimmunization in pregnancy. Transplantation 25:216–220

Sonnenberg A, Moddermann PN, Hogervorst F (1988) Laminin receptors on platelets is the integrin VLA-6. Nature 336:487–489

Stanisz AM (1994) Neuroimmunomodulation in the gastrointestinal tract. Ann N Y Acad Sci 741:64–72

Stanisz AM, scicchitano R, Dazin P, Bienenstock J, Payan DG (1987) Distribution of substance P receptors on murine spleen and Peyer's patch T and B cells. J Immunol 139:749–754

Starkey PM (1991) Expression on cells of early human pregnancy decidua, of the p75, IL-2 and P145, IL-4 receptor proteins. Immunology 73:64–70

Starkey PM, Sargent IL, Redman CWG (1988) Cell populations in human early pregnancy decidua: characterization and isolation of large granular lymphocytes by flow cytometry. Immunology 65:129–134

Stead RH, Bienestock J (1990) Cellular interactions between the immune and peripheral nervous system. A normal role for mast cells? In: Burger MM, Sordat B, Zinkernagel RM (eds) Cell to cell interaction. Karger, Basel, pp 170–187

Stewart IJ, Mukhtard D (1994) A scanning electron microscopy study of interactions between mouse GMG and placental trophoblast cells in vitro. J Anat 184:153–156

Stray B, Stray-Pedersen S (1984) Etiological factors and subsequent reproductive performance in 195 couples with a prior y of habitual abortion. Am J Obstet Gynecol. 148:140–146

Stray-Pedersen B, Stray-Pedersen S (1988) Recurrent abortion: the role of psychotherapy. In: Beard RW, Sharp F (eds) Early pregnancy loss, mechanisms and treatment. Peacock, Ashton-under-Lyne, p 433

Szekeres-Bartho J, Varga P, Kinsky R, Chaouat G (1990) Progesterone-mediated immunosuppression and the maintenance of pregnancy. Res Immunol 141:175–181

Tabibzahdeh S, Satyaswaroop PG (1989) Sex steroid receptors in lymphoid cells of human endometrium. Am J Clin Pathol 91:656–663

Tachi C, Tachi S, Knyszynski A, Lindner HR (1981) Possible involvement of macrophages in embryo-maternal relationships during ovum implantation in the rat. J Exp Zool 217:81–92

Van Kaer L, Wu M, Ichikawa Y, Ito K, Bonneville M, Ostrand-Rosenberg S, Murphy DB, Tonegawa S (1991) Recognition of MHC TL gene products by γδcells. Immunol Rev 120:89–115

Wanger F, Fink R, Hart R, Dancygier H (1987) Substance P enhances γ-interferon production by human peripheral blood mononuclear cells. Regul Pept 19:355–358

Wegmann TG (1988) Maternal T cells promote placental growth and prevent spontaneous abortion. Immunol Lett 17:297–302

Wegmann TG, Waters CA, Drell DW, Carlson GA (1979) Pregnant mice are not primed but can be primed to fetal alloantigens. Proc Natl Acad Sci USA 76:2410–2414

Wegmann TG, Lin H, Guilbert L, Mosmann TR (1993) Bidirectional cytokine interactions in the maternal-fetal relationship: is successful pregnancy a TH_2 phenomenon? Immunol Today 14:353–356

Wood GW, Kamel S, Smith K (1988) Immunoregulation and prostaglandin production by mechanically-derived and enzyme-derived murine decidual cells. J Reprod Immunol 13:235–248

Zhang L, Miller RG (1993) The correlation of prolonged survival of maternal skin grafts with the presence of naturally transferred maternal T cells. Transplantation 56:918–924

Zhou Y, Damsky CH, Chiu K, Roberts J, Fisher SJ (1993) Preeclampsia is associated with abnormal expression of adhesion molecules by invasive cytotrophoblasts. J Clin Invest 91:950–960

Ontogeny of Human Natural and Acquired Immunity

M. ADINOLFI

1 Introduction

In many species, the integrity of the body against bacterial and viral infections is preserved during perinatal life by the development of specialized organs and differentiation of a variety of immunological competent cells together with the temporary acquisition of maternally derived antibodies. The ontogeny of the immune system is a complex process that requires the maturation of many cells with different biological functions and the synthesis of a large number of proteins acting, for example, as ligands, receptors, transport, or lytic molecules.

This chapter describes briefly the basic properties of the cells and molecules involved in the acquisition of immune responses. This is followed by an analysis of the role that maternal antibodies play in protecting fetuses and neonates against infections and by a review of the maturation of T and B cells, cytokines, components of complement and lysozyme. Although I concentrate on the ontogeny of

Galton Laboratory, University College London, 4 Stephenson Way, London NW1, UK acquired immunity in humans, some views are also based on results obtained from studies carried out using experimental animals.

2 Cell Interactions and Immune Responses

2.1 Antigen Presentation and Cell Interaction

The humoral (antibody-mediated) and cellular (cell-mediated) immune responses to foreign antigens are promoted and regulated by complex interactions among at least three major groups of cells, endowed with different biological properties and capable of producing and releasing a variety of proteins, some acting as membrane receptors and others as ligands (FOWLKES and PARDOLL 1989; CRABTREE 1989; JANEWAY 1992; JORGENSEN et al. 1992; GERMAIN and MARGULIES 1993; JANEWAY and BOTTOMLY 1994; SPRENT 1995). The system comprises the antigen-presenting (AP) cells, which include phagocytic elements such as macrophages, monocytes and dendritic cells besides the main subgroups of T helper (Th) and T cytotoxic cells and the B lymphocytes producing specific antibodies. These cellular elements express on their surface unique receptors and ligands that act as recognition molecules, coactivators or transmembrane and cytoplasmic transmitters. The detection of these molecules, as antigenic markers, allows the identification of the various subgroups of the immune cells. Since these molecules play an essential role in triggering specific immune responses, they start to be synthetized during fetal and perinatal life in order to provide the infant with an efficient, maternally independent immune protection.

Antigen presentation and processing require receptors for Ig (FcRs) that can recognize the Fc region of Ig molecules complexed with antigens (Fig. 1; ZIEGLER and UNANUE 1981; UNANUE 1984; LANZAVECCHIA 1985, 1988; BRODSKY and GUAGLIARDI 1991; STEINMANN 1991). Immune complexes that include components of complement (such as C3 or C5) are recognized by AP cells via complement receptors (CRs; ROSS and ATKINSON 1985). Finally, macrophages, for example, may directly interact with foreign antigens by a mechanism of protein-protein interactions. Thus AP cells do not display strict clonal specificity for antigens but recognize self from nonself antigens mainly *via* activated antibodies or components of complement. Once the macromolecular complexes are endocytosed, they are "processed", and selected peptides are then transported and presented on the surface of AP cells in association with the major histocompatibility (MHC) molecules (SCHWARTZ 1985; STRACHAN 1987; TROWSDALE 1987; STROMINGER 1987; KAUFMAN 1993; GERMAIN 1994).

Processing and cytoplasmic transport of peptides are mediated by several groups of molecules, including the transporter molecules (TAP; HILL and POEGH 1955) and the major histocompatibility complex (MHC) molecules (WEISS and BOGEN 1991; OWEN and CRUMPTON 1987; GERMAIN 1994). Extensive studies have

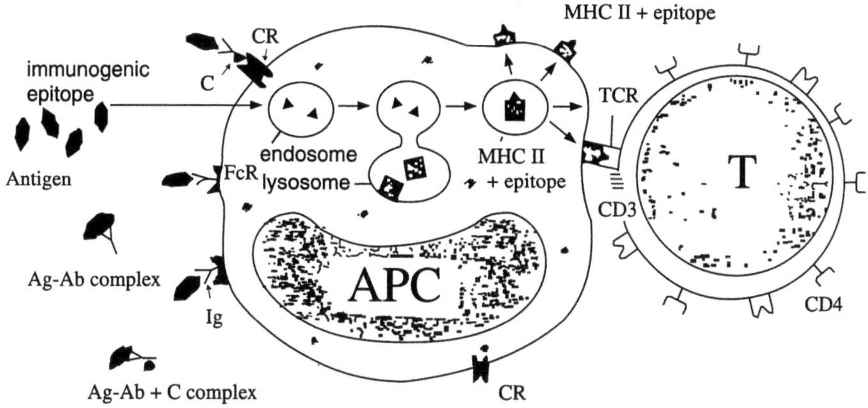

Fig. 1. Schematic representation of the uptake and processing of antigens by macrophages and other antigen-presenting cells (*APC*). Antigens are recognized after reacting with a specific antibody (*Ag-Ab complexes*) via FcR molecules or as Ag-Ab-complement complexes (*Ag-Ab-C*) by complement receptors (*CR*). After being processed, selected epitopes are transported by MHC molecules to the surface of the APCs and presented to T helper cell (*Th*) which recognize the MHC-Ag complex via TCR and CD3 molecules

been performed on the structure of the two classes of MHC molecules (KLEIN 1986; TOWSEND and BODMER 1989; RAMMENSEE et al. 1993). In humans MHC I (HLA-A,-B and -C) molecules are formed by a polymorphic and partially transmembrane heavy chain (44 kDa) associated with a 12-kDa subunit termed β_2-microglobulin (β_2m) that can be released in plasma. Structurally they belong to the immunoglobulin family (Fig. 2; WILLIAMS and BARCLAY 1988; KAUFMAN 1993). The extracellular portion of the heavy chain is divided into three domains, and the genes encoding these polymorphic proteins map to chromosome 6; the β_2m gene maps instead on chromosome 15 (OWEN and CRUMPTON 1987; TOWSEND and BODMER 1989; BJORKMAN and PERHAM 1990). High-resolution X-ray crystallography has shown that the first and second domains form a binding-site for processed antigens (BJORKMAN et al. 1987a,b), an observation that has greatly helped our understanding of the biological role of MHC molecules (GERMAIN and MARGULIES 1993). HLA class II molecules have a similar antigen-binding site and are formed by two chains noncovalently associated (BROWN et al. 1993).

HLA class I – together with viral antigens expressed on the surface of infected cells – are recognized by T cell receptors (TCRs) present on T cytotoxic cells, a phenomenon known as MHC-restricted recognition; they are also the target of antibodies and cytotoxic T cells during rejection of foreign transplants (ZINKERNAGEL and DOHERTY 1974; TOWSEND et al. 1985; TOWSEND and BODMER 1989). HLA class II molecules, associated with a processed antigen, are recognized by TCRs present on the surface of Th cells (Fig. 1). Thus, an important discovery in the field of immunology has been the demonstration that TCR molecules recognize simultaneously an endogenous antigenic determinant (e.g. a viral antigen) in association with class I or an exogenous epitope together with class II MHC mole-

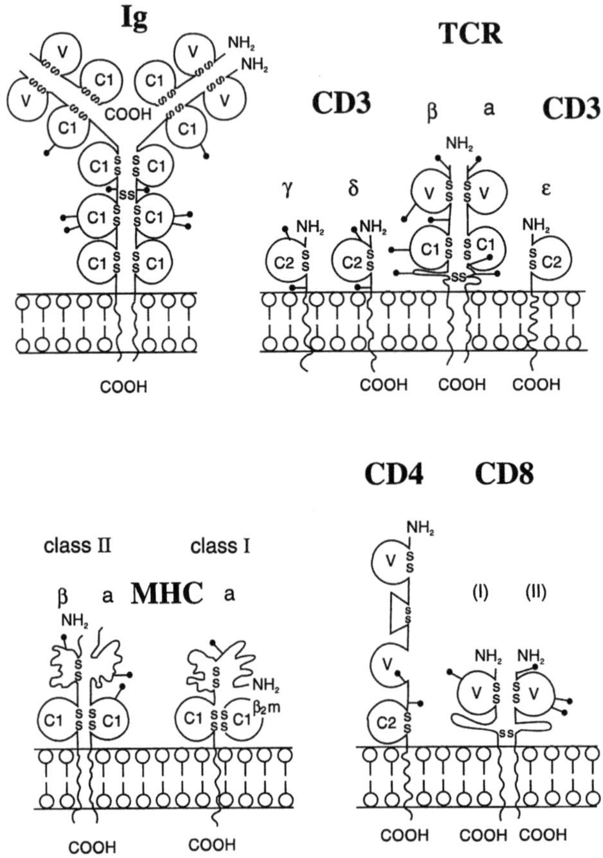

Fig. 2. Schematic structures of lg, TRC, CD3, MHC, CD4 and CD8 molecules, showing the various domains and their similarities

cules (Zinkernagel et al. 1978; Bjorkman et al. 1987a,b; Bjorkman and Perham 1990; Wade et al. 1993).

Two main types of TCRs are present in human cells (TCRγδ and TCRαβ); from the analysis of their amino acid sequences these molecules have been shown to be heterodimers and immunoglobulin (Ig)-like in structure (Fig. 2; Gascoigne et al. 1984; Brenner et al. 1986; Tonegawa et al. 1989). The assembly of the TCR genes is therefore similar to that of Ig genes (see next section). TCRs are formed by the activation and expression of genes controlling the variable (V) region, the joining (J) and diversity (D) regions and the constant (C) domains (Clevers et al. 1993; Jeneway and Bottomly 1994). Some mutations, in positions corresponding to the complementarity-determining regions (CDR) 1, 2 and 3, have been found to abolish T cell recognition. Thus, while the V-(D)-J region of the TCR molecules are responsible principally for the binding to peptides, the CDR1 and CDR2 loops contact the helices of the MHC molecules (Clevers et al. 1988, 1993; Chien and Davis 1993).

Many more molecules present on the surface of T cells regulate immune responses and their role in the interaction with B cells (PARKER 1993; CLARK and LEDBETTER 1994). Here their properties are mentioned briefly. CD3 is a complex of structurally distinct molecules, referred to as α, γ (26 kDa), δ (20 kDa), ε (20 kDa), ζ (a homodimer, 16 kDa) and *n* (28 kDa; Fig. 2; CLEVERS et al. 1988). CD2 has the distinction of being one of the first T cell markers to be described as an E-rosette receptor (BIERER et al. 1989). For many years, in fact, T-cells were recognized because they could bind ovine red cells. The ligand for CD2 has now been identified and classified as CD58 (LFA-3), a molecule present on many peripheral white cells and on epitelial cells.

Both CD4 and CD8 are members of the immunoglobulin family (Fig. 2; TRAVERS 1990). CD4 is a single-chain 60-kDa glycoprotein strongly expressed on Th cells, but also weakly present on monocytes and members of the macrophage family, such as microglial and dentritic cells (BIERER et al. 1989). CD4 is an essential molecule in the presentation of antigenic determinants and interaction with B lymphocytes (MICELI and PARNES 1993). The estimation of the blood levels of $CD4^+$ cells is an important diagnostic tool to evaluate the immune capability of an individual. Thus a deficit of $CD4^+$ cells is a valuable diagnostic sign of a partial immunodeficiency and a tendency to infections.

Cytotoxic T cells express on their surface CD8 heterodimeric molecules formed by an α and a β chain. Once again, structurally they belong to the immunoglobulin family (WILLIAMS and BARCLAY 1988; BIERER et al. 1989). Other specific molecules are present and characterize the biological properties of subclasses of lymphocytes; some of these are expressed during unique periods of development, such as CD10 (or common acute lymphoblastic leukaemia antigen; CALLA), a 100-kDa glycoprotein that, within the lymphoid lineage, allows identification of this population of pre-B cells. The term CALLA refers to the original observation of these molecules in pre-B acute leukaemias.

In recent years it has also become apparent that the commitment and differentiation of haemopoietic cells, including the T cells, involve a cascade of cytokines and nuclear transcription factors which regulate cellular phenotypes at each stage of their biological development (ROMAGNAMI 1989; WEISS and LITTMAN 1994). This cascade of molecular events does not evolve in an autonomous fashion but is triggered by signals transduced from cell-surface receptors interacting with a variety of ligands, such as adhesion molecules and growth factors. Transcription molecules for most genes, encoding the TCR-CD3 complex, have been identified as DNA-binding factors, some specific and some used by other types of cells (for references see CLEVERS et al. 1993). They are essential to control the commitment of lymphoid progenitor cells towards mature cell lineages.

Figure 3 shows the interaction between T and B cells, mediated by the complex system of molecules present on the cell surface. Details about these factors and their structural properties can be found in KANSAS and DAILEY (1989); KINKADE (1993) and WADE et al. (1993).

Again, it is important to stress that the synthesis of these molecules must start during fetal life in order to provide the infant with an efficient immune mechanism

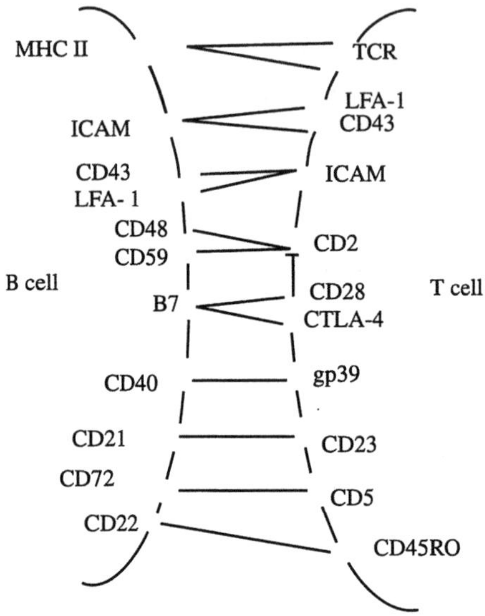

Fig. 3. The interaction between Th and B cells is mediated by many ligands and receptors which are essential for an efficient immune response. *LFA*, Leucocyte function antigen; *ICAM*, immune cell adhesion molecule

of defense against infections as soon as the passively transferred maternal antibodies have been catabolized.

2.2 Assembly of Ig and TCR Genes

The basic structure of the five classes of Ig present in human sera results from the fusion of two polypeptide heavy (H) chains with two light (L) chains. Each chain has an amino-terminal "variable" (V) region and a "constant" (C) region; the V regions of an H (VH) and a L chain (VL) interact to form the antibody combining site. Consequently an IgG molecule has two antibody sites while an IgM molecule, with five basic units, has ten antibody combining sites (HONJO 1983; BLACKWELL and ALT 1989).

The constant regions of the two L chains (κ and λ) consist of 107 amino acids and are unique for the two types of chains. The constant region (C) of the H chains are formed by distinct domains that distinguish the five classes of Ig molecules and characterize their unique biological properties, such as that of binding components of complement. In humans, the genes for the H chains map on chromosome 14, while those for the κ and γ chains map on chromosomes 2 and 22, respectively (HONJO 1983; BLACKWELL and ALT 1989).

The H and L chains are synthetized through the assembly of sets of genes that control the various domains (TONEGAWA 1983; ALT et al. 1992; DESIDERIO 1993). In the human genome, several VH and VL genes – subdivided into families – are present, and these are the primary sources of the extensive antibody heterogeneity. In early ontogeny the 3' end VH genes C most closely linked to the C genes are preferentially rearranged, but later other VH genes can replace the original segment. The repertoire of antibody specificities is further increased by the presence of DNA sequences (D and J genes) that are responsible for the assembly of the V and C domains.

The first step in the assembly of the heavy chain genes is the association of a D with a J gene followed by the rearrangement of one of the many V genes. The DNA sequence between the D and J genes forms a loop that is then released in the nucleus and deleted. Next, one of the many VH genes is translocated to form a continuous VDJ complex encoding an entire variable region of the heavy chain. This process of translocation changes the physical relation of the two regulatory gene sequences; it brings a promoter sequence – located upstream (5' end) of the leader sequence of the transposed VH – under the influence of the transcriptional enhancer, located between the JH and Cm genes (Tonegawa 1983; Lieber 1992; Lewis 1994).

The rearrangement of the V-D-J genes does not necessarily produce a functional unit; a further rearrangement may take place. The V-H-J complex then assembles with the a C gene, usually the genes of the μ and δ chains. Subsequently a new rearrangement may occur, leading to a switch from one class to another and thus, for example, to the synthesis of IgA or IgG molecules (Shimuzu and Honjo 1984; Weissman 1994).

The assembly of the light chain genes is similar to that of the H genes, with the difference that the D sequences are not present; thus the final assembly consists of single V, J and C (κ or λ) genes (Alt et al. 1987, 1992; Lewis 1994).

The repertoire of the antibody molecules is further increased by the presence of unique DNA sequences consisting of three elements: a heptameric sequence, a spacer region and a nonameric sequence (Honjo 1983; Alt et al. 1992; Lewis 1994). While the heptameric and nonameric sequences are conserved, the spacer regions – which fall within the DNA sequences of the 12 and 23 base pairs – are subject to variations during recombination of the V, D and J genes, thus increasing the heterogenity of the Ig molecules and their specificity.

The correct rearrangement of genes controlling the heavy and light chains occurs in only one of the two homologous chromosomes (allelic exclusion), thus ensuring that a single B cell produces only one type of antibody molecule (clonality). If the assembly preserves the reading frame, it is said to be productive; out-of-frame rearrangements result in non-productive genes (Rolink and Melcher 1991; Lewis 1994). The corresponding cell dies in situ, within the primary organ.

Another important source of heterogeneity – which greatly increases the repertoire of antibodies and affects their affinity and, occasionally, specificity – is the high frequency of somatic mutations, a phenomenon physiologically limited to the Ig genes (Tonegawa 1983; Tonegawa et al. 1989; Alt et al. 1992; Lewis 1994).

It has long been known that, following exposure to an antigen, the class of specific antibodies and their affinity change with time. Antibodies produced at an early stage are often of the IgM class; they can then switch to IgG or to other classes of Ig molecules; their affinity for a specific antigen increases by the selection of B lymphocytes whose Ig genes have gone through further rearrangements.

As mentioned above, the assembly of the TCR genes proceeds in a pattern similar to that of the Ig genes, with the exception of the absence of somatic mutations (GASCOIGNE et al. 1984; HOOD et al. 1985; MARRACK and KAPPLER 1987). This suggests that, while a small amount of auto-antibodies may be produced and tolerated by somatic mutations of the Ig genes, the accidental synthesis, by somatic mutations, of TCR molecules reacting against self-antigens does not occur in order to avoid harmful immune reactions.

In recent years it has been shown that two specific recombinase (RAG1 and RAG2) and several other enzymes are involved in the assembly of the Ig and TCR genes (OETTINGER et al. 1990; OETTINGER 1992; LIN and DESIDERIO 1993).

3 Transfer of Maternal Immunoglobulins

The route and the degree with which the various classes of maternal immunoglobulins are transferred to the offspring vary in different species (Table 1; FEDRA 1962; BRAMBELL 1970; WILD 1973, 1975, 1981; HEMMINGS and WILLIAMS 1976). Not all types of maternal antibodies enter the fetal circulation since the transfer is not regulated by the thickness of the placental or intestinal membranes but depends upon the capacity of cells forming such membranes to allow proteins to cross them by an active process of endocytosis (BRAMBELL 1966, 1970; WILD 1975, 1981).

In humans the transmission of Ig molecules occurs mainly by way of the chorio-allantoic placenta (GITLIN et al. 1964; BRAMBELL 1966; GITLIN 1974; HEMMINGS and WILLIAMS 1976), and selection is one of its most remarkable features. It should be appreciated that while in humans only IgG cross the placenta, in some species, such as in rabbit, maternal IgM molecules are also transported to the fetus. This means that the mechanisms that select the transfer of Ig operate independently of the molecular size of the proteins but depend on the presence of specific ligands and cell membrane receptors. In fact, the transfer of IgG across the human placenta has been elucidated with the demonstration that these molecules express unique sequences on their Fc region, and that trophoblastic cells produce specific Ig receptors (FcRs; MATRE et al. 1975; JENKINSON et al. 1976; WILD 1975, 1981).

Table 1. Major routes of transmission of maternal antibodies in different species

Human	Placenta	Prenatal
Primates	Placenta	Prenatal
Rabbit	Yolk sac	Prenatal
Guinea pig	Yolk sac	Prenatal
Rat, mouse	Yolk sac (milk)	Pre-and Postnatal
Horse, pig	Gut (milk)	Postnatal

FcRs are a diverse family of membrane glycoproteins that bind the carboxy-terminal part of the constant region of Ig molecules and direct their transport across cellular membranes. These receptors are present on many types of cells (e.g. trophoblasts, macrophages, red cells) and therefore play different biological functions (RAVETCH and KINET 1991). On haematopoietic cells FcRs are responsible for the production of antibodies (including IgE mediated allergic reactions), the uptake of immunocomplexes and the triggering of cytotoxic responses. FrRII and FcRIII – present respectively on placental endothelium and syncytiotrophoblastic cells and therefore responsible for the transport of human maternal IgG to the fetus – are heterodimeric molecules whose heavy chains are similar in sequence to the heavy chain of MHC class I molecules; the light chain is the same as that of β_2 microglobulin used by MHC class I (STORY et al. 1994; BURMEISTER et al. 1994; RAVETCH and MARGULIES 1994).

The transport of IgG across the placenta (or the intestinal epithelium in some species) occurs via the formation of a complex (e.g. FcR IgG) transcytosed into the blood and later dissociated (WILD 1981; RAVETCH and MARGULIES 1994).

Evidence that the great majority of immunoglobulins present in the fetal and newborn circulations is derived from the maternal IgG molecules is based on the following observations: (a) Maternal IgG antibodies against blood groups, bacterial or viral antigens are readily detectable in cord sera while IgM are absent (VAHLQUIST 1958; HITZIG 1959; FREDA 1962; DE MURALT 1962; see also: ADINOLFI 1974). (b) In early studies labelled IgG injected intravenously into pregnant women were detected in fetal and cord blood (DU PAN et al. 1959). (c) Most IgG molecules in fetal and cord sera express allotypic specificities similar to those present in the corresponding maternal blood (GRUBB and LAURELL 1956; LINNET-JEPSEN et al. 1958; ADINOLFI 1974, 1981a).

Maternal IgG molecules start to cross the placenta after about 6 weeks of gestation. Around 10 weeks, if the mother is RhD negative and produces anti-Rh(D) antibodies, the fetal RhD-positive cells may react with an antiglobulin test, thus revealing the presence of maternal IgG antibodies (MOLLISON 1951).

The rate of active transport of IgG varies during the course of normal pregnancy; after around 10–16 weeks of gestation the concentrations of IgG range between 100 and 200 mg/100 ml; after 20–22 weeks of pregnancy the transfer of maternal IgG increases rapidly and, at about 26 weeks the fetal levels are similar to those present in the corresponding maternal peripheral blood samples (GITLIN 1974; ADINOLFI 1974). It has been claimed that the transfer of IgG subclasses is selective, and that at 16 weeks the majority of the transferred maternal molecules are IgG1; at 22 weeks all subclasses cross the placenta.

At time of delivery the concentration of IgG in cord sera may be slightly higher than that in the corresponding maternal sample. Infants born to mothers with immunodeficiencies have low serum levels of IgG, while those born to mothers with chronic infections (e.g. malaria) have high concentrations; this indirectly confirms the maternal origin of this class of immunoglobulins (for references see ADINOLFI 1974, 1981a).

Maternal antibodies associated with IgM, IgA and IgE are not present in sera from normal infants (for references see ADINOLFI 1974, 1981a). If these classes of Ig are detectable in newborn samples, they are produced by the fetuses (see next section).

In some species the main source of maternal antibodies during perinatal life derives from colostrum and milk (Table 1). In humans most of the Ig molecules present in colostrum, milk and other body fluids are secretory IgA. Maternal antibodies present in milk are claimed to play an important role in protecting the neonate against necrotizing enteroclitis and the development of allergic reactions (HANSON et al. 1987). In addition to IgA, human colostrum and milk contain many other factors that can protect the infant against infection, including lysozyme and components of complement (ADINOLFI and GLYNN 1979; HANSON et al. 1987).

The induction of tolerance by oral immunization is also a well-recognized phenomenon (ANDRE et al. 1975; SANSOREMO 1995), and it has been suggested that maternal milk may perform a similar function (BRAMBELL 1970).

The biological advantages of breast feeding on infant morbidity and mortality have been repeatedly emphasized, but social and economic pressures render any scientific discussion on this topic ineffectual.

4 Synthesis of Immunoglobulins During Fetal Life

The levels of IgG, measured in infants bled at intervals soon after birth, decline during the first 3 months of life. For many years this decrease was interpreted as evidence of a slow catabolism of the maternal IgG antibodies. However, in 1959 TREVORROW showed that the decline in IgG levels is also due to the expanding fetal plasma volume, and that, if this phenomenon is taken into consideration, the concentrations of IgG in sera from normal infants are relatively constant. On the basis of this observation TREVORROW first suggested that the catabolized maternal IgG molecules are replaced by antibodies produced by the fetus and the newborn. This hypothesis was in agreement with previous observations that documented the presence of plasma cells, albeit in low numbers, in normal fetuses during the last period of gestastion and showed that their incidence increases in liver, lung and spleen of newborns with congenital syphilis or toxoplasmosis (PORCILE 1904; PUND and VON HAAM 1957). These findings were later confirmed by SILVERSTEIN and LUKES (1962), who detected plasma cells in 16 fetuses with congenital syphilis and in three with toxoplasmosis.

Following infections during fetal life, abnormally high levels of IgM have been detected in sera from fetuses or infants with congenital rubella, cytomegalic inclusion disease or infections with *Toxoplasma gondii* (ALFORD 1965; MCCRACKEN and SHINEFIELD 1965; REMINGTON and MILLER 1966; STIEHM et al. 1966; ALFORD et al. 1967; ADINOLFI 1974; AHO et al. 1987). According to SOOTHILL et al. (1966), long-sustained antigenic stimulation during fetal life may affect and reduce the synthesis of IgG while increasing the levels of IgM.

Low levels of IgM (ranging between 5%–10% of the values in adult samples) have been detected in sera from normal infants occasionally these IgM have the characteristics of auto-antibodies, but they may react against blood group or bacterial antigens (GARDNER and ADINOLFI 1968; see also ADINOLFI 1974; BUTLER et al. 1987).

Evidence supporting the fetal synthesis of immunoglobulins includes:

- Presence in normal cord sera of IgM antibodies – not derived from the maternal circulation – with specificities against:
- I blood groups (cold agglutinins)
- κ-chain epitopes
- Trypsinised human red blood cells
- A and B blood groups
- Gram-negative bacteria and *Listeria*
- Viruses and bacteria following in utero infections
- Detection of IgG genetic variants (Gm groups) produced under the control of paternal genes
- In vitro synthesis of IgG and IgM immunoglobulins using fetal spleen and lymph nodes

EPSTEIN (1965) has shown that some cord sera contain antibodies directed against antigenic determinants expressed on the light (κ) chains. IgM anti-I cold agglutinins, present in almost all sera from normal adults, are also detectable in cord sera (ADINOLFI 1965). Occasionally, IgM anti-A or anti-B agglutinins, which cannot be derived from maternal blood, are present in newborn sera (for references see ADINOLFI 1974). Many investigators have shown that human neonatal B cells are capable of producing IgM antibodies reactive with several auto-antigens after appropriate stimulation or spontaneously (ROMAGNANI et al. 1980; RUUSKANEN et al. 1980; LYDYARD et al. 1990; LEVINSON et al. 1987; BARBOUCHE et al. 1992; HAMET et al. 1992).

Early studies using in vitro cultures of fetal tissues have also conclusively demonstrated that immunoglobulins are synthesized during fetal life (VAN FURTH et al. 1965; ADINOLFI and WOOD 1969). Following the incubation of fetal tissues in media containing labelled amino acids and the analysis of the culture fluids by immunoelectrophoresis and autoradiography, newly produced IgM and IgG molecules were detected in culture media from spleen and lymph nodes. The same studies showed by immunostaining that large and medium-sized cells from fetal spleen express IgM and IgG molecules on their surface.

These findings are in agreement with later observations that B lymphocytes – bearing specific markers and expressing Ig molecules – can be detected at early stages of embryonic development. Using fluroescein-labelled antibodies against different classes and subclasses of Ig molecules and by investigating the assembly of Ig genes, a clear picture of the maturations of B cells during fetal life has now emerged. At their early stages of maturation pre-B (null) cells begin to assemble the

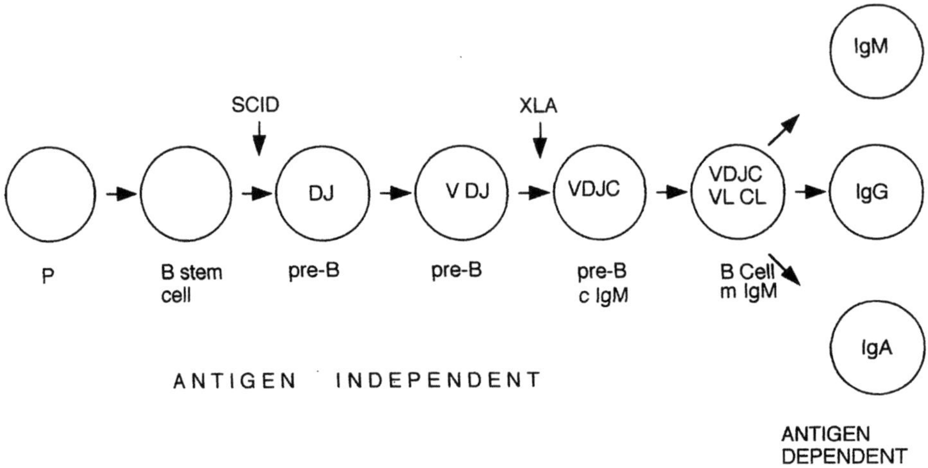

Fig. 4. Model of the maturation of B cells that starts with the transformation of precursors (*P*) into more differentiated stem cells and then pre-B cells, which show rearrangements of a D a J and then one of the V genes of the lg heavy chains. Genes for the domains of a light chain are also rearranged, resulting in the synthesis of cytoplasmic (*clgM*) and later surface lgM. This leads to the antigen-dependent production of mature B cells expressing lgM, lgG, lgA or lgE

Ig genes, starting with the activation and joining of a D and a J sequence followed by the rearrangement of a V gene (Fig. 4). It is claimed that in human fetuses about 7.5 weeks old liver cells (approximately 0.1%) start to synthesise Ig molecules; after around 12 weeks pre-B cells containing cytoplasmic IgM are present in bone marrow, from which location they generate B lymphocytes throughout life. The rearrangement of the Ig genes progresses and in fetuses 9.5–12.5 weeks old the first peripheral blood B lymphocytes expressing surface IgM ($sIgM^+$) appear; their incidence increases to around 6% after about 16.5 weeks. B cells producing IgD have been detected in fetuses 12 weeks old; after about 15 weeks of fetal life around 50% of $sIgM^+$ also express IgD molecule.

The generation of a large repertoire of different B cell clones through the assembly of the Ig genes, which culminates in the maturation of single cells producing only one class of Ig molecules with a unique specificity, is antigen-independent (Fig. 4). B lymphocytes that encounter an antigen complementary to their antibody combining sites and receive help from Th cells undergo a series of changes leading to their division, the release of large quantities of antibodies and the production of memory cells.

As mentioned above, B cells express on their surface a wide assortment of cells receptors that play an important role in governing their responses. Receptors for components of C, interferon (IFNs) interleukin (IL) 2 and 4, and many other cytokines must be synthesized during fetal development to provide the newborn with the ability of producing circulating antibodies. Pre-B (null) cells lack receptors for the components of C or FcRs but express HLA class II molecules. Pre-B cells have also been found to produce a surrogate L chain (Sakaguchi and Melchers

1986; KUDO and MELCHERS 1987; ROLINK and MELCHERS 1991) Although the newborn produces a large number of B cells with different specificities, the full array of antibody responses is reached only a few years after delivery by the gradual esposure to bacteria and viruses and the acquisition of memory cells.

Humoral responses to different types of antigens are also genetically and sequentially acquired (SILVERSTEIN 1964; ADINOLFI 1974). Usually B cell responses to protein antigens, requiring Th cells, can be readily induced in newborns; in contrast, antibody responses to polysaccharides are acquired later in life (COWAN et al. 1978; ANDERSON 1985).

When SMITH et al. (1964) immunized newborn infants with *Salmonella* strains against which they lacked maternal antibodies, marked differences from the immune responses seen in adults were observed. Antibodies to the protein H were readily detected, but they were persistently associated with IgM, while in adults a switch to IgG was noticed within 5–15 days. The polysaccharide O antigen did not induce antibodies in the newborns. On the other hand, an excellent immune response to hepatitis B vaccine has been reported in young infants by LEE et al. (1983).

B lymphocytes constitute 15%–20% of mononuclear cells in cord blood at full term; the majority of these cells express IgM and IgD on their membrane (ANDERSON et al. 1981; ANDERSON 1985, 1987; RACADOT 1993). According to BARBOUCHE et al. (1992), about 15% of human neonatal B lymphocytes form a subset of $sIgM^+$, $sIgD^+$, $CD23^+$, $CD16^+$ and $CD5^+$ cells responsible for the production of autoantibodies; this subset is not detectable in normal adults.

5 T Cell Development

At early stages of fetal growth, when spleen and lymph nodes are still poorly developed, the thymus is already an active organ. The human thymus, which originates from the ectoderm of the third branchial anlage, reaches its maximum size in relation to body weight at the time of delivery and then declines. For many years a controversy has surrounded the origins of thymocytes. In 1879 KOLLIKER suggested that thymic lymphocytes are derived from the transformation of epithelial cells intrinsic to the thymic anlage. Only in 1910 did HAMMAR and MAXIMOV propose an extrinsic origin of thymocytes (quoted in HAMMAR 1921, 1936). This claim was confirmed by MOORE and OWEN (1967) and MOORE and METCALF (1970) who, using chromosome markers, demonstrated an inflow of primordial cells from the yolk sac into the mouse thymus around the tenth day of fetal life. A similar process of migration, which culminates in the development of the lymphoid system, has also been demonstrated in avians (LE DUARIN and JOTEREAU 1975) and in humans (OWEN and JENKINSON 1981; ROSENTHAL et al. 1983; for references see also ADINOLFI 1974, 1988).

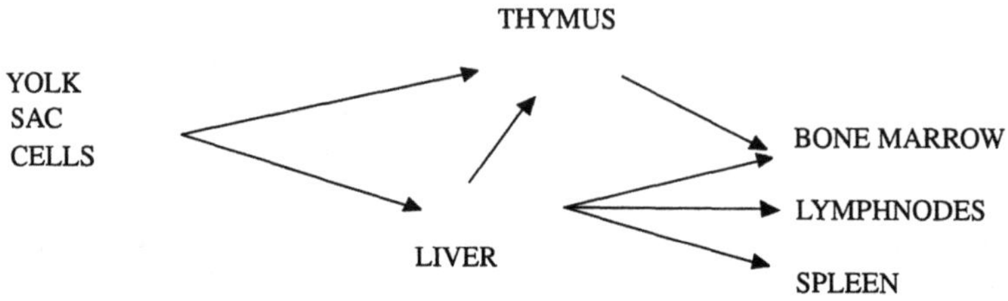

Fig. 5. Haematopoietic stem cells derived from the yolk sac reach the thymus and/or the liver to migrate into the bone marrow, lymph nodes and spleen to differentiate into mature T or B cells (see text)

In mouse embryos haematopoietic stem cells appear in the yolk sac blood island after 7–8 days of fetal life and start to colonize the thymus at day 10 (Fig. 5; EDDY et al. 1981; OWEN and JENKINSON 1981). It is generally believed that migration of yolk sac primordial cells starts in human fetuses about 5 weeks old; lymphocyte precursors have been observed in fetal livers after about 7 weeks and in the thymus after 10 weeks. The events leading to the dissemination of the pluripotential haematopoietic yolk sac cells include the seeding of these cells in various organs, initial differentiation into specific types of cells under the influence of local inductive factors and further relocation of the released cells into other organs (e.g. spleen, lymph nodes), which culminate in their definitive differentiation (LASSILA 1981; HAYNES 1984; STUTMAN 1985, 1987; HAYNES et al. 1988, 1989).

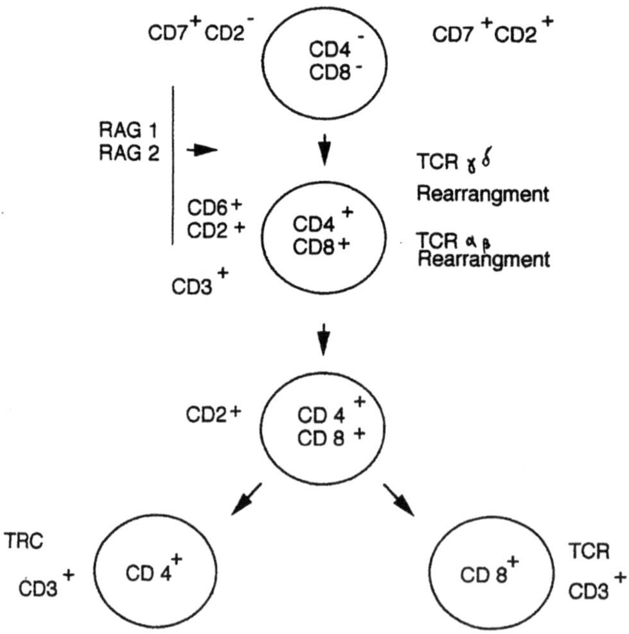

Fig. 6. Maturation of T cells from precursors $CD7^+$, $CD4^-$, $CD8^-$, into double-positive $CD4^+$, $CD8^+$ cells which also express TCR molecules and CD3. These cells then produce $CD4^+CD8^-$ or $CD4^-$ $CD8^+$ mature T cells (see text)

Table 2. Expression of TCR and CD3 molecules on fetal thymocytes (modified from McVay et al. 1991)

	Ages of fetuses				
	13 weeks	16 weeks	17 weeks	19 weeks	6 months
TCRα	15	23	21	34	55
TCRβ	2	1.5	1.6	1.4	1.1
TCRγ	16	1.2	1.3	1	n.d.
$CD3^+$	34	37	30	47	64

In mouse embryos and in avian a second site of hematopoietic activity has been identified in the aorta-gonadmesonephron region. This is claimed to be a major source of definitive hematopoiesis in adult mammals (for references see Adinolfi 1988; Medivinsky and Dzierzak 1996).

Intrathymic T-cell development requires a continuous input of precursor cells from either the fetal liver or, as in adults, the bone marrow (Fowlkes and Pardoll 1989; Haynes et al. 1989; Boyd and Hugo 1991; Boyd et al. 1993). Studies in human and rodent fetal thymuses have shown that subsequent differentiation eventually leads to the production of mature, self-tolerant, self-MHC-restricted T cells (Fig. 6; Raulet et al. 1985; Boyd and Hugo 1991; Clevers and Owen 1991; Godfrey and Zlotnik 1993; Ritter and Boyd 1993). This process can be summarized as follows: after about 8–9 weeks of gestation about 50% of the thymocytes are $CD7^+$ $CD2^+$ and the remaining cells $CD7^+$ $CD2^-$. These precursor cells are $CD3^-$, $CD4^-$, $CD8^-$ ("triple negative") and do not contain rearranged TCR genes (Fig. 6; Haynes et al. 1988, 1989; Kearse et al. 1995). After around 10 weeks thymocytes start to produce CD3 mRNA (Haynes et al. 1988, 1989; Clevers et al. 1993); the intrathymic prethymocytes are cells that express all CD3 genes and have initiated but not completed the rearrangement of the TCR genes in an orderly fashion. According to McVay et al. (1991), in human fetuses between 11 and 22 weeks old all V and V genes are rearranged and expressed with the possible exception of Vd4. Vd2 appears to be the most conspicuously expressed Vd gene is fetal thymus. As ontogeny proceeds, the frequency of TCRγδ cells declines while that of TCRαβ increases (Table 2). The early population of $CD4^-$, $CD8^-$ "double negative" cells encompasses T lymphocytes that can be $CD3^+$ and start to express TCR molecules. These double-negative cells then give rise to $CD3^+$, $CD4^+$, $CD8^+$ cells (double positive), which then down regulate their CD4 or CD8 genes and mature into functional $CD4^+$, $CD8^-$ or $CD4^-$, $CD8^+$ T cells.

There are still uncertainties about the maturation of TCRαβ and TCRγδ molecules and particularly about the derivation of T cells TCRαβ from cells that have rearranged the γ and δ chains. As shown in Fig. 7, evidence has been produced in favour of an early rearrangement of the γ and δ chains followed by an rearrangement of α the β and α chains. Alternatively, failure to rearrange the γ and δ chains may result in the correct expression of the α and β genes. A third possibility is that the TCR genes are arranged at random (Kronenberg and Brines 1993).

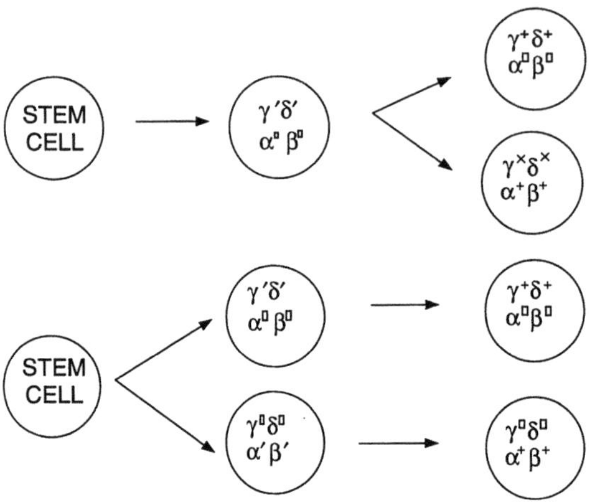

Fig. 7. T cells expressing TCR $\gamma\delta$ molecules are thought to be derived from cells which have successfully rearranged the γ and δ genes while unproductive rearrangements of these genes result in the activation of the α and β genes and expression of TCR$\alpha\beta$ molecules. Alternatively, it has been suggested that the rearrangement is random, resulting in the production of distinct T cell lines. *o*, *r* and *x*, germline, successful and unsuccessful rearranged genes

However, it is clear that T cells expressing TCRγδ genes appear before TCRαβ cells and that TCRγδ thymocytes are differentially located in various tissues (Ito et al. 1989; Konenberg and Brines 1993; Roth and DeFranco 1995).

In pre-TRC cells the TCR β chain is covalently associated with a 33-kDa glycoprotein termed pre-Ta (Groettrup et al. 1993) and a pre-V chain. This pre-TCR complex is postulated to induce rearrangement and expression of the $CD4^+$ $CD8^+$ (double positive) T cells. A striking feature of the pre-TCR complex is its similarity to the pre-B complexes with the five light chain and pre-V domains (Sakagushi and Melcher 1986; Chien and Joves 1995; Roth and DeFranco 1995).

The maturation of T cells requires the sequential expression of several factors, including RAG-1 and RAG-2, Lck and ZAP-70 (Weiss and Littman 1994; Chan et al. 1994). Defective ZAP-70 genes have been detected in patients with T cell immunodeficiency (Chan et al. 1994). Studies in mice with mutations of either RAG-1, RAG-2 or individual TCR genes (Mombaerts et al. 1992; Shinkai et al. 1992; Godfrey and Zlotnik 1993) and investigations in transgenic mice (von Boehmer 1992) have shown that these genes are essential for the development of T cells. Mutations of these genes arrest T cells at the triple-negative stage and induce absence of TCR expression, ultimately being responsible for severe immunodeficienses (Rosen et al. 1995).

Investigations in athymic (nude) mice have also revealed the existence of alternative, extrathymic developmental pathways (Rocha et al. 1992). In these rodents lymphocytes expressing the CD3-TCR complex can be detected in spleen, lymph nodes, gut, liver and skin. They appear relatively late in ontogeny and increase in numbers only with aging (for references Rocha et al. 1992). The T cells of athymic mice may express either types of TCR molecules, but the incidence of TCR γδ or TCR αβ varies greatly in different organs and between and within the same strains of mice. In nude mice, the vast majority of TCR^+ cells do not express the Thy1 antigen.

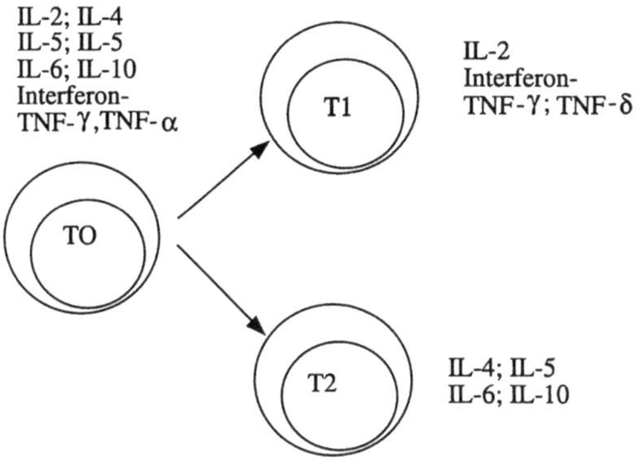

Fig. 8. Maturation of lymphocytes t0 into two subclasses (T1 and T2) expressing different types of cytokines

Investigations in rodents have also documented the interdependence of T cells and the surrounding stromal thymic cells (Ritter and Boyd 1993). Data from several naturally occurring and experimental situations suggest that without mature medullary thymocytes there is no or little development of thymic stromal cells. The dialogue between the different types of cells is, again, mediated by a large number of ligands and receptors, including several cytokines.

Upon antigenic stimulation $CD4^+$ T cells differentiate into two distinct populations, Th1 and Th2, each producing its own set of cytokines and able to mediate separate effector functions (Fig. 8; Mossmann and Coffman 1989; Paul and Seder 1994). Th1 cells produce IL-2, tumor necrosis factors α and β and IFN-δ, thereby activating macrophages and inducing delayed-type hypersensitivity responses. Th2 cells produce IL-4, IL-5, IL-6 and IL-10. Since, in addition to $CD4^+$ cells, also $CD8^+$, $CD4^-CD8^-$ and cells expressing TCRγδ secrete different types of cytokines, it has been suggested that the two populations of T cells should be referred to as T1 and T2, and as derived from a precursor T0 (Swain 1995). The differentiation of T cells into these two subtypes (Fig. 8) has important biological implication in terms of susceptibility or resistance to diseases (Kuchroo et al. 1995).

In the human fetal thymus $CD44^+$, cells are present after about 10–11 weeks of gestation. The $CD44^+$ cells can be found in both cortex and medulla (Wu et al. 1993; Owen 1993; Ruiz et al. 1995). This molecule belongs to a family of transmembrane glycoproteins which are generated as multiple isoforms by the differential splicing of pre-mRNA. Each isoform exhibits highly specialized patterns of expression in various tissues, and lymphopoiesis is regulated by the presence of selectively and temporarily expressed CD44 molecules together with other cell adhesion proteins (Adams and Watt 1993; Ruiz et al. 1995).

Antibodies against CD44 have been shown to inhibit thymus repopulation by bone marrow progenitor cells (Wu et al. 1993). Although much remains to be learned about the biological role of CD44 molecules, it seems that these glycoproteins are indispensable for the development and differentiation of many lymphopoietic cells. In fact, CD44 also defines two populations of bone marrow B cells that differ 10-to 15-fold in the levels of CD44 expression (KANSAS and DAILEY 1989). The early pre-B cells (CD19$^+$ CD10$^+$) have CD44-low phenotype, with the transition to the CD44-high phenotype occurring relatively late in development when the cells become immature IgM$^+$ (see KINCADE 1993).

6 Ontogeny of AP and NK Cells

Macrophages monocytes and dentritic cells have been detected in human fetuses from the second trimester of gestation (for references see ADINOLFI 1974, 1981; HOFMAN et al. 1984). The presence of these cells has been investigated using MAbs or the expression of unique proteins (e.g. lysozyme) and HLA antigens.

Since 1971 HLA antigens have been detected in selected cells (e.g. monocytes, peripheral blood lymphocytes, spleen and thymic cells obtained from human fetuses more that 12 week old (CROME et al. 1971; CEPPELLINI et al. 1971). Macrophages and Payer cells from fetuses over 9 weeks old have been shown to stain specifically when tested with antisera against lysozyme (KLOCKARS et al. 1977). This is in agreement with the demonstration that lysozyme is present in sera from fetuses 9 week old (GLYNN et al. 1970; ADINOLFI et al. 1971).

Using specific MAbs, macrophages and monocytes have been detected in human fetuses as early as at 12 weeks of gestation, but the expression of specific surface markers varies qualitatively and quantitatively with increasing gestational age (BHOOPAT et al. 1986). Although it has been claimed that fetal or neonatal AP cells are functionally immature, the lower capacity to induce immune responses is probably due to reduced expression of antibodies and receptors responsible for the recognition of foreign antigens more than to an intrinsic incapacity to process.

NK cells are a subpopulation of lymphocytes that have the capacity to lyse certain cancer or virus-infected cells without requiring the presence of MHC class I or II in order to recognize their targets (TRINCHIERI 1989). NK cells do not rearrange TCR genes and do not express CD3; they can be identified as being phenotypically CD3$^-$, CD16$^+$ and CD56$^+$ (FcRIII; LANIER et al. 1986).

Functional NK cells have been detected in human fetal liver at early stages of embryonic development (TOIVANEN et al. 1981) and in neonates (MACCARIO and BURGIO 1987). Freshly isolated fetal NK cells can mediate MHC-unrestricted cytotoxicity against sensitive target cells and acquire the ability to lyse NK-resistent cancer cell after overnight incubation with IL-2 (PHILLIPS et al. 1992). Unlike adult NK cells, freshly isolated fetal cells – and clones derived from them – are found to express substantial levels of CD3 in the cytoplasm.

The postnatal expansion of NK cells has been documented by ABO et al. (1982) using MAb against CD56 (NHK-1), a heavily glycosilated isoform of the neural cell adhesion molecule.

7 Immune Tolerance

During fetal development the immune system acquires tolerance towards self antigens through a variety of complex mechanisms. The idea that the immune system "learns" what is antigenically "self" was first suggested by OWEN et al. (1945) from studies of dizygotic twins in cattle. The offspring were found to be chimeric, having in their circulation erythrocytes of the twin as well their own. This chimerism – arising from blood vessel anastomoses in the placenta and reciprocal transfer of the haematopoietic stem cells – suggested that tolerance is induced during fetal life. This hypothesis was later tested by injecting murine spleen cells of one strain into fetuses or newborns mice of another strain (BILLINGHAM et al. 1953). The treated mice were then shown not to reject grafts taken from the donor strain, while they were still capable of rejecting grafts from a third strain of mice. Similar results were obtained in avians in which the circulatory systems of two embryos were joined (parabiosis; Hasek and Hraba 1955 quoted in HASEK et al. 1961). In more recent experiments tetraparental (allophenic) mice derived from the fusion of two heterozygous eight-cell embryos have been shown to be tolerant to tissues grafted from the parents (MINTZ and SILVERS 1967, quoted in HASEK et al. 1961). In 1961 MILLER also demonstrated that mice, thymectomized as newborns, accept histoincompatible grafted tissues, thus confirming that immunotolerance is a phenomenon controlled by the thymus (MILLER 1961a,b, 1994).

These and other experiments support the hypothesis, advanced by BURNET and FENNER (1949; BURNET 1962), that exposure of the developing immune system to foreign antigens induces specific tolerance. According to the clonal theory of BURNET and TALMAGE, individual clones of lymphocytes with receptors for self-antigens are deleted or inactivated during development (LEDERBERG 1959; TALMAGE 1969). Although physical deletion of antibody producing cells has been observed, in most instances antigen-reactive cells can still be detected in tolerant animals and in humans (for references see NOSSAL 1983, 1994). These observations argue for the concept of clonal anergy, whereas T and B cells are functionally inactivated without being physically deleted (NOSSAL and PIKE 1980; HARRIS et al. 1982; SCHWARTZ 1989; GOODNOW et al. 1990, 1991; BLACKMAN et al. 1990).

The present view is that, during development in the thymus, T lymphocytes undergo selective events of negative and positive selections mediated by the expression of MHC molecules (ZINKERNAGEL et al. 1978; MARRACK and KAPPLER 1987, 1993; TEH et al. 1988; SPRENT et al. 1988, 1990; SCHWARTZ 1989; HUGO et al. 1993; VON BOEHMER 1992; MILLER and MORAHAN 1992; NOSSAL 1994). Many theories have been proposed to explain the two opposite mechanisms. The premise is that selection operates at the level of thymocytes initially expressing the whole spectrum of TCR molecules that these cells are genetically capable of encoding. Negative selection occurs with the engagement of TCRs with MHC molecules bound to self-antigens, presented by thymic stromal elements and bone marrow derived AP cells. It is suggested that the tolerigenic effect is mediated by the high antigenic affinity of the self-reactive clones. The positive selective process presumes that thymocytes with TCRs reactive with foreign antigens have low affinity for self-MHC; these are the T cells that later expand (NIKOLIC-ZUGIC and BEVAN 1990; ASHTON-RICHARDT et al. 1994; TRAVERS 1993).

According to the so-called "instructive" hypothesis, the interaction between TCR and MHC molecules with CD4 or CD8 correctors is essential for the development of the double-positive T cells into cells expressing only CD4 or CD8. Accordingly, a T cell engagement with an MHC class II receptor induces the expression of CD4 while suppressing CD8 gene; engagement with MHC class I, on the other hand, suppresses the expression of CD4, allowing the cells to be $CD8^+$. The contrasting stochastic theory proposes, instead, that the double-positive CD4, CD8 cells randomly repress one of the coreceptor's gene.

Recent studies also suggest that antigenic determinant (peptides) per se play an important role in T cells selection. Peptides with similar structure may act as agonists (that fully stimulate the TCRs) or antagonists, according to how closely they fit to TCR molecules. Antagonistic peptides reduce or abrogate specific immune responses toward agonistic peptides. In order to survive during development T cells must be stimulated by the interaction with self-peptide and self-MHC. If they interact too strongly, they die or become anergic, thus eliminating potentially dangerous self-reactive T cells. Those reacting weakly survive and later expand under the stimulation of foreign antigens. The interaction of the TCRs and self-antigens, leading to tolerance, is also regulated by the complex set of other cell surface molecules (e.g. CD3; MARX 1995).

8 Ontogeny of Complement

The complement (C) system consists of over 30 plasma and membrane-associated proteins which, upon interaction with each other, acquire new biological properties (MÜLLER-EBERHARD 1986). Therefore a characteristic of many components of C is the ability to generate, upon activation, fragments endowed with the capacity to bind other components of C for at least a short period of time.

The activation of C occurs as a cascade of reactions that proceeds via two pathways (Fig. 9; OSLER and SANDBERG 1973; ROTHER and ROTHER 1986; MÜLLER-EBERHARD 1986). The classical activation is initiated by the interaction of an antibody-antigen complex with the first components (C1 q, r, s), followed by the interaction with C4 and C2 that binds the surface of the antigens (e.g. bacteria or red blood cells). The activated fragments of C4 and C2 acts as a C3 convertase that then cleaves C3 (Fig. 9). C3 can also be activated by components of the alternative pathway, which include factor B and factor D. Most components of C are molecules formed by two or more polypeptyde chains whose genes have been mapped. C4, C2 and factor B genes are located on chromosome 6 between MHC class I and class II genes. C3 maps on chromosome 19, and it is synthesized as a single-chain precursor (pro-C3) which is then processed by proteolytic enzymes into two sub

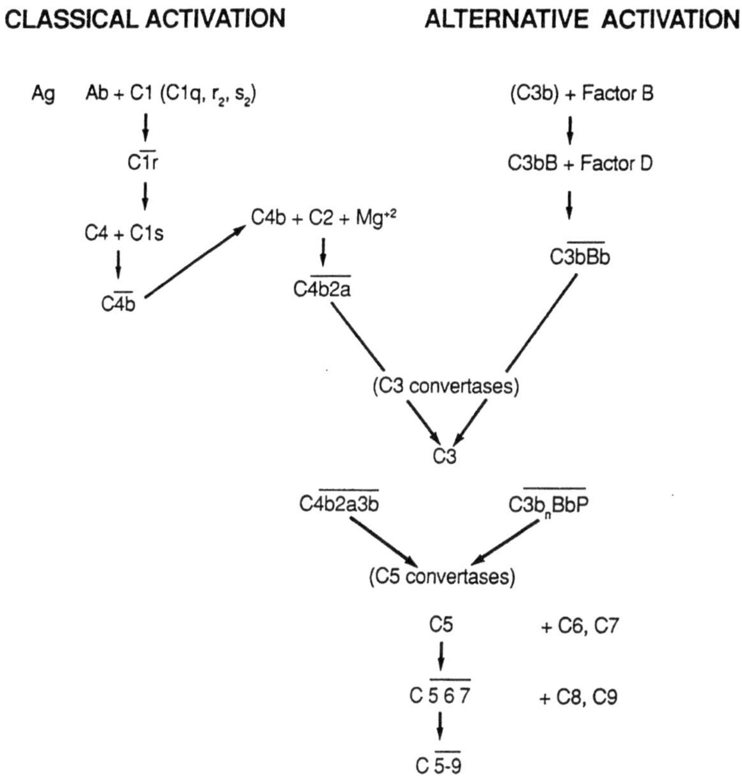

Fig. 9. Classical and alternative pathways of C activation. The classical pathway usually starts with the interaction of C1 with the Ag-Ab complexes, while the alternative pathway is activated by bacterial or fungal cell wall polysaccharides. The resulting C3 convertase induces activation of the late components of C

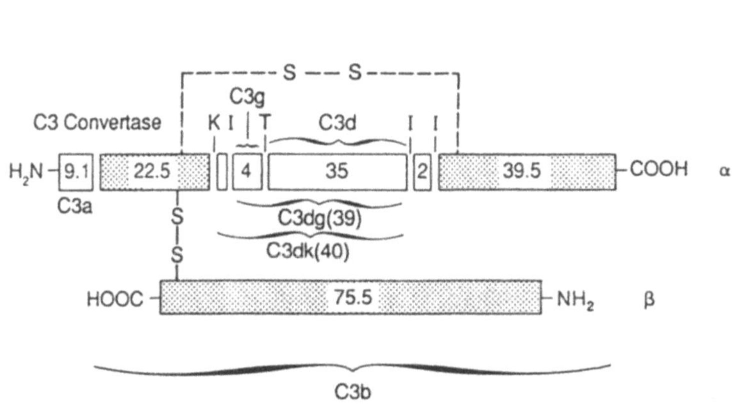

Fig. 10. Upon activation C3 molecules are sequentially degraded and produce fragments with different biological activities, some (e.g. C3d) with strong influence on the production of antibodies

Table 3. Major steps in the maturation of immune responses during fetal life

Weeks		
4–5	Yolk sac pluripotent cells	Synthesis of C1-INH
6	Thymus rudiment appears	
7	Lymphopoiesis in liver	
8	First B cells in liver	
9	$CD7^+$, $CD2^+$ in thymus	lysozyme in fetal sera
10	$CD3^+$;HLA antigens	Maternal IgG in fetal sera
11		C3 and C2 in fetal sera
12	TCRγδ; TCRαβ; IgM and IgG^+ B cells	
13		
14	Lymphocytes in peripheral blood	CR1, CR3 (complement receptros)
15	IgM in sera	Lysozyme in Paneth cells
16		
17–18		
19–20	Marked increase HLA II^+ cells	All components of C in fetal sera
22		Increased transfer maternal IgG

units (Fig. 10; Müller-Eberhard 1975; Sottzup-Jensen et al. 1985). In this final form C3 is thus composed by two polypeptide chains α and β, with approximate molecular masses of 120 and 75 kDa, respectively. As a result of activation by either the classical or alternative convertases, the α chain is cleaved into several fragments with different biological properties.

The basic structure of C3, also observed in other components of C (for example, C5), is reported here to illustrate how the activation of many components of C proceeds, and how a variety of fragments are produced which have different biological properties. In fact, the biological activities of C are not limited to the lysis of bacteria or red cells but include immune adherence, viral neutralization, chemotaxis, release of histamine, production of antibodies, bone metabolism and cell proliferation (for references see Adinolfi 1993a). Several components of C also play a very important role as "acute-phase proteins" during infections (Adinolfi and Lehner 1988).

The C system includes many proteins with regulatory functions and several types of cells receptors. The activation of C needs to be controlled at each step in order to avoid self-damage; thus, activated components of C must be inhibited after a short period of time. Furthermore, fragments of various components of the classical or alternative pathways need to react with receptors present on the surface of AP cells, red blood cells or bacteria (Ross and Atkinson 1985; Rother and Rother 1986; Cooper et al. 1988).

CRs that recognize C1q are present on neutrophils, monocytes and B cells (Feron and Wong 1983; Ross and Atkinson 1985; Tenner and Cooper 1981; Table 3). Four proteolytic fragments of C3 – C3b,i C3b, C3d and C3d,g – have been shown to interact with three types of CR molecules present on the membrane of several cells (Bianco et al. 1970; Dobson et al. 1981; Fearon and Wong 1983; Ross and Atkinson 1985).

Many CR molecules have been investigated in detail and their genes mapped (see Adinolfi 1993a). For example, four codominantly expressed CR1 genes have been identified. The molecular size and gene frequencies of CR1 are: A, 190 kDa (0.83); B, 220 kDa (0.16); C, 160 kDa (0.01) and D, 250 kDa (less than 0.01). (Ross and Atkinson 1985). The number of these receptors expressed on erythrocytes is also genetically controlled by two autosomal codominant alleles for high and low frequency of CR1 per red cell. Thus homozygotes for the "high" genes have 800 000 receptors per erythrocyte whereas homozygotes for the "low" alleles have only 200 000 CR1 molecules per cell (Fearon and Wong 1983; Wilson et al. 1982). An association between high and low levels of CR1 molecules and disease has been observed; for example, while only 12% of normal individuals are homozygous for the "low" allele, 53% of those with systemic lupus erythematosus are homozygous for this gene (Miyakawa et al. 1981; Fearon and Wong 1983).

Since many components of C are produced in excess of the minimal amounts required, and alternative activations are possible, some deficiency of C is well tolerated. However, an efficient immune response during perinatal life depends on at least a partial maturation of the entire system (Adinolfi 1993a).

Several approaches have been employed to establish the onset and site of synthesis of the various components of C during fetal life in humans and experimental animals (Adinolfi 1972, 1977, 1993a; Colten 1973, 1976). One of the first studies on maturation of the C system was published in 1932, when Hyde demonstrated that sera of newborn guinea pigs delivered by mothers with a deficiency in a component of C had normal lytic activities. He also demonstrated that the maternal component of C did not cross the placenta and could not be found in newborns with a specific deficiency.

Since 1940 studies in humans have documented the presence of total lytic activities in sera from normal neonates, although at levels near half of those present in maternal samples (Wasserman and Alberts 1940; Traub 1943; Arditi and Nigro 1957). In 1961 Fishel and Pearlman observed that all four components of C known at the time could be detected in cord sera. Further investigations have confirmed that all plasma components of C are detectable in cord blood when their presence was studied using either functional assays or immunoprecipitation techniques (see Adinolfi 1993a). The mean levels of most components of C in newborn sera are near half the values of those detected in maternal samples, with the exception of C9 which is present at low concentrations (Adinolfi 1993a).

As shown in Fig. 11, C3 and C4 start to be detectable in sera from fetuses 9–10 weeks old, and their levels increase with gestational age (Adinolfi et al. 1968; Fireman et al. 1969; Sawyer et al. 1971; Adinolfi 1993a). C1q has been detected in sera of fetuses more that 20 weeks old while C5 was found in samples obtained from fetuses 5 weeks old (Adinolfi 1972, 1993a). C7 is already present at 14 weeks of gestation, and its levels increase to values between 30% and 75% of those detectable in sera from normal adults (Fig. 12; Adinolfi and Beck 1976; Adinolfi 1993a). Most regulatory components C, such as C1-INH and factors I and H, have also been detected in fetal and cord sera (for references see Adinolfi 1993a).

Due to the different techniques employed, there are some discrepancies about the levels of the various components of C in newborn samples, but the published results show that all components of C are produced in fetal life and are detectable

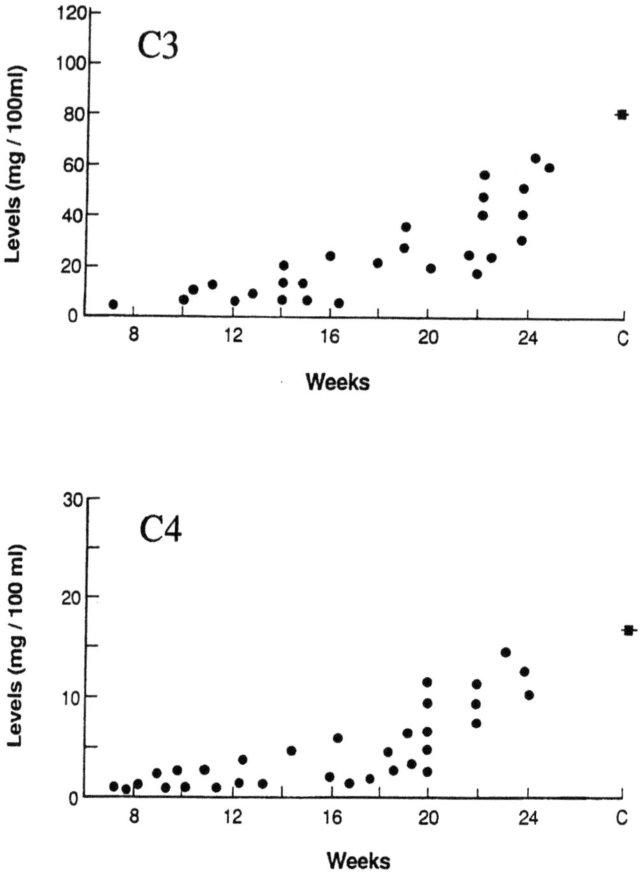

Fig. 11. Individual levels of C3 and C4 in sera from human fetuses at different ages of gestation and newborns at term. (From ADINOLFI 1993)

in cord sera, reaching levels nearly 50%–75% of those in normal adults, with the exception of C9 (Fig. 12; ADINOLFI 1993).

The site of synthesis of many components of C has been investigated using fetal tissues incubated in media containing radiolabelled amino acids. The proteins synthesized in the in vitro cultures were then analysed by immunoelectrophoresis and autoradiography of the immunoplates (THORBECKE et al. 1965; ADINOLFI et al. 1968; ADINOLFI 1972; COLTEN 1976).

Since many components of C show high genetic polymorphism, the detection of different phenotypes in pairs of maternal fetal or cord sera allows one to establish without any doubt their ontogeny. For example, in 1968 PROPP and ALPER demonstrated discordant C3 phenotypes in pairs of maternal and cord samples. In the following years various genetic variants of C4, C6 and factor H have also been detected in pairs of maternal and cord sera (for references see ADINOLFI 1993).

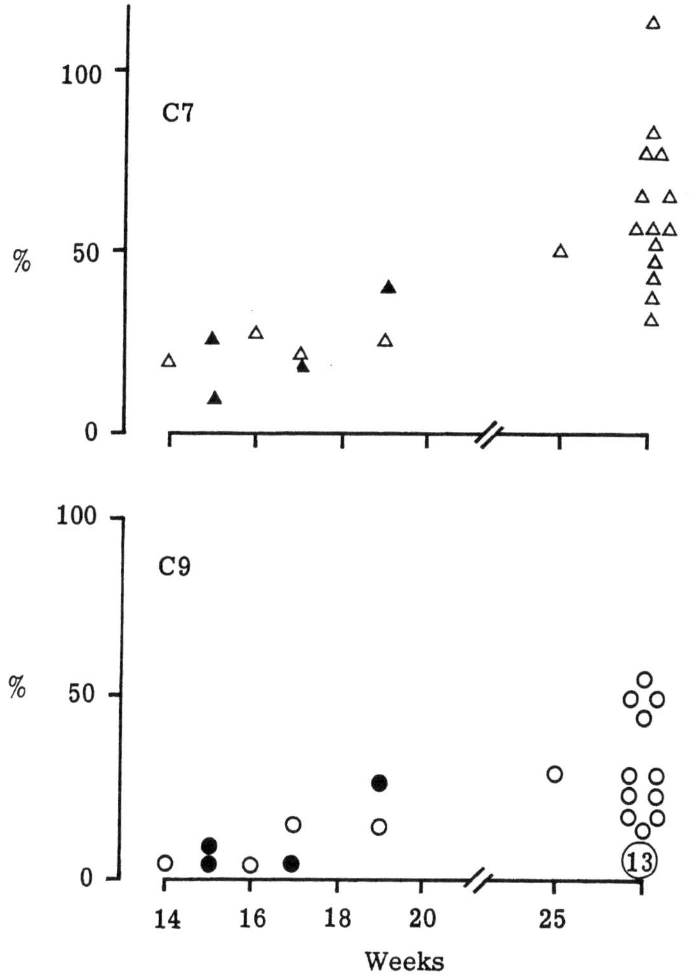

Fig. 12. Levels of C7 and C9 in fetal and cord sera, expressed as percentages of the mean levels in sera from normal adults. (From ADINOLFI 1993)

Studies of infants born to mothers with deficiencies in single components of C have also provided useful information about the ontogeny (ADINOLFI 1993).

With regard to complement receptors, CR3 has been detected in about 30% of pre-B cells present in human fetal bone marrow. The expression of these molecules increases with the maturation of B cells so that 90% of IgM^+, D^+ cells are $CR3^+$ (TEDDER et al. 1983; ADINOLFI et al. 1988; ADINOLFI 1993). CR1 has been detected on peripheral monocytes and neutrophils obtained from fetuses more that 14 weeks old and from subpopulations of cells from fetal bone marrow, spleen and thymus (ADINOLFI et al. 1988). CR2, which appears on the membranes of B cells at their early stages of maturation and synthesis of IgM (COOPER et al. 1988), is also present on monocytic cells in cord blood (ADINOLFI, unpublished observations).

9 Conclusions

During fetal development the immune system emerges as a constantly evolving network of interacting cells and molecules capable of differentiating self- from nonself-antigens and of protecting the infant from infections by bacteria, viruses, fungi and protozoa. In recent years it has been possible to elucidate many of the developmental and genetic mechanisms responsible for the maturation of the immune cells and their complex interactions (Table 3). The genes responsible for the control of these processes start to be activated early during fetal life, thus providing the newborn with an efficient immunological protection as soon as the maternally transferred antibodies are catabolized. In normal infants any gap in the immune responses probably does not result from intrinsic deficiencies in B or T cells but rather from a lack of immunlogical experience (ADINOLFI 1974; BUTLER et al. 1987).

Specific immunodeficiencies are instead the result of unique genetic defects affecting the maturations of single types of cells or proteins (ROSEN et al. 1995). It is beyond the scope of this review to describe the different forms of immunodeficiencies that can arise as a result of a block or anomaly in maturation of T and/or B cells. Of the many (over 50) genetic immune deficiencies that have been recognized in humans the X-linked disorders are among the most frequent (STIEM 1993; ROSEN et al. 1993). Mutations to at least seven loci on chromosome X have so far been identified (for references see CONLEY 1994; BELMONT 1995). These include the Wiskott-Aldrich syndrome (WAS), the X-linked form of hyper-IgM disorder (XHM), the severe combined immune deficiency (XSCID) and the X-linked agammaglobulinaemia (XLA). Properdin deficiencies and a lymph proliferative syndrome are also X-linked conditions.

These recent findings show that studies of the ontogeny of immunoglobulins, T cell receptors, components of complement and the various factors responsible for the maturation of an efficient immune responses have entered the realm of clinical medicine, in addition to being the object of interest of specialized groups of immunologist and biologists.

Another area of increasing interest is the recently documented interdependence between the nervous and immune systems (REICHLIN 1993). Several endorphins, enchephalins, cytokines and other mediators or receptors have biological influences on lymphocytes and neurons. Several cytokines produced and released by lymphocytes have been shown to act as trophic, growth or differentiation factors when tested on brain cells using in vitro cultures. It has also been observed repeatedly that some members of the cytokine family are synthetized by brain cells and can affect immune responses (for references see REICHLIN 1993).

It has been suggested that cytokines – produced during infections by lymphocytes, monocytes and macrophages – may affect brain cells. These effects may be even more pronounced and permanent if triggered by infections occurring during pregnancy (ADINOLFI 1993b). Such effects on the developing fetal brain could ultimately be responsible for the pathogenesis of some as yet unclassified encephalopathies, behavioural disorders and selected cases of mental retardation.

Studies of the ontogeny of acquired immunity and the demonstration that humoral and cellular immune responses start to develop during fetal life have also raised important questions about the mechanisms that protect the fetus against the immunological attack of the mother. For example, it has often been suggested that immunosuppressive factors play an major role in modulating fetal and maternal responses.

The observation that cord blood lymphocytes inhibit alloantigen and mitogen-induced proliferation (OLDING et al. 1974; LAWLER et al. 1975) suggests a possible suppressor role of the fetal cells in the maternofetal relationship. A remarkable feature of this phenomenon is that it does not seem to affect cell division of allogeneic neonatal cells (OLDING and OLDSTONE 1976; OLDING et al. 1976). If cells from male neonates and maternal lymphocytes are kept in cultures and analysed, the great majority of metaphases show a chromosome complement 46, XY (ADINOLFI 1976). However, since the existence of suppressor T cells has now been challenged (see MÖLLER 1988), it has been suggested that these in vitro observations may not reflect in vivo properties of fetal T cells (ANDERSON 1987). This topic is analysed in detail by OLDING et al., this volume.

Also controversial are claims that α-fetoprotein has immunosuppressive properties. Following two early reports by MURGITA and TOMASI (1975a,b), α-fetoprotein has been claimed to suppress fetal and maternal immune responses. Yet other studies have not confirmed the immunosuppressive effects of α-fetoprotein and have shown that this protein does not play an important role in the maternal-fetal immune interaction (ADINOLFI 1982).

There are still many areas that remain to be investigated, the most promising being those in the field of immune tolerance and the detailed analysis of the genetic mechanisms controlling the activation of the genes responsible for the synthesis of the various proteins associated with the immune responses.

References

Abo T, Cooper MD, Bach CM (1982) Postnatal expansion of the natural killer and killer cell populations in humans identified by the monoclonal NHK-1 antibody. J Exp Med 155:321–326

Adams JC, Watt FM (1993) Regulation of development and differentiation by the extracellular matrix. Development 117:1183–1198

Adinolfi M (1965) Anti-I antibodies in normal human newborn infants. Immunology 9:43–52

Adinolfi M (1972) Ontogeny of components of complement and lysozyme. Ciba Found Symp, pp 65–81

Adinolfi M (1974) The development of lymphoid tissues and immunity. In: Davis JA, Dobbing J (eds) Scientific foundation of paediatrics. Heineman, New York, pp 333–348

Adinolfi M (1976) Inhibition of mitosis of maternal lymphocytes by fetal cells. Lancet i:97

Adinolfi M (1977) Human complement: onset and site of synthesis during fetal life. Am J Dis Child 131:1015–1023

Adinolfi M (1981a) The development of lymphoid tissues and immunity. In: Davis JA, Dobbing J (eds) Scientific foundations of paediatrics. Heinemann, London, pp 525–544

Adinolfi M (1981b) Ontogeny of complement, lysozyme and lactoferrin in man. In: Lambert HP, Wood CBC (eds) Immunological aspects of infections in the fetus and newborn. Academic, London, pp 19–52

Adinolfi M (1982) Two aspects of the materno-fetal relation: the immunosuppressive role of a-fetoprotein and the transfer of lymphocytes across the placenta. In: Shulman S, Doudero F, Nicotra M (eds) Immunological factors in human reproduction, Serono symposia 45. Academic, London, pp 199–219

Adinolfi M (1988) New and old aspects of the ontogeny of immune responses. In Stern CMM (ed) Immunology of pregnancy and its disorders. Kluwer Academic, New York, pp 33–59

Adinolfi M (1993a) Ontogeny and phylogeny of complement. In: Cooper EL, Nisbet-Brown E (eds) Developmental immunology. Oxford University Press, Oxford, pp 290-314

Adinolfi M (1993b) Infectious diseases in pregnancy, cytokines and neurological impairment: an hypothesis. Dev Med Child Neurol 35:549–558

Adinolfi M, Beck S (1976) Human complement C7 and C9 in fetal and newborn sera. Arch Dis Child 50:562–564

Adinolfi M, Glynn A (1979) The interaction of antibacterial factors in breast milk. Dev Med Child Neurol 21:808–819

Adinolfi M, Lehner T (1988) C9 and factor B as acute phase proteins and their diagnostic and prognostic value in disease. Exp Clin Immunogenet 5:123–132

Adinolfi M, Wood C (1969) Ontogenesis of immunoglobulins and components of complement in man. In: Immunology and development. Spastics International Medical, London, pp 27–61

Adinolfi M, Gardner B, Wood CBS (1968) Ontogenesis of two components of human complement. β1E and β1C-1A globulins. Nature 319:189–191

Adinolfi M, Martin W, Glynn A (1971) Ontogenesis of lysozyme in man and other mammals. In: Peeters H (ed) Protides of the biological fluids. Proceedings of the 18th colloquium, Bruges, 1970. Pergamon, New York, pp 91–93

Adinolfi M, Cheetham M, Lee T, Rodin A (1988) Ontogeny of human complement receptors CR1 and CR3: expression of these molecules on motocytes and neutrophils from maternal, newborn and fetal samples. Eur J Immunol 18:565–569

Aho K, Palosuo T, Andersson M, Turunen H, Terho P, Vesikari T, Leinikki P (1987) Raised acute-phase glycoprotein and IgM levels in cord serum. Gynecol Obstet Invest 24:50–55

Alford CA Jr (1965) Studies on antibody in congenital rubella infection. I. Physico-chemical and immunologic investigation of rubella neutralizing antibody. Am J Dis Child 110:455–463

Alford CA, Schaefer J, Blankenship WJ, Straumfjord JV, Cassidy G (1967) A correlative immunologic, microbiologic and clinical approach to the diagnosis of acute and chronic infections in newborn infants. N Engl J Med 277:437–449

Alt FW, Blackwell TK, Yancopoulos GD (1987) Development of the primary antibody repertoire. Nature 328:1079–1087

Alt FW, Oltz Em, Young F, Gorman J, Taccioli G, Chen J (1992) VDJ recombination. Immunol Today 13:306–314

Andersson U (1985) Development of B lymphocyte function in childhood. Acta Paediatr Scand 74:568–573

Andersson U (1987) Regulation of antibody synthesis in the neonate. In: Burgio GR, Hayson LA, Ungazio AG (eds) Immunology of the neonate. Springer, Berlin Heidelberg New York, pp 37–50

Andersson U, Bird AG, Britton S (1981) Humoral and cellular immunity in humans studied at the cell level from birth to two years of age. Immunol Rev 57:5–37

Andre C, Heremans JF, Vaerman JP, Cambiaso CL (1975) A mechanism for the induction of immunological tolerance by antigen feeding: antigen-antibody complexes. J Exp Med 142:1509–1519

Arditi E, Nigro N (1957) Ricerche sul comportamento serico nell'immaturo. Minerva Pediatr 9:921–928

Ashton-Rickardt PG, Bandeira A, Delaney JR, Van Kaer L, Pircher H-P, Zinkernagel RM, Tonegawa S (1994) Evidence for a differential avidity model of T cell selection in the thymus. Cell 76:651–663

Barbouche R, Forveille M, Fischer A, Avrameas S, Durandy A (1992) Spontaneous IgM autoantibody production in vitro by B lymphocytes of normal human neonates. Scand J Immunol 35:659–667

Belmont JW (1995) Insights into lymphocyte development from X-linked immune deficiencies. Trends Genet 11:112–116

Bhoopat L, Taylor CR, Hofman FM (1986) The differentiation of antigens of macrophages in human fetal liver. Clin Immunol Immunopathol 41:184–192

Bianco C, Patrick R, Nussenzweig V (1970) A population of lumphocytes bearing a membrane receptor for antigen-antibody-complement complexes: I. Separation and characterization. J Exp Med 132:702–720

Bierer BE, Sleckman BP, Ratnofsky SE, Burakoff SJ (1989) The biologic roles of CD2, CD4, and CD8 in T cell activation. Annu Rev Immunol 7:579–599

Billingham RE, Brent L, Medawar PB (1953) Actively acquired tolerance of foreign cells. Nature 172:603–606

Bjorkman PJ, Perham P (1990) Structure, function and diversity of class I major histocompatibility complex molecules. Annu Rev Biochem 59:253–288

Bjorkman PJ, Saper MA, Samraoui B, Bennett WS, Strominger JL, Wiley DC (1987a) Structure of the human class I histocompatibility antigen, HLA-A2. Nature 329:506–512

Bjorkman PJ, Saper MA, Samraoui B, Bennett WS, Strominger JL, Wiley DC (1987b) The foreign antigen binding site and T cell recognition regions of class I histocompatibility antigens. Nature 329:512–518

Blackman M, Kappler J, Marrack P (1990) The role of the T cell receptor in positive and negative selection of developing T cells. Science 248:1335–1341

Blackwell KT, Alt FW (1989) Mechanism and developmental program of immunoglobulin gene rearrangement in mammals. Annu Rev Genet 23:630–636

Boyd RL, Hugo P (1991) Towards an integrated view of thymopoiesis. Immunol Today 12:71–79

Boyd RL, Tucek CL, Godfrey DI, Izon DJ, Wilson TJ, Davidson NJ, Bean AGD, Ladyman HM, Ritter MA, Hugo P (1993) The thymic microenvironment. Immunol Today 14:445–454

Brambell FWR (1966) The transmission of passive immunity from mother to young and the catabolism of immunoglobulins. Lancet ii:1087–1093

Brambell FWR (1970) The transmission of passive immunity from mother to young. North Holland, Amstardam (Frontiers of biology, vol 18)

Brenner MB, McLean J, Dialynas DP, Strominger JL, SMith JA, Owen FL, Seidman JG, Ip S, Rosen F, Krangel MS (1986) Identification of a putative second T-cell receptor. Nature 322:145–148

Brodsky FM, Guagliardi LE (1991) The cell biology of antigen processing and presentation. Annu Rev Immunol 9:707–744

Brown JH, Jardetzky TS, Gorga JC, Stern LJ, Urban RG, Strominger JL, WIley DC (1993) The three-dimensional structure of the human class II histocompatibility antigen HLA-DR1. Nature 364:33–39

Burmeister WP, Gastinel LN, Simister NE, Blum ML, Bjorkman PJ (1994) Crystal structure of 2.2 Å resolution of the MHC-related neonatal Fc receptor. Nature 372:336–343

Burnet FM (1962) The role of the thymus and related organs in immunity. Br Med J 2:807–811

Burnet FM, Fenner F (1949) The production of antibodies, 2nd edn. Macmillan, London:

Butler JL, Suzuki T, Kubagawa H, Cooper MD (1987) Humoral immunity in the human neonate. In: Burgio GR, Hanson LA, Ugazio AG (eds) The immunology of the neonate. Springer, Berlin Heidelberg New York, pp 27–36

Ceppellini R, Bonnard GD, Coppu F, Miggiano VC, Pospisil M, Curtoni ES, Pellegrino M (1971) Mixed leukocyte cultures and HL-A antigens. I. Reactivity of young foetuses, newborns and mothers at delivery. Transplant Proc 3:58–71

Chan AC, van Oers NSC, Trans A, Turka L, Law C-L, Ryan JC, Clark EA, Weiss A (1994) Differential expression of ZAP-70 and sky protein tyrosine kinases and the role of this family of protein and tyrosine kinases in TCR signalling. J Immunol 152:4758–4765

Chien J-H, Jores R (1995) T cells with B-cell-like recognition properties. Curr Biol 5:1116–1118

Chien Y, Davis MM (1993) How αβ T-cell receptors "see" peptide/MHC complexes. Immunol Today 14:597–601

Clark EA, Ledbetter JA (1994) How B and T cells talk to each other. Nature 367:425–428

Clevers H, Alarcon B, Wileman T, Terhorst C (1988) The T cell receptor/CD3 complex: a dynamic protein ensemble. Annu Rev Immunol 6:629–662

Clevers HC, Owen MJ (1991) Towards a molecular understanding of T-cell differentiation. Immunol Today 12:86–91

Clevers HC, Oosterwegel MA, Georgopoulos K (1993) Transcription factors in early T-cell development. Immunol Today 14:591–596

Colten HR (1973) Biosynthesis of the fifth component of complement (C5) by human fetal tissues. Clin Immunol Immunopathol 1:346–352

Colten HR (1976) Biosynthesis of complement. Adv Immunol 22:67–118

Conley ME (1994) X-linked immunodeficiencies. Curr Opin Genet Dev 4:401–406

Cooper NR, Moore MD, Nemerow GR (1988) Immunology of CR2, the lymphocyte receptor for Epstein-Barr virus and the C3d complement fragment. Annu Rev Immunol 6:85–113

Cowan JM, Ammann AJ, Wara DW, Howie VM, Schultz L, Doyle N, Kaplan M (1978) Pneumococcal polysaccharide immunization in infants and children. Pediatrics 62:721–727

Crabtree GR (1989) Contingent genetic regulatory events in T lymphocyte activation. Science 243:355–360
Crome P, Moffatt B, Adinolfi M (1971) HLA-antigens in human foetuses. In: Peeters H (ed) Protides of the biological fluids.Proceedings of the 18th colloquium, Bruges, 1970. Pergamon, New York, pp 55–61
De Muralt G (1962) La maturation des immuno-globulines chez l'homme. Vox Sang 7:513–525
Desiderio SV (1993) Organization and assembly of immunoglobulin genes. In: Cooper EL, Nisbet-Brown E (eds) Developmental immunology. Oxford University Press, Oxford, pp 129–152
Dobson NJ, Lambris JD, Ross GD (1981) Characteristics of isolated erythrocyte complement receptor type one (CR1, C4b-C3b receptor) and CR1 specific antibodies. J Immunol 126:693–698
du Pan RM, Wenger P, Koechli S, Scheidegger JJ, Roux T (1959) Etude de passage de la γ-globuline marqueé à travers le placenta humain. Clin Chim Acta 4:110–115
Eddy EM, Clark JM, Gong D, Fenderson BA (1981) Origin and migration of primordial germ cells in mammals. Gamete Res 4:333–362
Epstein WV (1965) Specificity of macroglobulin antibody synthesised by the normal human fetus. Science 148:1591–1592
Fearon DT, Wong WW (1983) Complement ligand-receptor interactions that madiate biological responses. Annu Rev Immunol 1:243–271
Fedra VJ (1962) Placental transfer of antibodies in man. Am J Obstet Gynecol 84:1756–1760
Fireman P, Zuchowski DA, Taylor PM (1969) Development of human complement system. J Immunol 103:25–31
Fishel CW, Pearlman DS (1961) Complement components of paired mother-cord sera. Proc Soc Exp Biol Med 107:695–699
Fowlkes BJ, Pardoll DM (1989) Molecular and cellular events of T cell development. Adv Immunol 44:207–264
Gardner B, Adinolfi M (1968) Serological and physicochemical characteristics of antibodies against Listeria monocytogenes in normal human sera. Guys Hosp Rep 117:19–30
Gascoigne NRJ, Chien Y, Becker DM, Kavaler J, Davis MM (1984) Genomic organization and sequence of T-cell receptor β-chain constant and joining-region genes. Nature 310:387–391
Germain RN (1994) MHC-dependent antigen processing and peptide presentation: providing ligands for T lymphocyte activation. Cell 76:287–299
Germain RN, Margulies DH (1993) The biochemistry and cell biology of antigen processing and presentation. Annu Rev Immunol 11:403–450
Gitlin D (1974) Protein transport across the placenta and protein turnover between amniotic fluid, maternal and fetal circulations. In: Moghissi KS, Hatze ESE (eds) The placenta: biological and clinical aspects. Thomas, Springfield, pp 151–191
Gitlin D, Kumate J, Urrusti J, Morlaes C (1964) The selectivity of the human placenta in the transfer of plasma proteins from mother to fetus. J Clin Invest 43:1938–1951
Glynn AA, Martin W, Adinolfi M (1970) Levels of lysozyme in human foetuses and newborns. Nature 225:77–78
Godfrey DI, Zlotnik A (1993) Control points in early T-cell development. Immunol Today 14:547–553
Goodnow CC, Adelstein S, Basten A (1990) The need for central and peripheral tolerance in the B cell repertoire. Science 248:1373–1379
Goodnow CC, Brink R, Adams E (1991) Breakdown of selftolerance in anergic B lymphocytes. Nature 352:532–536
Griffiths-Chu S, Patterson JAK, Berger CL, Edelson RC, Chu AC (1984) Characterization of immature T cell subpopulations in neonatal blood. Blood 64:296–300
Groettrub M, Ungewiss K, Azogni O, Palacios R, Owen MY, Hayday AC, von Boehmes H (1993) A novel disulfide-linked heterodimer on pre-T-cells consists of the T cell receptor β chain and 33 kd glycoprotein. Cell 75:283–294
Grubb R, Laurell AB (1956) Hereditary serological human serum groups. Acta Pathol Microbiol Scand 39:390–398
Hamet I, Erkeller-Tuksel F, Lydyard P, Deneys V, DeBruyere M (1992) Developmental and maturational changes in human blood lymphocyte populations. Immunol Today 13:215–218
Hammar JA (1921) The new views as to the morphology of the thymus gland and their bearing on the problem of the function of the thymus. Endocrinology 5:543, 731
Hammer JA (1936) Die normal-morphologische Thymus-forschung imletzten Vierteljahrhundert. Barth, Leipzig

Hanson LA, Adlerberth I, Carlsson B, Dahlgren U, Jalil F, Khan SR, Zaman S, Larsson P, Mellander L, Sheikh AK, Soderstrom T, Wold AES (1987) The ontogeny of the immune response: the role of maternal factors. In: Burgio GR, Hanson LA, Ugazio AG (eds) The immunology of th neonate. Springer, Berlin Heidelberg New York, pp 51–58

Harris DT, Schumacher MJ, Locascio J, Besencon FJ, Olson GB, DeLuca D, Shenker L, Bard J, Boyse EA (1982) Phenotypic and functional immaturity of human unbilical cord blood lymphocytes. Proc Natl Acad Sci USA 89:10006–10010

Hasek M, Leugerova A, Vojtiskova M (1961) Mechanisms of immunological tolerance. Proceedings of the Prague Symposium, 8–10 Nov 1961. Academic, London

Haynes BF (1984) The human thymic microenvironment. Adv Immunol 36:87–142

Haynes BF, Martin ME, Kay HH, Kurtzberg J (1988) Early events in human T cell ontogeny: phenotypic characterization and immunohistologic localization of T cell precursors in early human fetal tissues. J Exp Med 168:1061–1080

Haynes BF, Denning SM, Singer KH, Kurtzberg J (1989) Ontogeny of T-cell precursors: a model for the initial stages of human T-cell development. Immunol Today 10:87–91

Hemmings WA, Williams EW (1976) The attachment of IgG to cell components of the transporting membrances. In: Hemmings WA (ed) Materno foetal transmission of immunoglobulins. Clinical and experimental immunoreproduction, vol 2. Cambridge University Press, Cambridge, pp 91–111

Hill A, Ploegh H (1995) Getting the inside out: the transporter associated with antigen processing (TAP) and the presentation of viral antigen. Proc Natl Acad Sci USA 92:341–343

Hitzig WH (1959) Über die transplacentare Übertragung von Antikörper. Schweiz Med Wochenschr 89:1249–53

Hofman FM, Danilovs JA, Taylor CB (1984) HLA-DR (Ia)-positive dendritic-like cells in human fetal nonlymphoid tissues Transplantation 37:590–594

Honjo T (1993) Immunoglobulin genes. Annu Rev Immunol 1:499–528

Hood L, Kronenberg M, Hunkapiller T (1985) T cell antigen receptors and the immunoglobulin supergene family. Cell 40:225–229

Hugo P, Kappler JW, Marrack PC (1993) Positive selection of TCR αβ thymocytes: is cortical thymic epithelium an obligatory participant in the presentation of major histocompatibility complex protein? Immunol Rev 135:133–155

Hyde RR (1932) The complement deficient guinea pig: a study of an inheritable factor in immunity. Am J Hyg 15:824–836

Ito K, Bonneville M, Takagaki Y, Nekanishi N, Kanagawa O, Kucko EG, Tonegawa S (1989) Different T-cell receptors are expressed on thymocytes at different stages of development. Proc Natl Acad Sci USA 86. 631–635

Janeway CA (1992) The T cell receptor as a multicomponent signalling machine: CD4/CD8 coreceptors and CD45 in T cell activation. Annu Rev Immunol 10:645–674

Janeway CA, Bottomly K (1994) Signals and signs for lymphocyte responses. Cell 76:275–285

Jenkinson EJ, Billington WD, Elson J (1976) Detection of receptors for immunoglobulin on human placenta by EA rosette formation. Clin Exp Immunol 23:456–461

Jorgensen JL, Reay PA, Ehrich EW, Davis MM (1992) Molecular components of T cell recognition. Annu Rev Immunol 10:835–873

Kansas GS, Dailey MO (1989) Expression of adhesion structures during B-cell development in man. J Immunol 142:3058–3062

Kaufman J (1993) Ontogeny and phylogeny of MHC molecules. In: Cooper EL, Nisbet-Brown E (eds) Developmental immunology. Oxford University Press, Oxford, pp 53–84

Kearse KP, Roberts JD, Wiest CL, Singer A (1995) Developmental regulation of αβ T cell antigen receptor assembly in immature CD4+CD8+ thymocytes. Bioessays 17:1049–1054

Kincade PW (1993) Cell adhesion mechanisms utilized for lymphoporesis. In: Shimizu (ed) Lymphocyte adhesion molecuses. Texas: Landes, Austin, pp 249–279

Klein J (ed) (1986) Natural history of the major histocompatibility complex. Wiley, New York

Klockars M, Reitamo S, Adinolfi M (1977) Ontogeny of human lysozyme. Distribution in fetal tissues. Biol Neonate 37:243–249

Kronenberg M, Brines R (1993) Developmental control of T cell antigen receptor gene rearrangement and expression. In: Cooper EL, Nisbet-Brown E (eds) Developmental immunology. Oxford university Press, Oxford, pp 153–173

Kuchroo VK, Das MP, Brown JA, Ranger AM, Zamkl SS, Sobel RA, Weiner HL, Kobari N, Glimcher LH (1995) B7-1 and B7-2 costimulatory molecules activate differentially the Th1/Th2 developmental pathways: application to autoimmune disease therapy. Cell 80:707–718

Kudo A, Melchers F (1987) A second gene, Vpre-B in the γ5 locus of the mouse which appears to be selectivley expressed in pre-B lymphocytes. EMBO J 6:2267–2272
Lanier LL, Le AM, Cirin CI, Loken MR, Phillips JH (1986) The relationship of CD16 (Leu-ii) and Leu-19 (NHK-1) antigen expression on human peripheral blood NK cells and cytotoxic T lymphocytes. J Immunol 136:4480–4485
Lanzavecchia A (1985) Antigen-specific interaction between T and B cells. Nature 314:537–539
Lanzavecchia A (1988) Clonal sketches of the immune response. EMBO J 7:2945–2951
Lassila O (1981) Embryonic differentiation of lymphoid stem cells. Dev Comp Immunol 5:403–414
Lawler SD, Ukaljiofa EO, Reeves BR (1975) Interaction of maternal and neonates cells in mixed lymphocyte culture. Lancet ii:1185–1187
Lederberg J (1959) Genes and antibodies: do antigens bear instructions for antibody specificity or do they select cell lines that arise by mutation? Science 129:1649–1653
LeDouarin NM, Jotereau FV (1975) Tracing of cells of the avain thymus through embryonic life in interspecific chimeras. J Exp Med 142:17–40
Lee CYG, Hwang LY, Beesly RP, Chen SH, Lee TY (1983) Immunogenicity of hepatitis B virus vaccine in healthy Chinese infants. J Infect Dis 148:526–529
Levinson AI, Dalal NF, Haidar M, Tar L, Orlow M (1987) Prominent IgM rheumatoid factor production by human cord blood lymphocytes stimulated in vitro with Staphyloccus aureus cowan I. J Immunol 139:2237–2241
Lewis SM (1994) The mechanisms of V(D)J rejoining: lessons from molecular, immunological, and comparative analysis. Adv Immunol 56:27–149
Lieber MR (1992) The mechanism of V(D)J recombination: a balance of diversity, specificity, and stability. Cell 70:873–876
Lin W-C, Desiderio S (1993) Regulations of V(D)J recombination activator protein RAG-2 by phosphorylation. Science 260:953–959
Linnet-Jepsen P, Galatius-Jensen F, Hauge M (1958) On the inheritance of Gm serum group. Acta Genet 8:164–196
Lo D, Sprent J (1986) Identity of cells that imprint H-2 restricted T cell specificity in the thymus. Nature 319:672–675
Lydyard PM, Quartey-Papafio R, Broker B, MacKenzie L, Jonquan J, Blaschek MA, Steele J, Petrou M, Collins P, Isenberg D, Youinou PY (1990) The antibody repertorire in early human B cells. Scand J Immunol 31:33–43
Maccario R, Burgio GR (1987) T and NK lymphocyte subpopulations in the neonate. In: Burgio GR, Hanson LA, Ugazio AG (eds) The immunology of the neonate. Springer, Berlin Heidelberg New York, pp 120–129
Marrack P, Kappler J (1987) The T cell receptor. Science 238:1073–1087
Marrack P, Kappler JW (1983) How the immune system recognizes the body. Science 222:49–55
Marx J (1995) The T cell receptor begins to reveal its many facets. Science 267:459–460
Matre R, Tonder O, Endresen C (1975) Fc receptors in human placenta. Scand J Immunol 4:741–745
McCracken GH, Shinefield HR (1965) Immunoglobulin concentrations in newborn infants with congenital cytomegalic inclusion disease. Pediatrics 36:933–937
McVay LD, Carding SR, Bottomly K, Haydoy AC (1991) Regulated expression and structure of T cell receptor γ/δ transcripts in human thymic ontogeny. EMBO J 1:83–91
Medivinsky A, Dzierzak E (1996) Definitive haematopoiesis is autonomously initiated by the AMG region. Cell 86:897–906
Miceli MC, Parnes JR (1993) Role of CD4 and CD8 in T cell activation and differentiation. Adv Immunol 53:59–122
Miller JFAP (1961a) Analysis of the thymus influence in leukaemogenesis. Nature 191:248–249
Miller JFAP (1961b) Immunological function of the thymus. Lancet ii:748–749
Miller JFAP (1994) The thymus: maestro of the immune system. Bioessays 16:509–513
Miller JFAP, Morahan G (1992) Peripheral T cell tolerance. Anna Rev Immunol 10:51–70
Miyakawa Y, Yamada A, Kosaka K, Tsuda F, Mayumi M (1981) Defective immune-adhernce (C3b) receptor on erythrocytes from patients with systemic lupus erythematosus. Lancet ii:494–497
Möller G (1988) Do suppressor T cells exist? Scand J Immunol 27:247–250
Mollison PL (1951) Blood transfusion in clinical medicine. Blackwell, Oxford:
Mombaerts P, Iacomini J, Johnson RS, Herrup K, Tonegawa S, Papaiannou VE (1992) RAG-1-deficient mice have no mature B and T lymphocytes. Cell 68:869–877
Moore MAS, Metcalf D (1970) Ontogeny of the haemopoietic system: yolk sac origin of *in vivo* and *in vitro* colony forming cells in the developing mouse embryo. Br J Haematol 18:279–296

Moore MAS, Owen JJT (1967) Experimental studies on the development of the thymus. J Exp Med 126:715–726
Mossman TR, Cottman RL (1989) Th 1 and Th 2 cells: different patterns of lymphokine secretion lead to different functional properties. Annu Rev Immunol 7:145–173
Müller-Eberhard HJ (1975) The complement system. In: Putnam FW (ed) The plasma proteins, vol 1. Academic, New York, pp 394–432
Müller-Eberhard HJ (1986) The membrane attack complex of complement. Annu Rev Immunol 4:503–528
Murgita RA, Tomasi TB (1975a) Suppression of the immune response by a-fetoprotein. I. The effect of mouse a-fetoprotein on the primary and secondary antibody responses. J Exp Med 141:269–286
Murgita RA, Tomasi TB (1975b) Suppression of the immune response by a-fetoprotein. II. The effect of mouse a-fetoprotein on mixed lymphocyte activity and mitogen-induced lymphocyte transformation. J Exp Med 141:440–452
Nikolic-Zugic J, Bevan M (1990) Role of Self-peptides in positively selecting the T cell repertoire. Nature 344:65–67
Nossal GJV (1983) Cellular mechanisms of immunological tolerance. Annu Rev Immunol 1:33–62
Nossal GJV (1994) Negative selection of lymphocytes. Cell 76:229–239
Nossal GJV, Pike BL (1980) Clonal anergy: persistence in tolerance mice of antigen-binding B lymphocytes incapable of responding to antigen or mitogen. Proc Natl Acad Sci USA 77:1602–1608
Oettinger MA (1992) Activation of V(D)J recombination by RAG1 and RAG2. TIG 8:413–416
Oettinger MA, Schatz DG, Gorka C, Baltimore D (1990) RAG-1 and RAG-2, adjacent genes that synergistically activate V(D)J recombination. Science 248:1517–1523
Olding LB, Oldstone MBA (1976) Thymus-derived peripheral lymphocytes from human newborns inhibit division of their mother's lymphocytes. J Immunol 116:682–686
Olding LB, Bernishke K, Oldstone MBA (1974) Inhibition of mitosis of lymphocytes from human adults by lymphocytes from human newborns. Clin Immunol Immunopathol 3:79–84
Osler AG, Sandberg AL (1973) Alternate complement pathways. Prog Allergy 17:51–92
Owen JJT, Jenkinson EJ (1981) Embryology of the lymphoid system. Prog Allergy 29:1–34
Owen MJ (1993) T-cell differentiation under control. Curr Biol 3:780–782
Owen MJ, Crumpton MJ (1987) The role of class I and II antigens in T cell recognition. Br Med Bull 43:228–240
Owen RD (1945) Immunological consequences of vascular anastomoses between bovine twins. Science 102:400–401
Parker DC (1993) T cell-dependent B-cell activation. Annu Rev Immunol 11:331–360
Paul WE, Seder RA (1994) Lymphocyte responses and cytokines. Cell 76:241–251
Phillips JH, Hori T, Nagler A, Bhat N, Spits H, Lanier LL (1992) Ontogeny of human natural killer (NK) cells: fetal NK cells mediate cytolytic function and express cytoplasmic CD3E, εδ proteins. J Exp Med 175:1055–1066
Porcile V (1904) Untersuchungen über der Herkunft der Plasmazellen in der Leber. Beitr Pathol Anat 36:375–381
Propp RP, Alper CA (1968) C3 synthesis in the human fetus and lack of transplacental passage. Science 162:672–673
Pullen AM, Marrack P, Kappler JW (1988) The T-cell repertoire is heavily influenced by tolerance to polymorphic self-antigens. Nature 355:796–801
Pund ER, Von Haam E (1957) Spirochetal and venereal disease. In Anderson WAD (ed) Pathology. Mosby, St Louis, pp 264–266
Racadot E (1993) Cord-blood lymphocyte population. Immunol Today 14:189–190
Rammensee H-G, Falk K, Rötzschke O (1993) Peptides naturally presented by MHC class I molecules. Annu Rev Immunol 11:213–244
Raulet DH, Garman RD, Saito H, Tonegawa S (1985) Developmental regulation of T-cell receptor gene expression. Nature 314:103–107
Ravetch JV, Kinet J-P (1991) Fc receptors. Annu Rev Immunol 9:457–492
Ravetch JV, Margulies DH (1994) New tricks for old molecules. Nature 372:323–324
Reichlin S (1993) Neuroendocrine-immune interactions. N Engl J Med 329:1246–1253
Remington JS, Miller MJ (1966) 19S and 7S antitoxoplasma antibodies in the diagnosis of acute congenital and acquired toxoplasmosis. Proc Soc Exp Biol 121:357–363
Ritter MA, Boyd RL (1993) Development in the thymus: it takes two to tango. Immunol Today 14:462–469

Rocha B, Vassalli P, Guy-Grand D (1992) The extrathymic T-cell development pathway. Immunol Today 13:449–453
Rolink A, Melchers F (1991) Molecular and cellular origins of B lymphocyte diversity. Cell 66:1081–1094
Romagnani S (1989) Cytokines involved in activation, growth and differentiation of human B cells. J Immunol Res 1:41–51
Romagnani S, Del Prete GF, Maggi E, Falagiani P, Ricci M (1980) T-cell independence of immunoglobulin synthesis by human peripheral blood lymphocytes stimulated with SpA-containing staphylococci. Immunology 41:921–927
Rosen FS, Cooper MD, Wedgwood RIP (1995) The primary immunodeficiencies. N Engl J Med 7:431–440
Rosenthal P, Rimm IJ, Umiel T, Griffin JD, Osathanondh R, Schlossman SF, Nadler LM (1983) Ontogeny of human hematopoietic cells: analysis utilizing monoclonal antibodies. J Immunol 131:323–327
Ross GD, Atkinson JP (1985) Complement receptor structure and function. Immunol Today 6:115–119
Roth PE, DeFranco AL (1995) Intrinsic checkpoints for lineage progression. Curr Biol 5:349–352
Rother K, Rother U (1986) Biological functions of the complement system. Prog Allergy 39:24–100
Ruiz P, Schwarzler C, Gunthert U (1995) CD44 isoforms during differentiation and development. Bioessays 17:17–24
Ruuskanen O, Pittard WB, Miller K, Pierce G, Sorensen RU, Polmar SH (1980) Staphylococcus aureus cowan I-induced immunoglobulin production in human cord blood lymphocytes. J Immunol 125:411–413
Sakaguchi N, Melchers F (1986) γ5, a new light chain-related locus selectively expressed in pre-B lymphocytes. Nature 324:579–582
Sansoremo W (1995) A review of the mechanisms of oral tolerance and immunotheraphy. J R Soc Med 88:14–17
Sawyer MK, Forman MJ, Kuplic L, Stiehm ER (1971) Developmental aspects of the human complement system. Biol Neonate 19:148–162
Schwartz RH (1985) T-lymphocyte recognition of antigen in association with gene products of the major histocompatibility complex. Annu Rev Immunol 3:237–261
Schwartz RH (1989) Acquisition of immunological self-tolerance. Cell 57:1073–1081
Shimuzu A, Honjo T (1984) Immunoglobulin class switching. Cell 36:801–803
Shinkai Y, Rathbun G, Lam K-P, Oltz EM, Stewart V, Mendelsohn M, Charron J, Datta M, Young F, Stall AM, Alt FW (1992) RAG-2-deficient mice lack mature lymphocytes owing to inability to initiate V(D)J rearrangements. Cell 68:855–867
Silverstein AM (1964) Ontogeny of immune response. Science 144:1423–1425
Silverstein AM, Lukes RJ (1962) Fetal response to antigenic stimulus. I. Plasma-cellular and lymphoid reactions in human fetus to intrauterine infection. Lab Invest 11:918–932
Smith RT, Eitzman DV, Catlin MC, Wirtz OE, Miller BE (1964) The development of the immune response. Characterization of the response of the human infant and adult to immunization with Salmonella vaccines. Pediatrics 68:163–183
Smith LG, Weissman IL, Heimfeld S (1991) Clonal analysis of haemotopoietic stem cell differentiation in vivo. Proc Natl Acad Sci USA 88:2788–2792
Soothill JF, Hayes K, Dudgeon JA (1966) The immunoglobulins in congenital rubella. Lancet i:1385–1386
Sottzup-Jensen L, Stepanik TM, Kristensen T et al (1985) Common evolutionary origin of a_2-macroglobulin and complement C3 and C4. Proc Natl Acad Sci USA 82:9–13
Sprent J (1995) Professional and amateurs. Curr Biol 5:1095–1097
Sprent J, Loh D, Gao EK, Rpn Y (1988) T cell selection in the thymus. Immunol Rev 101:173–190
Sprent J, Gao E-K, Webb SR (1990) T cell reactivity to MHC molecules:immunity versus tolerance. Science 248:1357–1363
Steinman RM (1991) The dendritic cell system and its role in immunogenecity. Annu Rev Immunol 9:271–296
Stiehm ER, Amnann AJ, Cherry JD (1966) Elevated cord macroglobulins in the diagnosis of intrauterine infections. N Engl J Med 275:971–977
Sties DP, Fudenberg HH (1974) Ontogeny of cellular immunity in the human fetus. Development of responses ot phytohemagglutinin and to allogeneic cells. Cell Immunol 11:257–271
Story CM, Mikulska JE, Simister NE (1994) A major histocompatibility complex class I-like Fc receptor cloned from human placenta: possible role in transfer of immunoglobulin G from mother to fetus. J Exp Med 180:2377–2381

Strachan T (1987) Molecular genetics and polymorphism of class I HLA antigens. Br Med Bull 43:1–14
Strominger JL (1987) Structure of class I and class II HLA antigens. Br Med Bull 43:81–93
Stutman O (1985) Ontogeny of T cells. Clin Immunol Allergy 5:191–234
Stutman O (1987) T-cell development. In: Burgio GR, Hason LA, Ugazio AG (eds) The immunology of the neonate. Springer, Berlin Heidelberg New York, pp 5–26
Swain SL (1995) who does the polarizing? Curr Biol 5:849–851
Talmage DW (1969) The nature of the immunological response. In: Adinolfi M (ed) Immunology and development. Spastics International Medical Publications, London, pp 1–26
Tedder TF, Fearon DT, Garland GL, Cooper MD (1983) Expression of C3b receptors on human B cells and myelomonocytic cells but not natural killer cells. J Immunol 130:1688–1673
Teh H-S, Kisielow P, Scott B, Kishi H, Uematsu Y, Blutmann H, von Boehmer H (1988) Thymic MHC antigens and the αβ T cell receptor determine the CD4/CD8 phenotype of T cells. Nature 335:229–233
Tenner AJ, Cooper NR (1981) Identification of types of cells in human peripheral blood that blind Clq. J Immunol 126:1174–1179
Thorbecke GJ, Hochwald GM, van Furth R, Müller-Eberhard HJ, Jacobsent ER (1965) Problems in determining the sites of synthesis of complement reactions. Ciba Found Symp, pp 99–114
Toivanen P, Uksila J, Leino A, Lassila O, Hirvonen T, Ruuskanen O (1981) Development of mitogen responding T cells and natural killer cells in the human fetus. Immunol Rev 57:89–105
Tonegawa S (1983) Somatic generation of antibody diversity. Nature 302:575–581
Tonegawa S, Berns A, Bonneville M, Farr A, Ishida I, Ito K, Itohara S, Janeway CA, Kanagawa O, Katsuki M, Kubo R, Lafaille J, Mombaerts P, Murphy D, Nakanishi N, Takagaki Y, Van Kaer L, Berbeek S (1989) Diversity, development, ligands, and probable functions of γδ T cells. Cold Spring Harb Symp Quant Biol LIV:31–44
Townsend A, Bodmer H (1989) Antigen recognition by class I restricted T lymphocytes. Annu Rev Immunol 7:601–624
Townsend AR, Gotch FM, Davey J (1985) Cytotoxic T cells recognize fragments of the influenza nucleoprotein. Cell 42:457–467
Traub M (1943) The complement activity of the serum of healthy persons, mothers and newborn infants. J Pathol Bacterial 55:447–452
Travers P (1990) One hand clapping. Nature 348:393–394
Travers P (1993) Immunological agnosia. Nature 363:117–118
Trevorrow VE (1959) Concentration of gamma-globulin in the serum of infants during the first 3 months of life. Paediatrics 24:746–751
Trinchieri G (1989) Biology of natural killer cells. Adv Immunol 47:187–376
Trowsdale J (1987) Genetics and polymorphism: class II antigens. Br Med Bull 43:15–36
Unanue ER (1984) Antigen-presenting function of the macrophage. Annu Rev Immunol 2:395–428
Vahlquist B (1958) The transfer of antibodies from mother to offspring. Adv Pediatr 10:305–325
van Furth R, Schuit HRE, Hijmans W (1965) The immunological development of the human fetus. J Exp Med 122:1173–1188
von Boehmer H (1992) Thymic selection: a matter of life and death. Immunol Today 13:454–458
von Boehmer H (1994) Positive selection of lymphocytes. Cell 76:219–228
Wade WF, Davoust Y, Salemero J, André P, Watts TH, Combier J-C (1993) Structural compartmentalisation of MHC class II signaling function. Immunol Today 14:539–546
Wasserman P, Alberts E (1940) Complement titre of blood of the newborn. Proc Soc Exp Biol Med 45:563–564
Weiss A (1991) Molecular and genetic insights into T cell antigen receptor structure and function. Annu Rev Genet 25:487–510
Weiss A, Bogen B (1991) MHC class II-restricted presentation of interacellular antigen. Cell 64:767–776
Weiss A, Littman DR (1994) Signal transduction by lymphocyte antigen receptors. Cell 76:263–274
Weissman IL (1994) Developmental switches in the immune system. Cell 76:207–218
Wild AE (1973) Transport of immunoglobulins and other proteins from mother to young. In: Dingle JT (ed) Lysosomes in biology and pathology. University of Chicago press, Chicago, pp 495–514
Wild AE (1975) Role of the cell surface in selection during transport of proteins from mother to foetus and newly born. Phil Trans R Soc Lond 271B:395–410
Wild AE (1981) Endocytic mechanisms in protein transfer across the placenta. Placenta [Suppl] 1:165–186
Williams AF, Barclay AN (1988) The immunoglobulin superfamily: domains for cell surface recognition. Annu Rev Immunol 6:381–405
Wilson JG, Wong WW, Schur PH, Fearon DT (1982) Mode of inheritance of decreased c3b receptors on erythrocytes of patients with systemic lupus erythematosus. N Engl J Med 307:981–986

Wu L, Kincade PW, Shortman K (1993) The CD44 expressed on the earliest intrathymic precursor population functions as a thymus homing molecule but does not bind to hyaluronate. Immunol Lett 38:69–75

Ziegler K, Unanue ER (1981) Identification of a macrophage antigen-processing event required for I-region-restricted antigen presentation to T-lymphcytes. J Immunol 127:1869–1875

Zinkernagel RM, Doherty PC (1974) Restriction of ; in vitro T cell medicated cytotoxicity in lymphocytic choriomeningitis within a syngeneic or semi-allogenic system. Nature 248:701–702

Zinkernagel RM, Callahan G, Althage A, Cooper S, Klein P, Klein J (1978) On the thymus in the differentiation of H-2 self-recognition by T cells: evidence for dual recognition. J Exp Med 147:882–896

Maternal T Cell Reactivity in Pregnancy?

G. CHAOUAT and E. MENU

1 Introduction: An Allograft?

This review deals with maternal T cell reactivity in pregnancy. Since other chapters consider recurrent spontaneous abortion in human, we focus (very briefly) only on data in such situations when they cast light on maternal T cell status in normal human pregnancy. It is necessary, however, to deal with abortion models in mice since these are models for study of T cell reactivity during gestation.

Since Peter Medawar's original proposition that there are indeed some "immunological and endocrinological problems raised by the evolution of viviparity in vertebrates," the fetus has been viewed as "nature's allograft" (MEDAWAR 1953). Therefore viviparity has been viewed by most as an immunological paradox. Indeed, it appears as a semiallogenic graft, and even in cases of oocyte and semen donation and embryo transfer in humans and animals, respectively, it is a fully allogeneic or even xenogeneic graft since in some species, such as the horse, fully xenogeneic pregnancies have been achieved with few, or even no immunomanip-

Bâtiment de Gynécologie/Obstétrique, Hôpital Antoine Béclère. Avenue de la Porte de Trivaux, Clamart 92140, France

ulation. [ALLEN et al. (1986) have successfully transferred zebra embryos into mares and horse embryos in donkeys and obtained fully xenogeneic live offspring.]

The placenta expresses paternally derived histocompatibility antigens in cells in contact with maternal blood in many types of placentation. It should be recalled that anatomical and histological variations exist between the placentation in rodent, equine, porcine, and primate species which render the "maternal exposure" different in each species. This exposure often results in a confrontation between maternal immune cells at recognition and effector stages in the decidua with paternal alloantigens expressed on the placenta. In no species do the trophoblast layers express class I alloantigens, and it has been postulated that this is an important feature of pregnancy success. Indeed, expression of class II on trophoblasts induced by azacytidine resulted in regular abortion in mice (ATHANASSAKIS VASSILIADIS and PAPAMETTHEAKIS 1991). According to the authors, this finding has been extended to humans by examination of products of spontaneous early abortion (ATHANASSAKIS et al., personal communication, 1996), but controversy exists since these findings are not seen in rats (GILL, personal communication, 1995).

Unfortunately, no study has been conducted on the consequences of such class II antigen expression on maternal T cell status in vivo. It has only been shown that whereas, as described by many, normal placental cells are relatively poor stimulator cells in a mixed lymphocyte reaction, trophoblast obtained from azacytidine-treated mice are efficient stimulators of a mixed lymphocyte reaction, as assessed by an efficient [^{3}H]thymidine incorporation (JENKINSON and OWEN 1980). No studies, however, have been carried out to ascertain the effect of azacytidine on the secretion of placental suppressor factors, and a facile alternative explanation to the findings is that azacytidine merely interferes with the pathway leading to the production of such important immunoregulators.

Regarding class I expression, polymorphic MHC alloantigens are expressed on porcine, equine, and rodent trophoblast. For example, in mice convincing experiments have rather surprisingly demonstrated that while the labyrinth does not express MHC antigens (as expected from cells which would interface an antigenically neutral barrier between the mother and the fetus), the outer layer of the placenta, the spongiotrophoblast, does express (as do the annexes) MHC class I (H-2 K, D, L in mice) in detectable amounts. The material can be detected at membrane level in situ or on isolated trophoblasts, and proper mRNA transcripts are readily detectable. These class I MHCs are in direct contact with maternal circulation and are accessible to monoclonal antibodies of the relevant antipaternal specificity, quickly degraded once bound to the placenta in smaller peptidic fragments. This has been called the paternal strain immunoadsorbant status of the placenta (JENKINSON and OWEN 1980; SINGH et al. 1983; REDLINE and LU 1990; CHATTERGEE-HASROUNI and LALA 1982; WEGMANN et al. 1979b).

In the rat the same is true: spongiotrophoblast expresses class I MHC, the RT1a antigens, and monomorphic MHC antigens, termed Pa1 and Pa2 (allelic forms), are expressed on the rat placenta. Evidence obtained by elegant embryo transfer experiments show that their expression is under the influence of genomic imprinting, biased only towards repression of MHC expression of maternally derived class I (BILLINGTON et BURROWS 1986; KANBOUR et al. 1987; KANBOUR-SHARIR et al. 1990). This implies that maternal immune cells are confronted with cells of foreign MHC haplotype and should react to them. It is the basis of the allograft paradox that this is often associated with allopregnancy.

In man, no polymorphic MHC antigens are expressed on the trophoblasts, and class I expression is restricted to HLA-G (ELLIS et al. 1986; KOVATTS et al. 1990, 1991; ELLIS 1990). Whereas a certain degree of diversity may exist among some HLA-G molecules (KOVATTS et al. 1991; VAN DER VEN and OBER 1993; LOKE, personal communication), the current, albeit fragile, consensus – challenged by such emerging notion that there is some polymorphism in HLA-G as well as HLA-C expression is that trophoblasts in humans offer an antigenically neutral barrier, apparently minimizing the paradox of the "allo" graft.

However, as stated above, in most species the placenta is not at all a neutral barrier, and the alloantigens are expressed in such species such as mice and rats "as if" purposely to confront the maternal immune system. Furthermore, supporters of the barrier theory forget that even in humans there are other types of confrontation between maternal immune cells and fetal cells. First, trophoblast cells migrate regularly into maternal blood and are detectable in mice and humans, where their presence, although not sufficiently reproducible for routine prenatal diagnosis, has been ascertained by various techniques (FACS, isolation on Percoll gradients, separation via magnetic beads, etc.). These cells are of course MHC class II negative, but some are weakly HLA class I positive, possibly as a result of differentiation, as observed by some workers in vitro, although most do express HLA-G. (HLA-G has been used to sort them from maternal blood; this process is now patented; SOCIÉ et al., personal communication.)

More importantly, however, fetal nucleated erythrocytes, which express classical polymorphic class I MHC antigens, are detected and have been sorted (HERZENBERG et al. 1979; BRUCH et al. 1991; SCHRODER 1975; DOUGLAS et al. 1959; BIANCHI et al. 1990, 1991, 1992, 1993). Erythroid-specific antibodies enhance detection of fetal nucleated erythrocytes in maternal blood.

Comparison of the situation with existing induced alloimmunization schedules, therefore leads to the concept that even in the case of a "neutral trophoblast" barrier such as in humans and primates the maternal immune system is in a situation resembling repeated microtransfusions at minimal exposure to only a class I disparate allograft in most cases. This situation offers a unique case to study T cell reactivity in a "physiological" allogeneic challenge.

2 General Overview of the Problem

Unfortunately, very few such studies have been conducted, and this review is therefore brief and sometimes influenced by the lack of appropriate controls. Such a situation is regretable when one considers what is known from artificial alloimmunization studies. In particular, very little is known about modifications, expansions and repression of the T cell repertoire as such, and hence this review centers on T cell reactivity during pregnancy.

The reasons for such a bias are numerous. First, emphasis has been placed on local suppression by well-defined experiments that have confirmed positive or negative regulation of peripheral T cells to have probably no crucial effect on pregnancy. The fetus survives and thrives in a T cell depleted host, such as the nude mouse and T cell depleted normal animals. As considered below, only placental weight, fetal weight, and the number of implants are decreased. These have lead to a semiconfirmation of the immunotrophic theory (Ahanassakis et al. 1991; Wegmann et al. 1991, 1993a; Wegmann 1984).The second reason is that the fetus survives and even thrives better in either a forcibly alloimmunized host or in a suppressor cytotoxic T cell depleted host (Mitchison 1953; Lanman et al. 1962; Monnot and Chaouat 1984; Mattison and Holmdal 1987; Beer et al. 1975). Since the initial studies were conducted to test the concept that T cell suppression is important in the maintenance of pregnancy, emphasis was placed on local, nonspecific, placental, or decidual suppression while the predominant concept was still that of a "tolerated allograft." The third reason is that T cell suppression is often associated with the suspicion of artifacts since none of the many papers in the 1970s dealing with soluble, specific and nonspecific factors involved in the suppression circuits considered molecular status. Indeed, the I-J enigma and the fact that the suppression of mixed lymphocyte reaction (MLR) is associated with the defunct I-C region both for pregnancy-associated and non-pregnancy-associated suppressor factors in mice have cast doubts for the general immunologist about the validity of the studies.

However, as highly reproducible as the transfer experiments with lymphocytes from tolerant animals are, such as those from allotransplanted kidney recipients in rats, both pregnancy-associated suppression and alloimmunization-induced suppression, which share several pathways, are also perfectly reproducible, provided care is taken to follow the original protocol.

While writing this review, we were teased by the curiosity to have a student reproduce alloimmunization and multiple allopregnancy-induced allosuppression in MLR experiments, and both experiments were easily repeated at an almost 20-year interval. Despite attempts in 1987 no serious explanations now exist for the I-J phenomenon, and the fact that the region does not map inside the MHC does not in itself mean that all observed phenomena were "constructed" results. The final interpretation of the I-J data is still lacking. As far as MLR suppression (see below) is concerned, the phenomenon remains valid if one interprets I-C as being in fact I-E.

3 "Classical" Signs of T Cell Priming?

Notwithstanding these considerations, data show that maternal T cells are indeed primed to fetal alloantigens. These include the observation that the mother mounts in many species an alloantibody response which, although restricted to discrete epitopes in the rat (SMITH et al. 1982a,b), are definitely detectable, including alloantibodies directed against paternal alloantigens in "responder" mice (KALISS and DAGG 1964; VOISIN and CHAOUAT 1974; CHAOUAT et al. 1977, 1979; BELL and BILLINGTON 1980, 1983).

A similar immune response is observed in humans (BEER et al. 1983a,b), and lack of such a response is often referred as a concomitant of immune abortions due to "improper maternal recognition of the conceptus (GENETET 1988; REZNIKOFF-ETIEVANT et al. 1985; REAGAN and RAUDE 1987). Such responses are also observed in a third model of placentation, the equines (ALLEN et al. 1987, 1990; ANTCZACK and ALLEN 1984).

Such data, together with the observation of nonspecific enhancement of third-party or unrelated antigen antibody response (DRESSER 1991; MATTSON 1982), imply specific maternal, antipaternal T cell priming, although one can evoke the role of non-T derived, placental secreted factors (MATTISON 1982; DUC et al. 1986).

Based on the general "enhancement facilitation" concept of tolerance of VOISIN (1962, 1971), which postulated at that time the existence of primed, active cells blocked in vivo by enhancing antibodies as the general mechanism of allo- and self-tolerance, attempts were made to detect such signs of priming. [The concept itself was rejected when it was discovered that tolerance to self-proteins is MHC restricted, and it is obvious that antibodies are not MHC restricted. We are not associated in this respect with the claim that reproductive immunology must teach general immunologists that they are wrong, because pregnancy demonstrates the general validity of the facilitation concept].

In this conceptual framework it has been shown that allopregnancy mice are tolerant to paternal-strain tumor cells from allopregnant mice transferred in relatively small numbers to naive recipients, promoting an acceleration of paternal-strain tumor allografts (VOISIN 1971; CHAOUAT et al. 1979). Recently TAFURI et al. (1995a) obtained very similar data in a transgenic mouse system, showing that mice bearing a K^b-specific T cell receptors were nevertheless specifically tolerant to a K^b-positive tumor during pregnancy with a K^b but nor with a K^d or K^k father.

In retrospect, we do not find the growing rejection data very impressive, despite statistical significance. In contrast, WEGMANN et al. (1979a) reported that pregnant mice were not primed but could be primed to fetal alloantigens. Most mice do not show antipaternal antibody responses, and only a fraction of primiparous women show antibody against paternal alloantigens. As reported by WEGMANN, it is possible to prime the mother against paternal antigens both locally (and in such a case pregnancy induces a recall flare reaction in para-aortic draining lymph nodes; BILLINGHAM 1988; BEER and BILLINGHAM 1974; HOGARTH 1982) and systematically, without adversely affecting the fetus. In such cases one can detect specific priming by the existence of accelerated rejection of paternal (tumor) grafts and specific antipaternal CTLs. (MITCHISON 1953; LANMAN 1962; MONNOT and CHAOUAT 1984). However, the fetus survives, and the weight of the conceptus is higher than in control animals.

On the other hand, the induction of specific T cell tolerance to the paternal alloantigens results in a reduction in placental weight (BEER et al. 1975). This ambiguous phenomenon was not properly interpreted until the immunotrophic theory (WEGMANN 1984; and see below). This observation doomed the original facilitation theory since antibodies directed against paternal antigens should not distinguish between a distant paternal strain allograft and the placenta. Furthermore, let us recall that the pregnancy is perfectly normal in B cell depleted mice (MATTSON et al. 1985; RODGER 1985), and, as noted above, that self-tolerance is MHC restricted. This directed studies away from the general concept of the facilitation reaction.

Nevertheless, it is worth mentioning that, based on the observation that there have been very few cases in humans of maternally acquired runt disease (BEER and BILLINGHAM 1973) attempts were made to demonstrate the presence of actively expanded T ("sensitized") cells directed against paternal alloantigens of demonstrating that maternal T cells are able to induce runting in newborns. Indeed, the authors of this study claimed that they observed significant runting, and that they were able to inhibit it by maternal (antipaternal?) alloantibodies (VOISIN et al. 1986). A report in 1980 claimed the induction of runting by immunization against paternal alloantigens using a paternal-strain tumor (DOSNE PASQUALINI and MATUSEVITCH 1980). This is akin to the induction of abortion by immunization against a syngeneic tumor, attributed to excess local nonspecific tumor necrosis factor (TNF) secretion, as reported by TARTAKOWSKY and GORELIK (1986a,b) rather that entering in the facilitation reaction scheme.

4 Suppressor T Cells?

Consensus emerged in the 1970s and 1980s (BILLINGHAM 1988; HART 1988; HOGARTH 1982; HOLLAND et al. 1984) that in murine, primate – including humans – equine, and porcine species one can observe an alloantibody response of varying magnitude and isotype (see below), in some cases restricted to some isotypes. However, there is no demonstration in any species or strain under physiological circumstances of what would be predicted from the confrontation with class I positive cells, for example, active cytotoxic T cells.

The cellular immunity appeared even rather depressed, as judged by a decrease in natural killer (NK) activity (BARRET et al. 1982; LUFT and REMINGTON 1984). Similarly, it has long been known that and the data of Tafuri et al. are a mere repetition, cell-mediated immunity in mice towards paternal skin grafts or fetal alloantigens is specifically decreased (BAINES et al. 1980; BREYERE and BARRET 1976; O'HEARN and HILARD 1981) as it is in guinea pigs (DAVID and VOLKRINGER, personal communication) and in rats (BREYERE and BARRET 1976).

Such studies, in a period when suppressor T cells had only recently been uncovered and extended to allograft situation in vivo by BRENT, led us to propose investigation of whether one could observe such paternal-specific suppressor T cells by in vivo adoptive transfer. The in vivo results were clearcut. Transfer of splenocytes from multiparous mice in large number led unequivocally to hyporesponsiveness to paternal-strain allografts (CHAOUAT 1977, 1979).

These data were confirmed independently in an allograft situation by BAINES et al. (1980b), and a very high efficiency of such suppressor cells was noted by SMITH and POWELL (1977) who observed a transfer of permanent tolerance to the H-Y (male) antigen by injection of T cells from multiparous mice in naive recipients subsequently challenged with male skin grafts. Importantly, independent studies on H-Y antigen and mechanisms of the induction of its tolerance confirmed that multiparity induces such a state of tolerance to male skin grafts and its transfer by suppressor (T) cells (CHANDLER et al. 1980).

As regards in vitro studies the results are more conflicting. We conducted studies in 1% NMS and observed MLR suppressor T cells induced by *multiparity* that were both alloantigen specific and of the CD8 phenotype. The cells acted via soluble suppressor factor which was studied in detail (CHAOUTAT and VOISIN 1979, 1980, 1981a,b,c). We independently produced data that were strikingly similar to those obtained using footpad immunization by RICH and RICH (1976), for example, an apparent 1-C 1-E MHC restriction. In agreement with data obtained by NELSON et al. (1980) in a tumor system, we also found suppressor cells active at the effector stage (ZAGURY et al. 1979; Chaouat et al. 1980b; CHAOUAT and VOISIN 1982), for example, blocking CTL activity. It is fair to say that as far as in vitro studies in mice are concerned these data were controversial. Data from SMITH (1981), SMITH et al. (1978), BARG et al. (1978), STERN and KAHAN (1980), and FABRIS et al. (1977) were completely or partially confirmatory. On the other hand, PAVIA and STITES (1979) and GOTTESMAN and STUTMAN (1980a,b) failed to observe such MLR suppressor T cells.

However, we carried our studies without nonspecific stimulation by use of 1% mouse serum as described by PECK and BACH (1973), and we believe that this explains the discrepancy, since we found variation in detection of MLR suppressor cells if performed in FCS according to the batch used. Suppressor cells have also been observed in rats (KOVITAVONG and DOSSETOR 1981) and in humans (GENETET et al. 1982; LIBURD and DOSSETOR 1982). An in vitro study obtained strikingly similar results in mice concerning suppression specificity for stimulators, for example, paternal alloantigens and apparent MHC restriction of suppression (ENGLEMAN et al. 1978). It is beyond the scope of this review to detail studies on the mechanism of suppressor T cell induction, but studies carried out in mice and human show that it is under influence of soluble factors from the placenta (BARG et al. 1978; BOBE et al. 1984; CANEPA 1985; CHAOUTAT et al. 1980a; CHAOUAT and CHAFFAUX 1981; HAMAOKA et al. 1983; KHRIHSNAN et al. 1991).

In conclusion, there is reasonably good evidence that suppressor T cells acting in a paternal antigen specific fashion most likely via soluble factors do exist in mice, rats, and humans during allopregnancy. However, as far as their role is concerned, clearcut evidence is lacking that they are mandatory for successful pregnancy

(Monnot and Chaouat 1984; Mattson and Holmdal 1987). That they may be useful is evidenced by murine abortion models (see below).

5 Immune Rejection of the Fetus?

The first abortion putatively due to immune malfunction was the *Mus caroli/Mus musculus*: transfer of *M. caroli* embryos into the uterine horns of the laboratory mouse *M. musculus* failed. The abortion/resorbtion process starts by day 9.5–10, and by day 11–12 all *M. caroli* embroys are dead/resorbed, while cotransferred *M. musculus* embryos proceed further until delivery. *M. caroli* embryos are subjected to a massive lymphocytic infiltrate.

In embryonic injection chimeras Rossant et al. (1982) have shown in a series of elegant experiments that even though the internal cell mass ICM/future embryo could be *M. caroli,* if the external cell mass (ECM)/ECM-derived placenta is of *M. musculus* genotype, a successful pregnancy across the species barrier is possible. This demonstrates a crucial role for trophoblast-decidua interactions. Since then, similar injection chimeras as well as aggregation chimeras have been used in the sheep/goat system, also giving birth to chimeras across the species barrier, the unique and spectacular "unicornlike" offspring being the cover page of *Nature* (Meinecke Tillmann and Meinecke 1984).

The *M. caroli* model, however, has its weaknesses. The *M. musculus* mice are naturally hyper reactive, as if sensitized to *M. caroli* antigens. More importantly, it is now accepted that rejection of *M. caroli* embryos in *M. musculus* uterus is not immunologically initiated, although immunological mechanisms are involved later in embryonic rejection (Clark et al. 1986a; Croy et al. 1985).

It was originally discovered by Clark et al. (1980) that if one mates CBA/J (H-2^k) with DBA/2 males (H-2^d), this mating leads to a high rate of spontaneous resorptions (about 40%). This is not seen in other H-2^k × H-2^d combinations, such as the C3H × DBA/2, the C3H × BALB/c, and, more interestingly the CBA × BALB/c (also k × d), nor do high resorption rates in CBA × CBA, DBA/2 × DBA/2, and DBA/2 × CBA/J behave "normally." The "abortifacient trait" is recessive; for example, CBA × (BALB/c × DBA/2) F1s are not prone to high rates of resorbtion (Chaouat 1983, 1987).

What is important for us is that immunization with BALB/c spleen cells correct resorption rates. The model involves minor loci differences in the same MHC (H-2k × H-2d) combination since BALB/C are H-2d as DBA/2. In the same vein, B10 mated with B10.A exhibit an abnormally high resorption rate, not seen in B10 × B10.Br or B10 × B10.D2 matings (Chaouat et al. 1987, 1988b). The latter model is a mirror image of CBA × DBA/2, involving subtle MHC disparity on the same (B10) genetic background. The "MHC effect" certainly involves presentation/interactions, and self-peptide competition, since B10.A is H-2a, H-2a being a recombinant haplotype between H-2^d (B10.D2) and H-2^k (B10.Br). The two models share several characteristics: resorptions increase with aging, and there is a local deficiency in suppressor activity in paraortic draining lymph nodes of CBA × DBA/2 (CHAOUAT et al. 1988b,c) and in decidua-associated suppressor cells near embryos that would be resorbed (CLARK 1985; CLARK et al. 1986b).

Indirect evidence for T cell involvement comes first from the fact that repeated pregnancies with the "wrong" father enhance resorption (CHAOUAT et al. 1988; CLARK et al. 1986b), highly suggestive of a memory phenomenon. The resorbing embryos are infiltrated first by NK-lineage cells (CHAOUAT 1986; CHAOUAT et al. 1988), probably deriving from the early local accumulation around embryos at the early implantation period in mice (DE FOUGEROLLES and BAINES 1988; GENDRON and BAINES 1988). Modulation of NK activity, and NK accumulation at implantation sites is correlated with abortion: in vivo elimination of asialo-GM1 positive cells reduces resorptions (CHAOUAT et al. 1987; DE FOUGEROLLES and BAINES 1988). On the other hand, activation of NK cells results in increased abortion, whether by POLYIC12U or other Ds RNAs (CHAOUAT et al. 1987, 1990c; DE FOUGROLLES and BAINES 1988; KINSKY et al. 1990), interferon (IFN) inducer, or IFN-γ (which also induces class I MHC expression on trophoblast in vivo (CHAOUAT et al. 1990c, 1991a; MATTSON et al. 1989, 1991). IFN and Ds RNA systems work in any strain of mice, as do lipopolysaccharides and recombinant TNF to induce abortion (CHAOUAT et al. 1990c; KINSKY et al. 1990).

Decidua of "naturally" aborting combinations contain more IFN-γ and TNF-α than normal matings (CHAOUAT et al. 1991a; TANGRI and RAGHUPATHY 1993). Since lymphokine-activated cells are involved, it is tempting to use interleukin (IL)2. Reports of very low doses of IL-2 as abortifacient, or the combination of IL-2 and indomethacin have not been confirmed (TEZABWALA et al. 1989). Direct evidence for a role of T cells in regulating abortion rates comes from immunization studies: injection of of CBA/J prior to DBA/2 mating against BALB/c splenocytes, but not with DBA/2 ones, correct resorption rates (CHAOUAT et al. 1983, 1985).

What matters here is that the effect is transferable by cells or serum, and, most importantly purified T cells transfer the protective effect. The abortion rate is also correlated with decreased systemic Ts acitivity, and it was observed in the initial description that immunization is correlated with a recovery of such activity (CHAOUAT et al. 1988b,c). Similarly, immunization with DBA/2 cells or mating with DBA/2 males is correlated with low alloantibody production, but such production could be reestablished by immunization. Similar effects in another strain combination have been observed by CHAVEZ et al. (1987). Using other H-2^d strains and recombinants between BALB/c and DBA/2, it has been shown that the effects are very restricted to the CBA anti BALB/c immunization. Other H-2^d strains are not such efficient immunogens.

The use of recombinants allow segregation of the "beneficial" trait, and it has been shown that this was a single group of genes or a single gene. Recombinants, as well as H-2^d congenics, rule out the role of the minor loci system (Mls) as the immunogenic locus (BOBE et al. 1986; BOBE and KIGER 1987; CHAOUAT et al. 1988b,c). Furthermore, this also allowed the determination that there is no correlation between systemic suppression, alloantibody production, and antiabortive effects.

It has been claimed that T cells recognize a macrophage determinant present on BALB/c cells (Bobe et al. 1986; Bobe and Kiger 1987), but such studies have not been confirmed by independent investigators. When one injects a repressor tumor in C57BL/6 mice, one obtains a real abortion (with bleeding and expulsion, not merely a resorption). However, no data exist on T cell subsets versus NK lineage involvement in such systems (Dosne Pasqualini and Matusevitch 1980; Tartakowsky and Gorelik 1986a,b).

6 Immunotrophism?

In the CBA × DBA/2 model a striking observation was made by Kolb (Chaouat et al. 1983) and Wegmann (1984) when we described the effect of alloimmunization in correcting resorption rate. Jean Pierre had observed that after alloimmunization one sees an increase in placental weight. This coupled with the lack of definite correlation between peripheral suppression and antiabortive effects lead Wegmann (1984) to propose that the protection against abortion is due to immunostimulation rather than to immunosuppression. This was the initial formulation of the immunotropism theory. In it final form it did not exclude immunosuppression, suggesting than lymphokines are involved *in optimal* placental growth.

Anti-L3T4 plus anti-CD8 treatment does indeed reduce placental size and weight in a variety of strains (Athanasskis et al. 1990) and, most importantly, enhances abortion rates in the CBA × DBA/2 matings (Chaouat et al. 1987, 1988a-c). It also reduces placental weight even in fully congenic isogenic inbred matings, although less than in semiallogenic ones. It also reduces trophoblast phagocytic activity.

We then tested this treatment in cases of abnormal placental functions and growth induced by autoimmunity. We used MRL/lpr mice, an autoimmune strain that develops excessive colony-stimulating factor (CSF) secretion and antibodies of anti-idiotypic activity to IL-3 receptor endowed with IL-3-like activity as a consequence of autoimmunity. The reasons for autoimmunity are beyond the scope of this study, but there is T cell involvement. What matters here is that they show gross excessive placental weight, and hyperplacental phagocytic activity. As described above, anti-CD4 plus anti-CD8 treatment normalizes the excessive placental weight seen habitually as a correlative of the lpr trait and normalizes trophoblast phagocytic activity, MRL being H-2k as CBA/J. We transferred cells from lpr mice into CBA/j without obtaining immediate graft-versus-host or host-versus-graft reaction, and this was active in reducing resorption in the CBA × DBA/2 mating (Chaouat et al. 1988a).

In parallel, we have shown that anti-CD4 plus anti-CD8 treatment enhances drastically CBA × DBA/2 fetal loss and prevents fetal protection by alloimmunization (Athanassakis et al. 1987; Wegmann et al. 1988). In fact, anti-CD8 treatment alone in a single injection on day 7.5 prevents the beneficial effects: we observed for example, that, if one reduces resorption rates in CBA × DBA/2 from 28/65 (43.07%) to 5/61 (8.1%), such a single injection of anti-CD8 causes the resorption rate to remain at 29/61 (47.54%). We reasoned that the lpr transfer data are highly consistent with the effects observed in vitro of T cell derived cytokines of the CSF family as positive regulators of placental growth (Amstrong and Chaouat 1989; Athanassakis et al. 1987). We then tested directly the effects of such factors in CBA/J. IL-3 and granulocyte-macrophage CSF (GM-CSF) were indeed efficient in reducing resorption rates (Chaouat et al. 1990a,c).

7 Th1 Versus Th2?

On the other hand, it has been shown that IL-2 is abortifacient in mice (Chaouat et al. 1990c; Tezabwala et al. 1989). Similarly, it has long been known that TNF is abortifacient, a fact confirmed by several investigators (Parand and Chedid 1964; Gendron et al. 1989; Chaouat et al. 1990b, 1991a). It was also shown that there is excessive TNF and IFN-γ in the placenta and decidua of aborting CBA × DBA/2 (Tangri and Raghupathy 1993). This event was for the first time linked directly to both fetal abortion and "abnormal" T cell recognition since "mixed placental lymphocyte reactions" were performed between CBA/J cells and CBA × DBA/2 and CBA × BALB/c placental cells used as stimulators. The supernatants of such cultures contained much more TNF and INF-γ when CBA × DBA/2 were used instead of CBA × BALB/c placental cells, and the former products were abortifacient in vivo (Tangri et al. 1994).

Such data led to the concept that Th1 cytokines are nefast for placental growth and suggested, together with the above enhanced antibody production, isotypic regulation, for example, shift to IgG1 instead of IgG2 alloantibody production in mice, a decrease in delayed-type hypersensitivity reactions (Holland et al. 1984), a decrease in NK reactivity during pregnancy, and local and systemic decrease in certain patterns of antiparasitic activity (Bruce Chwatt 1983; Hart 1988; Laesen and Galask 1978; Redline and Lu 1988; van Zoorn 1986; Vleughels 1990; Weidanz 1982) which may involve the Th2 compartment.

Significant IL-10, IL-3, and IL-4 production was detected in the supernatants of placenta and dediduae (Chaouat et al. 1993b,c; Lin 1993). A shift towards Th2 production was also noted by Delassus et al. (1994), but production of IL-10 in the placenta is debatable. These data nevertheless led to the concept that "successful allopregnancy is a Th2 phenomenon" (Wegmann et al. 1993b).

IL-10 corrects abortion in the CBA × DBA/2 combination much more efficiently than any treatment that we have assayed before; anti-IL-10 enhances resorption rates. In contrast, anti-IFN-γ decreases resorption rates in synergy with pentoxyfillin. It is interesting to note that such effect is not observed in non-abortion-prone matings (Chaouat et al. 1994, 1995a). We noted that the CBA × DBA/2 fetal wastage can be prevented by in vivo a single pre-or peri-implantation injection of IFN-τ (ovine trophoblast protein, oTP). We wanted to assess whether this is due to induction by Recombinant oTP of the Th2 profile characteristic of successful pregnancy. Most interestingly, the induction of IL-10 production was indeed obtained in CBA × DBA/2 placentae by injection of recombinant ovine IFN-τ (Chaouat et al. 1995).

The significance of these data for a Th2 model of successful pregnancy is obvious. They suggest a key role for placental IFNs, which in addition to their cytostatic properties makes them ideal candidates for early pregnancy local suppression (one of the reasons for their important cross-species structural conservation. If τ-IFN acts not only as a local cytostatic agent and maintains the corpus luteum in a variety of species, devoid of chorionic gonadotrophin (CG), a single molecule (IFN-τ) could thus exert the functions of both endocrine signalization of early pregnancy (maternal recognition of pregnancy) and install the isotypic regulation and down-regulation of cellular immune responses characteristic of pregnancies before maternal allorecognition of the fetoplacental unit via IL-10 regulation of the effects. Production of the otherwise abortifacient cytokines TNF and INF-γ resolves the puzzling observation that in alloimmunized mice a shift towards IgG1 production is observed before classical T cell recognition of MHC antigens on the placenta occurs, i.e., before day 9.5 when MHC antigens are expressed for the first time on trophoblasts.

It remains to be determined whether the pathway acts exclusively on T cells or, more likely, on cells of the reproductive tracts as a part of their involvement in the gestational process secrete lymphokines involved in the implantation process as part of an immunoreproductive network. In this respect it is important to note that although INF-τ has not yet been completely convincingly demonstrated in humans, a candidate molecule (but which could be an ω one) has recently been cloned by Whaley et al. (1991a,b).

8 Endocrine Effects on T Cells?

Progesterone also plays an immunosuppressive role. It was first discarded as in vitro artifact since it is immunosuppressive in vitro on normal lymphocytes, but no progesterone receptors had then been demonstrated on resting T lymphocytes. However, both Szekeres Bartho and Beaman et al. observed that, upon pro gesterone treatment at physiological doses, alloactivated or pregnancy lymphocytes release at least two suppressor factors. The first one, still not purified or cloned, blocks NK cell mediated lysis: progesterone induced blocking factor (PIBF). This blocks NK action not only on classical K 562 NK targets but also on human embryonic fibroblasts. The physiological relevance is that in cases of immune abortion in mice within the placenta there are fibroblasts (SZEKERES-BARTHO et al. 1985). This factor is also endowed with other pleiotropic immunoregulatory activities: it blocks MLR, activates enhances absolute numbers of $CD8^+$, $D44^-$ T cells (Ts subset in humans) and the CD4 $2H4^+$, $TQ1^+$ (Ts inducer subset in human) in MLR (SZEKERES BARTHO et al. 1985, 1989b).

The second material is a T suppressor inducer factor, named J6B7, recently purified and cloned (LEE et al. 1990). It plays an integral role in pregnancy since well defined monoclonal antibodies raised against it are abortifacient in mice (BEAMAN and HOVERSLAND 1988; HOVERSLAND and BEAMAN 1990) without being by themselves teratogenic – a very important control indeed (HOVERSLAND and BEAMAN 1991), not shown in some studies using polyclonal antibodies of unchecked cross-reactivity and performed on a very low number of mice. The monoclonal antibody can be used to titrate the factor in lymphoid organs of pregnant mice (HOVERSLAND and BEAMAN 1990).

The release of such PIBF and probably that of J6B7 is blocked when one used RU 486, and similarly transcription of mRNAs for J6B7 is a progesterone-dependent event. The block of PIBF secretion after progesterone action on activated T cells is not seen with 43044 glucocorticoid blocker, specific for these, not acting on progesterone receptors.

Monoclonal antibodies specific for the N terminal part of the conventional progesterone receptor exists, developed by the Milgrom team and commercially available from Transbio (France) and Abbott (EIA Rpg kit). They react with activated T cells, those from phytohemagglutin and from concanavalin A stimulation, or MLR which mimics allorecognition as in the case in peripheral blood in pregnant women or in contact with class I positive cells or decidual antigen-presenting cells processed presented peptides from paternal MHC molecules. As far as in vitro assays are concerned in vivo, this is indeed the case of pregnancy, but more importantly of allotransplanted patients.

The presence of such receptors can be ascertained by immunohistochemical studies, enzyme/enzyme-linked immunosorbent assay, FACS analysis (which requires previous lysolecithin or saponin membrane permeation, a tricky technique but necessary since the receptors are nuclear ones. In rats their presence has been found by appropriate binding studies with the relevantly labeled materials (Philibert, Roussel Uclaf). However, their level in the first trimester is quite low (below 10 fmol/mg protein), the limit of sensitivity of the Abbott EIA being 1 fmol/mg protein (but it requires much care). The variance was, as expected , due to HLA variation between individuals in a randomly selected sample of an outbred wild primate population. In humans, this is too high for the assay to serve as a diagnostic tool to discriminate between aborter and normal first-trimester populations (a cell such as T47D or MCF7 displays 100–400 fmol/mg protein). The number of such receptors increases as a function of gestional age, and it was confirmed by an independent study which also reported a decrease in preeclampsia, not only in labor (VARGA and CHAOUAT 1989; SZEKERES BARTHO 1990; SZEKERES BARTHO and CHAOUAT 1990).

Polymerase chain reaction evidence has recently been obtained by PALDI et al. (1994) in cooperation with d'Auriol and Misrahi that it is a classical progesterone receptor. PIBF blocks TNF secretion by activated lymphocytes, and can also correct or prevent the effect of low doses of RU 486 in mice (SZEKERES BARTHO et al. 1993), suggesting an immune component in RU 486 activity that we have recently demonstrated (CHAOUAT et al. 1993a). This is of importance since the placenta is the only place where T cells can be simultaneously activated and confronted with progesterone in sufficient amounts to secrete immunomodulatory materials. These receptors of progesterones (Rpgs) show an abrupt disappearance during parturition or at the onset of threatened preterm delivery. They persist in cases of retardation of labor onset. Therefore it is possible that this event is associated with the induction of labor by allowing the release of TNF or TNF-like materials in the placental bed. Smooth muscle is a target, and once triggered by it, a further source of TNF which could increase its motricity and certainly also promotes vasoconstriction. In addition, TNF is a stop signal for placental growth, and it is cytotoxic for placenta at high doses.

It is therefore possible that immunoendocrine events are one of the (many) pathways involved in parturition and that some of them are regulated by T cells (LELAIDIER 1995). In addition, stress-mediated abortion or premature delivery can be prevented by alloimmunization, as in normal or artificial models of abortion (CHAOUAT et al. 1993a; ARCK et al. 1995), but it cannot prevent TNF induction of premature labor.

9 T Cell Recognition of the Fetoplacental Unit?

The data obtained in murine spontaneous abortion by immunization in mice and in aborting combinations (see above) that T cells are involved in protecting the fetoplacental unit (CHAOUAT et al. 1988a) either by suppressive activity locally (CLARK 1994) or in synergy with progesterone action acting on these T cells.

These data are somewhat contradicted by the early observation made in cooperation with our group and in our laboratory facilities of specific antipaternal CTLs in the blood of recurrent aborters in human (EDELMAN 1983). A Japanese group recently reported detection of specific (?) antipaternal CTLs expressing CD5, CD14, and CD16 markers and the excessive local accumulation of T cells of maternal origin in chorionic villi of placentae of recurrent aborters (LABARRERE and FAULK 1995; YOKOYAMA et al. 1995), suggesting maternal aggression of the placenta (CLARK 1995).

We have extensively studied such T cell recognition using the fact that maternal priming can prevent Ds RNA induced abortion (KINSKY et al. 1990). We have shown that immunization with MHC disparate cells and MHC-transfected L cells but not control, monomorphic MHC-transfected L cells prevent Ds RNA induced abortion. The protective effect was shown using immunization with lymphocytes from C57 BL/6 H-2^{bm} mutants specific for class I or class II mutation injected in correlation with immunizing strength of the immunizing cells (CHAOUAT et al. 1991b; KINSKY et al. 1991; MENU et al. 1995).

The immunization data show that paternal specificity is not required for effective protective effect because the effect is seen with alloimmunization of inbred crosses with allogeneic spleen cells. This is reminiscent of the work of Toder and colleagues, who showed the CBA × DBA/2 fetuses can be rescued from spontaneous resorption by footpad (but not intraperitoneal) injection of complete freund's adjuvant (TODER and SHOMER 1990; TODER et al. 1991). However, the use of L cells transfected with MHC presenting variations at discretely defined epitopes (ABASTADO et al. 1987) which were active as well as bm mutants allowed the effect to be attributed solely to MHC molecules alloantigenicity in our experimental conditions since monomorphic "37" transfected L cells (COCHET et al. 1989) did not have such effects (MENU et al. 1995).

Using such mutants, we (ABASTADO et al. 1987) showed that mutation on the surface of α-helices are indeed recognized as such and are beneficial for pregnancy in preventing Ds RNA induced abortion (CHAOUAT et al. 1993b). However, the fine pattern of allorecognition suggests that T cells are not involved in the effect. Based on accumulating evidence in other systems, it is clear that NK cells can exert allorecognition of mutate MHC. They can also recognize α-helices determinants (KURAGO et al. 1995).

It is our working hypothesis that most, if not all, allorecognition events attributed locally to T cells are in fact due to NK cell secretion of cytokines of differentiation activation into cytotoxic effectors by such allorecognition events. The events have so far been linked to T cells because allorecognition of defined MHC specificities by NK cells were not really suspected.

Our 1992 data, at that time attributed by us to T cell recognition, were probably the first indirect in vivo evidence of such a process. We are at present using allopregnancy as a tool to test the hypothesis that NK cells are a subset of cells that are primitive T cells, but already recognizing discrete MHC specificities, and that one of the pressures for polymorphism on α-helixes may be the advantage that allorecognition of MHC mutation on α-helices would afford to pregnancy.

This hypothesis shifts the major local role from T cells to non-T cells. This is more consistent with reports that classical T cells are sparse in the pregnant uterus after implantation (BULMER and RITSON 1998; MacMaster et al. 1992; NOUN et al. 1989; KACHKACHE et al. 1991) although classical T cells have been found by several authors, some of whom report a decreased expression of classical T cell receptors (MORI et al. 1993; CHERNISHOV et al. 1993).

An alternative hypothesis involves a major role of γ δ T cells. The presence of γ δ T cells is known in the decidua, and these cells are also known to recognize trophoblasts (HEYHORNE et al. 1994), but their action in pregnancy has so far not attracted the interest it deserves.

10 Epilogue

In keeping with data reviewed in this manuscript showing maternal mice and guinea pigs to be hyporesponsive to a paternal-strain allograft, Tafuri et al. (1995) have recently reported using mice trangenic for a specific TCR, namely K^b, and monoclonal antibodies specific for this clonotype (DES TCR mice). These were mated with C57BL/6 (H-2K^b), CBA/J (H-2^k), and ASW (H-2^s) mice. These Des K^b matings expressed a high clonotype level and a six to nine fold increase in the percentage of cells bearing the CD4/CD8 coreceptors, a fact not observed when mice were from the Des-H-2^k or H-2^s matings. This was observed in thymectomized animals. Furthermore, in agreement with our data, a vast majority of mice were unable during pregnancy to reject a K^b tumor only when coming from a Des-H-2^b mating and not in the control matings if grafted 3–5 days post coitum. All mice later rejected the tumor.

One explanation for this may be the action of Ts (see above) and/or placental and decidual (transforming growth factor β_2 -like) suppressive factors. We have recently succeeded in demonstrating that a low molecular weight placental suppressor factor induces a transient state of T cell anergy in T cells (De Smedt et al. 1996; Chaouat et al. 1995b).

References

Abastado JP, Jaulin C, Schutze M-P, Langlade-Denoyen P, Plata F, Ozato K, Kourilsky P (1987) Fine mapping of epitopes by intradomain K^d/D^d recombinants. J Exp Med 166:327–340

Allen WR, Kydd JH, Antczack DF (1986) Successful application of immunotherapy to a model of pregnancy failure in equids. In: Clark DA, Croy BA (eds) Reproductive immunology 1986. Elsevier Amsterdam, pp 253–261

Allen WR, Kydd J, Donaldson WL, Oriol JG, Antczak D (1987) Expression of immune response to fetal antigens in equine pregnancy. Coll INSERM 154:255

Allen WR, Kydd JH, Antczak DF (1990) Xenogeneic donkey-in-horse pregnancy created by embryo transfer: immunological aspects of a model of early abortion. In: Chaouat G (ed) The immunology of the foetus. CRC, Boca Raton

Amstrong DTA, Chaouat G (1989) Effects of lymphokines and immune complexes on murine placental cell growth in vitro. Biol Reprod 4:400–406

Antczack DF, Allen WR (1984) Invasive trophoblast in the genus Equus. Ann Immunol (Paris) 135 D:325–331

Arck PC, Merali FS, Manuel JS, Chaouat G, Clark DA (1995) Stress triggered abortion: inhibition of protective suppression and promotion of tumor necrosis factor alpha (TNF alpha) release as a mechanism triggering resorptions in mice. Am J Reprod Immunol 33(1):74–81

Athanassakis I, Bleackley RC, Paetkau V, Guilbert L, Barrp J, Wegmann TG (1987) The immunostimulatory effects of T cells and T cell lymphokines on murine foetally derived placental cells. J Immunol 138:37–44

Athanassakis I, Chaouat G, Wegmann TG (1990) The effects of anti CD4 and anti CD8 antibody treatment on placental growth and function in allogenic and syngenic pregnancy. Cell Immunol 129:13–21

Athanassakis vassiliadis I, Papamettheakis J (1991) Modulation of class II antigens on fetal placenta lads to fetal abortion. In: Chaouat G, Mowbray J (eds) Biologie cellulaire et moléculaire de la relation materno fétale. Libbey, Paris, pp 69–81

Athanassakis I et al. (1996) Am J Reprod Immunol (in press)
Baines MG, Speers EA, Pross HGF, Millar KG (1980a) Characteristics of the maternal lymphoid response in mice to paternal strain alloantigens induced by homologous pregnancy. Immunology 31:363–369
Baines MG, Millar KG, Pross HF (1980b) Allograft enhancement during normal murine pregnancy. J Reprod Immunol 2:141–148
Barg M, Burton RC, Smith JA, Luckenbach GA, Decker J, Mitchell GF (1978) Effect of placental tissues on immunological responses. Clin Exp Immunol 140:1588–1597
Barret DS, Rayfield LS, Brent L (1982) Suppression of natural cell mediated cytotoxicity in man by maternal and neonatal serum. Clin Exp Immunol 47:742–748
Beaman KD, Hoversland RC (1988) Induction of "spontaneous" abortion by blocking antigen specific suppression. J Reprod Fertil 82:135–139
Beer AE, Billingham RE (1973) Maternally acquired runt disease. Science 179:240–243
Beer AE, Billingham RE (1974) Host responses to intrauterine tissues, cellular and fetal allografts. J Reprod Fertil Suppl 21:59
Beer AE, Scott JR, Billingham RE (1975) Histocompatibility and maternal immunological status as determinants of foeto-placental size and litter weight in rodents. J Exp Med 142:180–198
Beer AE, Quebbeman JF, Semprini AE (1983a) Immunological aspects of recurrent abortions in humans. In: Edelmann P, Sureau C (eds) Immunologie de la Reproduction humaine. Sandoz, Basel
Beer AE, Quebbeman JF, Semprini AE, Smouse PE, Haines RF (1983b) Recurrent abortion: analysis of the role of parental sharing of histocompatibility antigens and maternal immunological responses to paternal antigens. In: Isojima S, Billington WD (eds) Reproductive immunology 1983. Elsevier, Amsterdam, pp 185–197
Bell SC, Billington WD (1980) Major antipaternal allo antibody induced by pregnancy is non complement fixing lgG1. Nature 288:387–388
Bell SC, Billington WD (1983) Anti fetal alloantibody in the pregnant female. Immunol Rev 75:5–30
Bianchi DW, Flint AF, Pizzimenti MF et al (1990) Isolation of fetal DNA from nucleated erythrocytes in maternal blood. Proc Natl Acad Sci USA 87:3279
Bianchi DW, Stewart JE, Garber MF et al (1991) Possible effect of gestationel age on the detection of fetal nucleated erythrocytes in maternal blood. Prenat Diagn 11:523
Bianchi DW, Mahr A, Zickwolf GK et al (1992) Detection of fetal cells with 47, XY, +21 karyotype in maternal peripheral blood. Hum Genet 90:368
Bianchi DW, Zickwolf GK, Yih MC et al (1993) Haploid-specific antibodies enhance detection of fetal nucleated erythrocytes in maternal blood. Prenat Diagn 13:293
Billingham RE (1988) Immunobiological aspects of the foeto maternal relationship. In: Lachman P, Peters D (eds) Clinical aspects of immunology, 4th edn. Blackwell, Oxford
Billington WD, Burrows FJ (1986) The rat placenta expresses paternal class I MHC antigens. J Reprod Immunol 9:155–160
Bobe P, Kiger N (1987) Immunogenetic aspects of feto maternal tolerance. Coll INSERM 154:235–247
Bobe P, Doric M, Kinsky RG, Voisin GA (1984) Modulation of mouse anti SRBC response by placental extracts. Cell Immunol. 89:355–364
Bobe P, Chaouat G, Stanislavski M, Kiger N (1986) Immunogenetics of spontaneous abortion in mice. II. Anti abortive effects are independent of systemic regulatory mechanisms. Cell Immunol 98:577–586
Breyere EJ, Barret MK (1976) Pregnancy induced hypo responsiveness to paternal alloantigens. II. Factors affecting altered expression of immunity in parous rats. Transplantation 34:258–263
Bulmer JD, Ritson A (1988) The decidua in early pregnancy. In: Beard RW, Sharp F (eds) Early pregnancy loss, mechanisms and treatment. 18th RCOG study group. Royal College of Obstetricians and Gynaecologists, London, pp 171–181
Bruce Chwatt LJ (1983) Malaria and pregnancy. Br Med J 286:1457
Bruch JF, Metezeau P, Garcia-fonknechten N et al (1991) Trophoblast-like cells sorted from peripheral blood using flow cytometry: a multiparametric study involving transmission electron microscopy and foetal DNA amplification. Prenat Diagn 11:787
Canepa S (1985) Properiétés immunologiques in vitro de surnageants de cultures de choriocarcinomes humains. DERBH University, Paris
Chandler P, Benjamin D, Simpson E (1980) Tolerance to H-Y antigens. In: Fougereau M, Dausset J (eds) 4th International Congress of Immunology, Paris 1980. Book of abstracts. Abstract 04 08 05
Chaouat G (1986) Placental infiltration of resorbing CBA × DBA/s embryos. J Reprod Immunol Suppl p 134

Chaouat G (1995) Low doses of LPS synergises with inflammatory cytokines in induction of murine resorbtions or labour. Alloimmunisation can prevent the abortifacient effects, but not the induction of pretern delivery. Cell Immunol 157:328–340
Chaouat G, Chaffaux S (1981) Induction by placental extracts of suppressor cells of the graft vs. host reaction. Am J Reprod Immunol 6(3):107–112
Chaouat G, Voisin GA (1979) Regulatory T cell subpopulations in pregnancy. I. Evidence for suppressive activity of the early phase of MLR J Immunol 122:1383–1388
Chaouat G, Voisin GA (1980) Regulatory T cells subpopulations in pregnancy. II. Evidence for suppressive activity of the late phase of MLR Immunology 39:239
Chaouat G, Voisin GA (1981a) Regulatory T cells in pregnancy. III. Evidence for the involvement of two T cell subsets. Immunology 44:393–399
Chaouat G, Voisin GA (1981b) Regulatory T cells in pregnancy. IV. Genetic characteristics and mode of action of early MLR suppressive population J Immunol 127:1335–1336
Chaouat G, Voisin GA (1981c) Regulatory T cells in pregnancy. V. Allopregnancy induced T cell suppressor factor is H-2 restricted and bears la determinants. Cell Immunol 62:186–195
Chaouat G, Voisin GA (1982) Regulatory T cells in pregnancy. VI. Evidence for T cell suppression of CTL generation. Cell Immunol 68:668–322
Chaouat G, Voisin GA, Daeron M, Kanellopoulos J (1977) Anticorps facilitants et cellules suppressives dans la réaction immunitaire maternelle anti-foetale. Ann Immunol (Paris) 128:21–24
Chaouat G, Voisin GA, Escalier D, Robert P (1979) Facilitation reaction (enchancing antibodies and suppressor cells) and rejection reaction (sensitised cells) from the mother to the paternal antigens of the conceptus. Clin Exp Immunol 35:13–24
Chaouat G, Chaffaux S, Voisin GA (1980a) Immuno-active products of placenta I. J Reprod Immunol 2:127–136
Chaouat G, Chaffaux S, Monnot P, Hoffmann M (1980b) Regulation of maternal cellular immunity to the conceptus. Am J Reprod Immunol 1:18
Chaouat G, Kiger N, Wegmann TG (1983) Vaccination against spontaneous abortion in mice. J Reprod Immunol 5:389–392
Chaouat G, Kolb JP, Kiger N, Stanislawski M, Wegmann TG (1985) Immunological concomitants of vaccination against abortion in mice. J Immunol 134:1594
Chaouat G, Lankar D, Kolb JP, Clark DA (1987) G.2 modèles d' avortements d' origine immunitaire chez la souris de laboratoire: mécanismes abortifs, modalités et mécanismes du traitement par l'immunisation contre un male relié ou non relié suivant les différences antigéniques père-mère. In: Chaouat G (ed) Immunologie de la relation féto-maternelle. Libbey, Paris, pp 243–255
Chaouat G, Menu E, Athanassakis I, Wegmann TG (1988a) Maternal T cells regulate placental size and fetal survival. Reg Immunol 1:143
Chaouat G, Clark DA, Wegmann TG (1988b) Immunogenetic studies of spontaneous abortion in mice. I. Preimmunisation of the mother with allogeneic spleen cells. J Immunol 134:2966–2972
Chaouat G, Clark DA, Wegmann TG (1988c) Genetics aspects of the CBA/J × DBA/2 J and B10 × B10. A models of murine spontaneous abortions and prevention by leukocyte immunisation. In: Allen WR, Clark DA, Gill TJ III, Mowbray JF, Robertson WR (eds) Early Pregnancy loss. Mechanisms and treatment. RCOG Press 89-105
Chaouat G, Menu E, Kinsky R, Dy M, Minkowski M, Delage G, Ming Nguy Thang, Clark DA, Wegmann TG, Szekeres Bartho J (1990a) Lymphokines and non specific cellular lytic effectors at the feto maternal interface affect placental size and survival. In: Mettler L, Billington WD (eds) Reproductive immunology 1989. 4th International Congress of Reproductive Immunology. Elsevier, Amsterdam, pp 283–290
Chaouat G, Menu E, Hoffman M, Dy M, Minkowski M, Clark DA, Wegmann TG (1990b) Lymphokines at the feto maternal interface affect fetal size and survival. Coll INSERM 199:133
Chaouat G, Menu E, Dy M, Minkowski M, Clark DA, Wegmann TG (1990c) Control of fetal survival in CBA × DBA/2 mice by lymphokine therapy. J Fertil Steril 89:447–458
Chaouat G, Menu E, Wegmann TG (1991a) Role des lymphokines de la famille du CSF, et du TNF, de l'interféron gamma, et de I'IL-2 sur la survie fétale et la croissance placentaire étudiées in vivo dans 2 modèles d'avortements immunitaires spontanés murins. In: Chaouat G, Mowbray J (eds) Biologie cellulaire et moléculaire de la relation materno fétale. Libbey, Paris, pp 91–101
Chaouat G, Menu E, David F, Szekeres Bartho J, Kinsky R, Dang DC, Kapovic M, Ropert S, Wegmann TG (1991b) Lymphokines, cytokines and immunoregulators involved in pregnancy success or perinatal AIDS. Periodicum Biol 93(1):49–54

Chaouat G, Menu E, Djian V, Delage G, Kinsky R, Assal-meliani A, Frydman R, Martal J (1993a) Lymphokines, cytokines, MHC allorecognition and successful early and late pregnancy. In: Dondero F, Lenzi D (eds) 5th International Congress on Reproductive Immunology. Serono symposia Raven, New York, p 107

Chaouat G, Menu E, David F, Djian V, Kinsky R (1983b) Reproductive immunology 1989–1992: some important recent advances about feto maternal relationship. In: Gergely J (ed) Progress in immunology 8. Springer, Berlin Heidelberg New York, p 825

Chaouat G, Menu E, Djian V, Delage G, Kinsky R, Assal-meliani A, Frydman R, Martal J (1993c) Lymphokines, cytokines, MHC allorecognition and successful early and late pregnancy. In: Dondero F, Lenzi D (eds) 5th International Congress on Reproductive Immunology. Serono symposia Raven, New York, p 107

Chaouat G, Menue E, Lelaidier C, Delage G, Moreauj F, Assal Meliani A, Djian V, Ropert S, David FJE, Wegmann TG, Lin Hui, Raghupathy R, Martal J, Frydman R (1994) Cytokines and immuno endocrine network as determinants of early pregnancy success or failure and in parturition. In: Mori T, Aono T, Tominaga T, Hiroi M (eds) Perspectives in assisted reproduction. Ares, Rome pp 227–235 (serono symposia)

Chaouat G, Assal meliani A, Martal J, Raghupathy R, Elliotj, Mossmann T, Wegmann TG (1995a) IL-10 prevents inflammatory cytokine-mediated fetal death and is inducible by tau interferon. J immunol 154(9):4261–4268

Chaouat G, Menu E, De smedt D, Khrishnan L, Lin Hui, Assal Meliani A, Martal J, Raghupathy R, Wegmann TG (19956) The emerging role of IL-10 in pregnancy. Am J Reprod Immunol 35:325–329

Chattergee-Hasrouni S, Lala PK (1982) Localisation of paternal H-2 antigens on murine trophoblast cells in vivo. J Exp Med 155:1679–1688

Chavez DJ, MacIntyre JA, Colliver JA, Page faulk WP (1987) Allogeneic matings and immunisation have different effects on nulliparous and multiparous mice. J Immunol 139(1):85–91

Chernishov VP, Sluvkin II, Bondarenko GI (1993) Phenotypic characterisation of CD7+, CD3+ and CD8+ lymphocytes from 1st trimester human decidua using two colour flow cyto fluorometry. Am J Reprod Immunol 295:17–21

Clark DA (1985) Maternal immune response to the fetus. Eos Rev Immunol Immunofarmacol 2:114–117

Clark DA (1995) Maternal aggression against placenta? Am J Reprod Immunol 31(4):205–207

Clark DA, McDermott M, Sczewzuk MR (1980) Impairment of host versus graft reaction in pregnant mice. II. Selective suppression of cytotoxic cell generation correlates with soluble suppressor activity and successful allogeneic pregnancy. Cell Immunol 52:106–118

Clark DA, Croy BA, Rossant J, Chaouat G (1986a) Immune presensitisation and local intrauterine defences as determinants of success or failure of murine interspecies pregnancies. J Reprod Fertility 77:633–643

Clark DA, Chaput A, Tutton B (1986b) Active suppression of host versus graft reaction in pregnant mice. VII. Spontaneous abortion of CBA × DBA/2 foetuses in the uterus of CBA/J mice correlates with deficient no-T suppressor cell activity. J Immunol 136:1668–1771

Clark DA, Banwatt D, Chaouat G (1983) Stress triggered abortion in mice is prevented by alloimmunisation. Am J Reprod Immunol 29(3):141–148

Clark DA, Chaouat G, Mogil R, Wegmann TG (1994) Prevention of spontaneous abortion in DBA/2 mated CBA/J mice by GM CSF involves CD8+ T cell dependent suppression of natural effector cells cytotoxicity against trophoblast target cells. Cell Immunol 154(1):143–153

Cochet M, Casrouge A, Dumont AM, Transy C, Baleux F, Lee Maloy W, Coligan John E, Cazenave PA, Kourilsky P (1989) A new cell surface molecule closely related to mouse class I transplantation antigens. Eur J Immunol. 19:1927–1931

Croy BA, Rossant J, Clark DA (1985) Effects of alterations in the immunocompetent status of Mus Musculus females on the survival of transferred Mus caroli embryos. J. Reprod. Fertil 74:479–489

De Fougerolles R, Baines M (1988) Modulation of natural killer activity influences resorption rates in CBA × DBA/2 matings. J Reprod Immunol 11(2):147

De Smedt et al (1996) Induction of transient T cell energy by low MW placental factor. Cell Immunology (in press)

Delassus S, Countinho GS, Saucier S, Darche S, Kourilky P (1994) Differential cytokine expression in maternal blood and placenta during murine gestation. J Immunol 152:2411–2420

Dosne Pasqualini C, Matusevitch R (1980) Induction of runting by pretreatment of the mother with paternal tumor antigens. In: Fougerean M, Paussel J (eds) 4th International Congress of Immunology, Abstract 165.11. Société Française d'Immunologie

Douglas GW, Thomas L, Carr M et al (1959) Trophoblast in the circulating blood during pregnancy. Am J Obstet Gynecol 78:960
Dresser DW (1991) The potentiating effect of pregnancy on humoral immune response of mice. J Reprod Immunol 20:253
Duc HT, Masse A, Bobe P, Kinsky RG, Voisin GA (1986) Deviation of humoral and cellular alloimmune reactions by placental extracts. J Reprod Immunol 7:27–39
Edelman P (1983) Cytotoxicité maternelle anti paternelle et avortement répétition. In: Edelmann P, Sureau C (eds) Immunologie de la reproduction humaine. Sandoz, Basel
Ellis SA (1990) HLA-G: at the interface. Am J Reprod Immunol 23:84–86
Ellis SA, Sargent IL, Redman CWG, McMichael AJ (1986) Evidence for a novel LA antigen found on human extravillous trophoblast and choriocarcinoma cell line. Immunology 59:595–601
Engleman EG, McMichael AJ, McDevitt HO (1978) Suppression of the mixed lymphocyte reaction in man by a soluble T cell factor: specificity of the factor for both the responder and the stimulator, J Exp Med 147:1037–1045
Fabris N, Painatanelli L, Muzzioli M (1977) Differential effects of pregnancy and gestagens on cell mediated immunity Clin Exp Immunol 28:306
Gendron RL, Baines M (1988) Infiltrating decidual natural killer cells are associated with spontaneous abortion in mice. Cell Immunol 113:261
Gendron RL, Nestel FP, Lapp WS, Baines MG (1989) Lipopolysaccharide induced fetal resorbtion involves embryo associated production of tumor necrosis factor 7th International Congress on Immunology Berlin Abstr 118/017
Genetet N (1988) Immunité cellulaire maternelle en grossesse. Communication la Société Franaise d'Etude de la Fertilité et de la Stérilité, Paris. PhD thesis, University of Rennes
Genetet N, Genetet B, Fauchet R (1982) Allogeneic responses in, vivo induced by feto maternal alloimmunisation. Am J Reprod Immunol 2:90
Gill TJ (1996) Am J Reprod Immunol (in press)
Gottesman S, Stutman O (1980a) Cellular immunity during pregnancy. Proliferative and cytotoxic activity of para aortic lymph nodes. Am J Reprod Immunol 1:10
Gottesman S, Stutman O (1980b) Cellular immunity during pregnancy. II. Response to T and B cell mitogens. Am J Reprod Immunol 1:57
Hamaoka T, Majusaki N, Itoh S, Tsuji Y, Izumi Y, Fujiwarah, Ono S (1983) Human trophoblast and tumor cell derived immunoregulatory factor. In: Billington WD, Isojima S (eds) Reproductive immunology III. Elsevier, Amsterdam, pp 103–107
Hamaoka T, Itoh K, Izumi Y, Ono S (1987) Selective Suppression of class II MHC-directed responses by soluble factors. In: Gill TJ, Wegmann TG (eds) Immunoregulation and fetal survival. Oxford University Press Oxford, pp 169–180
Hart CA (1988) Pregnancy and host resistance. Clin Immunol Allergy Allergy 2:735
Herzenberg LA, Bianchi DW, Schroder J et al (1979) Fetal cells in the blood of pregnant women: detection and enrichment by fluorescence-activated cell sorting. Proc Natl Acad Sci USA 76:1453
Heyhorne K, Fu YX, Nelson A, Farr A, O'Brien R, Born W (1994) Recognition of trophoblast by gamma delta T cells. J Immunol 153:2918–2926
Hogarth PJ (1982) Immunological aspects of mammalian reproduction. Blackie, Glasgow
Holland D, Bretscher P, Russel AS (1984) Immunologic and inflammatory responses during pregnancy. Clin Lab Immunol 14:177
Hoversland RC, Beaman KD (1990) Embryo implantation associated with increase in T cell suppressor factor in the uterus and spleen of mice. J Reprod Fertil 88:135–139
Hoversland RC, Beaman KD (1991) The lack of effect of a monoclonal antibody against murine T cell suppressor factor on murine embryo development in vitro. Am J Reprod Immunol 26:84–88
Jenkinson EJ, Owen V (1980) Ontogeny and distribution of major histocompatibility complex (MHC) antigens on mouse placental trophoblast. J Reprod Immunol 2:173–181
Kachkache M, Acker GM, Chaouat G, Noun A, Garabedian M (1991) Hormonal and local factors control the immunohistochemical distribution of immunocytes in the rat uterus before conceptus implantation: effects of ovariectomy, fallopian tube section and RU 486 injection. Biol Reprod 45:860
Kaliss N, Dagg NK (1964) Immune responses engendered in mice by multiparity. Transplantation 2:415–420
Kanbour A, Hong Nerg HO, Misra DN, MacPherson T, Kunz HW, Gill TJ (1987) Differential expression of MHC class I antigens on the placenta of the rat. A mechanism for the survival of the fetal allograft J Exp Med 166:1861

Kanbour-Sharir A, Zhang X, Rouleau A, Armstrong DT, Kunz HW, MacPherson TA, Gill TJ (1990) Gene imprinting and major histocompatibility complex class I antigen expression in the rat placenta. Proc Natl Acad Sci USA 87:444–448
Khrihsnan L, Menu E, Chaouat G, Talwar GP, Raghupathy R (1991) In vitro and in vivo immunosuppressive effects of supernatants from human choriocarcinoma. Cell Immunol 138:313–326
Kinsky R, Delage G, Rosin N, Thang MN, Hoffmann M, Chaouat G (1990) A murine model of NK cell mediated resorption. Am J Reprod Immunol 23:73
Kinsky R, Menu E, Delage G, Rosin N, Thang MN, Hoffmann M, Kapovic M, Jaulin C, Kourilsky P, Wegmann TJ, Chaouat G (1991) Murine NK cell mediated resorption and prevention by maternal alloimmunisation. In: chaouat G, Howbray J (eds) Biologie cellulaire et moléculaire de la relation materno fétale. Libbey, Paris, pp 245–261
Kinsky R, Kapovic M, Menu E, Jaulin C, Kourilksy P, Wegmann TG, Thank MN, Chaouat G (1993) The role of defined major histocompatibility antigens in preventing fetal death. In: Chaouat G (ed) The Immunology of pregnancy. CRC, Boca Ratou, pp 47–61
Kovatts S, Main EK, Libbrach C, Stublebline M, Fischer SJ, De Mars R (1990) A class I antigen, HLA-G, expressed in human trophoblasts. Science 248:220–223
Kovatts S, Librach C, Main EK, Sondel PM, Fischer SJ, De Mars R (1991) The role of non classical MHC class I on human trophoblast. In: Chaouat G, Mowbray J (eds) Biologie cellulaire et moléculaire de la relation materno fétale Libbey, Paris, pp 13–21, 41–51
Kovitavong T, Dossetor JB (1981) Suppressor T cells in rat pregnancy. In: Gill TG, Wegmann TG (eds) First Banff meeting. Banff, University of Alberta, Edmonton
Kurago ZH, Smith KD, Lutz CT (1995) NK cells recognition of MHC class I: NK cells are sensitive to peptide binding groove and surface alpha helical mutations that affect T cells. J Immunol 154(6):2631–2642
Labarrere C, Faulk WP (1995) Maternal cells in chorionic villi from placentae of normal and abnormal human pregnancies. Am J Reprod Immunol 33(1):54–60
Laesen B, Galask RP (1978) Host parasite interactions during pregnancy. Obstet Gynaecol surv 33:297
Lanman JT, Dinenstein J, Fikring S (1962) Homograft immunity in pregnancy. Lack of harm to foetus from sensitisation of the mother. Ann N Y Acad Sci 99:706–718
Lee CK, Ghoshal K, Beaman KD (1990) Cloning of a cDNA coding for a T cell molecule with putative immunoregulatory role. Mol Immunol 27:1134–1137
Lelaidier C (1995) Early embryo development, uterus preparation, and role of cytokines in implementation INSERM pp 182–198
Liburd J, Dossetor JB (1982) Suppressor cells in human pregnancy. In: Gill TG III, Wegmann TG (eds) First Banff meeting. Banff, University of Alberta, Edmonton
Lin H, Mossman TR, Guilbert L, Tuntipopipat S, Wegmann TG (1993) Synthesis of T helper -2 cytokines at the maternal fetal interface. J Immunol 151:4562
Luft, BJ, Remington JS (1984) Effect of pregnancy on augmentation of natural killer activity by Corynebacterium parvum and toxoplasma Gondii J Immunol 132:2375
MacMaster MT, Newton RC, Sudhanski KD, Andrews GK (1992) Activation and distribution of inflammatory cells in the mouse uterus during the preimplantation period. J Immunol 148:1699–1711
Mattson R (1982) Increase in the number of plaque forming cells with length of gestation in untreated pregnant mice. Dev Comp Immunol 6:339–348
Mattson R, Holmdal R (1987) Maintained allopregnancy in rats depleted of T cytotoxic/suppressor cells by OX8 monoclonal antibody treatment. J Reprod Immunol 12:23–24
Mattson R, Mattson A, Sulila P (1985) Allogeneic pregnancy in B cell depleted CBA/Ca mice. Effects on fetal survival and maternal lymphoid organs. Dev Comp Immunol 9:709–717
Mattsson R, Holmdahl R, Scheynius A, Bernadotte F, Mattsson L (1989) Allopregnancy in mice treated with recombinant rat interferon-gamma. J Reprod Immunol Suppl 151
Mattson R, Holmdahl R, Scheynius A, Bernadotte F, Mattsson L (1991) Placental MHC class I antigen expression is induced in mice following in vivo treatment with recombinant interferon gamma. J Reprod Immunol 19(2):115–129
Medawar PB (1953) Some immunological and endocrinological problems raised by the evolution of viviparity in vertebrates. Symp Soc Exp Biol 7:320–338
Meinecke Tillmann S, Meinecke B (1994) Experimental chimeras – removal of reproductive barrier between sheep and goat. Nature 307:637–638
Menu E, Chaouat G, Kinsky R, Delage G, Kapovic M, Thang MN, Jaulin C, Kourilsky P, Wegmann TG (1995) Alloimmunisation against well defined polymorphic major histocompatibility or class I MHC

transfected L cells can prevent POLY IC induced fetal death in mice. Am J Reprod Immunol 33:200–312

Mitchison NA (1953) The effect on the offspring of maternal immunisation in mice. J Genet 5:406–411

Monnot P, Chaouat G (1984) Systemic active suppression is not necessary for successful allopregnancy. Am J Reprod Immunol 6:5–8

Mori T, Nishikawa T, Saito S, Enomotop M, Ito A, Kurai K, Shimoayama T, Ichijo M, Narita N (1983) T cell receptors are expressed but down regulated on intra decidual T lymphocytes. Am J Reprod Immunol 29(1):1–5

Nelson K, Cory J, Hellstrom I, Hellsstrom K (1980) A suppressor T cell hybridoma. Proc Natl Acad Sci USA 7:2866

Noun A, Acker G, Chaouat G, Antoine JC, Garabedian M (1989) Macrophages and T lymphocyte bearing antigens bearing cells in the uterus before and during ovum implantation in the rat. Clin Exp Immunol 78:434–438

O'Hearn M, Hilard F (1981) Pregnancy induced alteration in graft versus host reactions of uterine and peripheral lymph nodes during towards fetal alloantigens. Transplantation 32:389

Paldi A, D'Auriol L, Misrahi M, Bakos A, Chaouat G, Szekeres Bartho J (1994) Expression of the gene coding for the progesterone receptor in activated human lymphocytes. Endocr J 2:317–319

Parand M, Chedid L (1964) Protective effects of chlorpromazine against endotoxin induced abortion. Proc Soc Exp Biol Med 116:906–915

Pavia CS, Stites DP (1979) Humoral and cellular immunity during pregnancy. J Immunol 123:2194–220

Peck AB, Bach FB (1973) A miniaturised mouse mixed lymphocyte culture in serum free and mouse serum supplemented media. J Immunol Methods 3:147

Reagan L, Raude PR (1987) Is paternal cytotoxic antibody a valid marker for the treatment of recurrent abortion. Lancet 2:280

Redline RW, Lu CY (1988) Specific defects in the anti listerial immune response in discrete regions of the murine uterus and placenta account for the susceptibility to infection. J Immunol 140:3497

Redline CW, Lu CY (1990) Localisation of fetal MHC antigens and maternal leukocytes in murine placenta. Lab Invest 61:27–38

Reznikoff-Etievant MF, Simonney N, Janaud A, Darbois Y, Netter A (1985) Treatment of recurrent spontaneous abortions by immunisation with paternal leukocytes. Lancet 1:1398

Rich SS, Rich RR (1976) Regulatory mechanisms in cell mediated immune responses III Region control of suppressor cell interaction with responder cells in mixed lymphocyte reactions. J Exp Med 140:1588

Rodger JC (1985) Lack of requirement for a maternal humoral immune response to establish or maintain a successful allogeneic pregnancy. Transplantation 40:372–375

Rossant J, Mauro VM, Croy BA (1982) Importance of trophoblast genotype for survival of interspecific murine chimeras. J Embryol Exp Morphol 69:141

Schroder J (1975) Transplacental passage of blood cells. J Med Genet 12:230

Singh B, Raghupathy R, Anderson DJ, Wegman TG (1983) The murine placenta as an immunological barrier between the mother and the fetus. In: Wegmann TG, Gill TG III (eds) Immunology of reproduction. Oxford University Press, New York (51st Banff conference)

Smith G (1981) Maternal regulator cells during murine pregnancy. Clin Exp Immunol 44:90–98

Smith JA, Burton RC, Barg M, Mitchell GF (1978) Maternal alloimmunisation in pregnancy. In vitro studies of T cell dependent immunity of paternal alloantigens. Transplantation 25:216

Smith RN, Powell AE (1977) The transfer of pregnancy induced hyporesponsiveness to male skin grafts with thymus dependent spleen cells. J Exp Med 156:899–911

Smith RN, Sternlicht M, Butler M (1982a) The alloantibody response in the allogeneically pregnant rat. I. The primary and secondary antibody response and the detection of Ir gene control. J Immunol 129:771–776

Smith RN, Margolies RT, Butler M (1982b) The alloantibody response in the allogeneically pregnant rat. II. Primary pregnancy induced anti RTI-A antibodies are not as cross reactive as secondary pregnancy induced or conventionally raised alloantibodies. J Immunol 129:777–782

Stern MM, Kahan MC (1980) Mixed lymphocyte reactivity and anti H-2 cytotoxicity during murine pregnancy. In: Fougereau M, Dausset J (eds) 4 th International Congress of Immunology, Paris 1980. Book of abstracts. Abstract 16.5.32. Societé Française d'Immunologie, Paris

Szekeres Bartho J, Chaouat G (1990) A T cell derived progesterone induced blocking factor correct resorbtions in a murine abortion system. Am J Reprod Immunol 23:26–29

Szekeres Bartho J, Kilar F, Falkay G, Csernu V, Torok A, Pacsa AS (1985) Progesterone treated lymphocytes release a substance inhibiting cytotoxicity and prostaglandin synthesis. Am J Reprod Immunol 9:15

Szekeres Bartho J, Reznikoff-Etievant M, Varga P, Pichon MF, Vargo Z, Chaouat G (1989a) Lymphocytic progesterone receptors in human pregnancy. J Reprod Immunol 16:239

Szekeres Bartho J, Autran B, Debre P, Andreu G, Denver L, Blot P, Chaouat G (1989b) Immunoregulatory effects of a suppressor factor from healthy pregnant women's lymphocytes after progesterone induction. Cell Immunol 122:281

Szekeres Bartho J, Szekeres G, Debre P, Autran B, Chaouat G (1990) Reactivity of lymphocytes to a progesterone receptor specific monoclonal antibody. Cell Immunol 125:273

Szekeres Bartho J, Kinsky R, Kapovic M, Chaouat G, Varga P, Csizar T (1993) The role of immuno endocrine mechanisms in pregnancy termination. In: Szekeres Bartho J (ed) Reproductive immunology. Raven, New York, pp 217–221 (Serono symposium 97)

Tafuri A, Alferink J, Moler P, Hämmerling G, Arnold B (1995) T cell awareness of paternal alloantigens during pregnancy. Science 270:630–633

Tamaki J, Arimura Y, Koda S, Fujimoto S, Fujino T, Wakisaka A, Kaminuma M (1993) Heterogeneity of HLA-G genes identified by polymerase chain reaction/single strand conformational polymorphism (PCR/SSCP). Microbiol Immunol 37:633

Tangri S, Raghupathy R (1993) Expression of cytokines in placenta of mice undergoing immunologically mediated fetal resorption. Biol Reprod 49(4):840–850

Tangri S, Wegmann TG, Lin H, Raghupathy R (1994) Maternal anti placental activity in natural, immunologically mediated fetal resorption. J Immunol 152:4903

Tartakowsky B, Gorelik E (1986a) Murine models of immunologically induced abortions. Coll INSERM 154:399

Tartakowsky B, Gorelik E (1986b) Murine abortion models. In: Wegmann TG, Gill TJ (eds) The placenta and the survival of the fetal allograft. Oxford University Press, (Reproductive immunology II) Oxford

Tartakowsky B, Gorelik E (1988) Immunisation with asyngeneic regressor tumor causes resorptions in allopregnant mice. J Reprod Immunol 13(2):113

Tezabwala BU, Jonhson PM, Rees RC (1989) Inhibition of pregnancy viability in mice following IL-2 administration. Immunology 67:115–120

Toder V Shomer B (1990) The role of lymphokines in pregnancy. Immunol Allergy Clin North Am 10(1):65–77

Toder V, Shepelovitch J, Carp H, Altaraz H, Strassburger D (1991) Cytokine function in immunopotentiated females. In: Chaouat G, Mowbray J (eds) Biologie cellulaire et moléulaire de la relation materno fêtale. Libbey, Paris, 263

Van der ven K, Ober C (1993) HLA-G polymorphism in African Americans. J Immunol 153:5628

Vanzoorn CJ (1986) Cortisol and malaria immunity during pregnancy. PhD thesis, University of Nijmegen

Vleughels AC (1990) Cerebral malaria immunity and pregnancy. PhD thesis, University of Nijmegen

Voisin GA (1962) Immunological tolerance to living cells. Homologus disease and immunological facilitation (enhancement phenomenon). A working hypothesis allowing a unified concept. In: Hasek M, Lengerova A, Vostiskova M (eds) Symposium on mechanism of immunological tolerance. Czechoslovakian Academy of Science, Prague, pp 435–455

Voisin GA (1971) Immunological facilitation. A broadening of the concept of the enhancement phenomenon Prog Allergy 15:328–485

Voisin G, Chaouat GA (1974) Demonstration, nature and properties of antibodies eluted from the placenta and directed against paternal antigens. J Reprod Fertili Suppl 21:89

Voisin JE, Monnot P, Voisin GA (1986) Maternal alloimmune reactions towards the conceptus and GVHR. I. Priming for antipaternal GVHR by gestation. J Reprod Immunol 9:73–81

Wegmann TG, Waters CA, Drell DW, Carlson GA (1979a) Pregnant mice are not primed but can be primed to fetal allo antigens. Proc Natl Acad Sci USA 76:2410–2412

Wegmann TG, Mossman TR, Carlson G, Olingk O, Singh B (1979b) The ability of the murine placenta to absorb monoclonal anti fetal H-2 K antibody from the maternal circulation. J Immunol 122:270–277

Wegmann TG (1984) Fetal protection against abortion: is it immunosuppression or immunostimulation? Ann Immunol (Paris) 135 D:309

Wegmann TG, Athanassakis I, Mogil R, Chaouat G (1988) Placental immunotrophism. Maternal T cells contribute to the growth and survival of the fetal allograft. In: proceedings VI World Congress on Human Reproduction, Elsevier, Amsterdam

Wegmann TG, Athanassakis I, Guilbert L, Branch D, Dy M, Menu E, Chaouat G (1989) The role of M-CSF and GM-CSF in fostering placental growth, fetal growth, and fetal survival. Transplant Proc 21(11):89, 566–569

Wegmann TG, Athanassakis I, Guilbert L, Branch D, Dy M, Menu E, Chaouat G (1991) Maternal T cell reactivity as a positive determinant of placental growth and fetal survival. In: Belissarion R, Mijezewski G (eds) Transplantation disorders. Prenatal detection, treatment and management. Liss, New York, pp 69–76

Wegmann TG, Lin H, Guilbert L, Mossman TH (1993) Bi-directional cytokines interactions in the materno fetal relationship: successful allopregnancy is a Th2 phenomenon. Immunol Today 14:353–355

Weidanz WP (1982) Malaria and alterations in immune reactivity. Br Med Bull 38:167

Whaley AE, Caroll RS, Nephew KP, Imakawa K (1991a) Molecular cloning of unique interferons from human placenta. In workshop of annual meeting of the International Society for Interferon Research. Nice (France). J Interferon Res 11 [Suppl] (abstract)

Whaley AE, Caroll RS, Imakawa K (1991b) Cloning and analysis of a gene encoding ovine interferon a-II. Gene 106:281–282

Yokoyama M, Sano M, Sonanda K, Nnozaki M, Nakamura G, Nakano H (1995) Cytotoxic cells directed against human placental cells detected in human habitual abortion by an in vitro terminal labelling assay? Am J Reprod Immunol 31(4):197–205

Zagury D, Chaouat G, Morgan DA, Voisin GA (1979) Participation aux mécanismes de suppression de la réaction immunitaire de cellules pouvoir cytotoxique en présence de lectines. CR Acad Sci [D] (Paris) 288:1343–1346

Immunobiology of the Trophoblast: Mechanisms by Which Placental Tissues Evade Maternal Recognition and Rejection

D.S. TORRY[1], J.A. MCINTYRE[2], and W.P. FAULK[2]

1 Introduction

The ability of women to gestate a fetus that is immunologically foreign has been the subject of intense study since the early 1950s. Indeed, an often-cited review of this problem was published in the 1960s by BILLINGHAM (1964), a colleague of Sir Peter Medawar. To this day the precise mechanisms supporting this phenomenon are still undefined, although several possibilities exist. The complexity of this problem is underpinned by the possibility that an immunobiological endeavor such as pregnancy probably does not, nor should not, rely on any one specific immune mechanism for success. It is well established that many pregnant women do not reject their embryos; what remains controversial, however, is to what extent an aberrant immune response to the pregnancy is responsible for those instances in which the fetus is lost. In fact, it is an assumption for us to discuss this problem as though it is

[1]Department of Obstetrics and Gynecology, University of Tennessee Graduate School of Medicine, 1924 Alcoa Highway, Knoxville, TN 37920, USA
[2]Center for Reproduction and Transplantation Immunology, Methodist Hospital of Indiana, Indianapolis, IN 46202, USA

essentially immunological, albeit this is our persuasion (FAULK et al. 1978; FAULK and MCINTYRE 1981, 1983; TORRY et al. 1989).

For successful pregnancy to occur in the fully immunocompetent woman the fetus must be able to evade either maternal immune recognition (the afferent arm) or immune rejection (the efferent arm). Conceivably, both mechanisms may be operative at the maternofetal interface. The end result of these processes is the same; a genetically foreign embryo is allowed to implant and develop for the duration of the gestation period. The mechanisms by which the fetus derives this privilege may be quite distinct. These range from modulation of maternal immune responses (for example, blocking antibodies) to the uniqueness and largely uncharacterized nature of characteristic trophoblast antigens (for example, HLA-G).

Essential to pregnancy and pivotal to the understanding of immune events at the maternal-fetal interface is the trophoblast. Because the trophoblast is thought to line all areas of contact between the fetus and mother, the trophoblast rather than the fetus per se must avoid being targeted by the maternal immune system. The ability of the trophoblast to evade immunological detection and /or rejection is the focus of this review, with the caveat that biochemical knowledge of the various types of so-called trophoblast antigens remains far from complete.

2 Evasion of the Afferent Arm of the Immune System

2.1 Role of Classical HLA Gene Expression

Perhaps the single most important facility that trophoblast possesses to evade maternal immune detection is the ability to suppress expression of conventional, polymorphic HLA class I and II antigens (reviewed by HUNT and ORR 1992). It is the lack of expression of classical histocompatibility antigens HLA-A, B, C, DR, DQ, and DP that separates placentation from other solid organ allografts. In addition to the lack of constitutive expression of classical HLA antigens, the trophoblast is thought to be resistant to cytokine-induced upregulation of these antigens (HUNT et al. 1987). This trait appears to be unique to trophoblast, for other somatic mammalian cells can be induced to increase expression of classical class I antigens (DAVID-WATINE et al. 1990).

The molecular mechanisms regulating HLA gene expression in trophoblast have received a great deal of investigative attention. What follows is an overview of the regulatory mechanisms thought to influence HLA expression in trophoblast. Readers are encouraged to examine a recent review of this subject published by LE BOUTEILLER (1995).

At the molecular level, the lack of expression of classical HLA class I antigens in trophoblast may result from both transcriptional and post transcriptional regulatory processes. Transcription of classical class I antigens in human trophoblast appears to be down-regulated by both *cis*-acting and *trans*-acting mechanisms. One prominent *cis*-acting regulatory mechanism is methylation of CpG islands near transcriptional start sites in genes. Typically such methylation results in decreased transcriptional activity of a particular gene (RAZIN and CEDAR 1991). Hypermethylation of CpG islands near the transcription start sites of human class I genes was found in the choriocarcinoma cell line JAR, a cell line known not to express HLA, A, B, C, F, or G (BOUCRAUT et al. 1993). Notably, methylation of CpG islands in HLA-E was not detected, and this class I gene is actively transcribed in these cells.

Curiously, methylation of CpG islands may not be uniquely responsible for controlling HLA class I expression in normal trophoblast (GUILLAUDEUX et al. 1995). No clear differences in CpG island methylation within HLA-A and –B loci were observed between in vitro differentiated syncytiotrophoblast and cytotrophoblast from term placenta, even though transcription was more active in the cytotrophoblast. Similarly, unmethylated HLA-G CpG islands were found in both cytotrophoblast and syncytiotrophoblast from term placenta, even though HLA-G expression is minimal in syncytiotrophoblast. This of course assumes that the classical morphological definitions of cytotrophoblast and syncytiotrophoblast are adequate to describe truly different populations, and at what point in their differentiation such differences become manifest. Nonetheless, alternative mechanisms of regulating gene expression or posttranslational regulation are active in trophoblast to repress HLA-A, -B, and -C expression.

Another regulatory mechanism known to influence expression of MHC class I molecules at the transcriptional level is the presence of a negative regulatory element upstream of the transcription start site of murine class I antigens (FLANAGAN et al. 1991). An identical sequence to that in mouse $H\text{-}2L^d$ is present in human HLA-A2 (CHIANG and MAIN 1994). Nuclear extracts from the HLA classical class I-negative choriocarcinoma cell lines JEG-3 and BeWo demonstrated specific binding to this negative regulatory element while extracts from control cells which express classical HLA gene products did not demonstrate significant binding. Importantly, the nonclassical MHC gene HLA-G lacks this consensus negative regulatory element, and this may enable expression of HLA-G in the enigmatic trophoblast.

In addition to regulation of HLA gene expression at the transcription level, there is evidence to support the idea that posttranslational mechanisms function in trophoblast to regulate HLA expression. Apparently, low level transcription of HLA-A and HLA-B genes exist in term villous cytotrophoblast, and the level decreases even more following in vitro differentiation to syncytiotrophoblast (GUILLAUDEUX et al. 1995). Despite low but detectable levels of transcription no surface HLA expression was detected. Similarly, HLA-G mRNA was detectable in villous cytotrophoblast, but cell-surface expression of the protein was not detected (CHUMBLEY et al. 1993; GUILLAUDEUX et al. 1995; HUNT and ORR 1992).

Expression of both chains of the class II MHC antigen DR α and β alleles may be regulated in a similar manner in first-trimester cytotrophoblast. These normal trophoblast displayed high levels of mRNA for HLA-DR and its invariant chain Ii although surface protein expression of these antigens was not detected (GIACOMINI et al. 1994). Furthermore, transcription of DR α, β, and Ii was inducible by interferon γ treatment of the trophoblast, although no surface antigen was detected. These data provide convincing evidence for a dissociation between mRNA production and protein expression that adds an additional level of regulation to the expression of conventional HLA class I and II antigens in trophoblast. Although the mechanisms postulated to down-regulate classical HLA gene expression in trophoblast are varied, the net result is that these highly polymorphic proteins are not expressed on the cell surface membranes of trophoblast.

2.2 Role of Other Allotypic Antigens

The presence or absence of polymorphic HLA antigens on trophoblast has attracted considerable attention in reproductive immunology, most likely because of the analogy often made between pregnancy and transplantation. In that the major hurdle in organ transplantation is HLA incompatibility, it is befitting that such attention has been emphasized concerning reproduction. However, other allotypic antigens have been proposed to be expressed by trophoblast. In light of the ability of the immune system to recognize and destroy "nonself" it is reasonable to assume that the maternal immune system is down-regulated to allotypic trophoblast antigens which can promote immune-mediated damage to the trophoblast. This statement is admittedly facile, although it appears to be true, at least in normal pregnancies.

2.3 Role of HLA-G

Within the MHC class I gene family there exists a large number of loci which encode class I molecules with the unifying trait of being oligomorphic (reviewed in SHAWAR et al. 1994). These genes are referred to as class IB genes to distinguish them from the conventional, highly polymorphic class IA gene products. One such member of the class IB family postulated to have a function in reproduction is HLA-G. Although HLA-G has been referred to historically as a non- or mono-polymorphic antigen, there is increasing evidence that a significant amount of polymorphism may exist (ALIZADEH et al. 1993; VAN DER VEN and OBER 1994).

One large study of HLA-G polymorphism in an African-American population showed that amino acid substitutions were clustered within the α_1 and α_2 domains, reminiscent of the polymorphism seen in classical HLA antigens (VAN DER VEN and OBER 1994). Additionally, the α_2 domain contained the most variability and was postulated, in this cohort of subjects, to be responsible for approximately 67% of these individuals' heterozygosity for HLA-G at the protein level. The peptide binding groove of HLA-G contains nine of the ten conserved amino acids in classical HLA class I antigens that are thought to be important for peptide binding and antigen presentation to T-cell receptors (reviewed in SCHMIDT and ORR 1993). It is clear from many studies that class IB antigens are capable of presenting antigen

(Shawar et al. 1994). At present it is not known whether HLA-G functions at the maternal-fetal interface to generate antigen-specific T cell responses. Also, the role of amplifying molecules such as intracellular cell adhesion molecule 1 (ICAM-1) is limited, although ICAM-1 has been identified on endovascular cytotrophoblasts of spiral arteries in certain abnormal pregnancies (Labarrere and Faulk 1995).

In the context of this review the functional properties of HLA-G are considered to be less important than the possibility that polymorphism in HLA-G protein may serve as a target for maternal antifetal immune responses, for limited polymorphism may be present in HLA-G, and single amino acid changes in class IA molecules are immunogenic (Klein 1990). It remains to be seen whether the polymorphism in HLA-G induces maternal immune responses. Ironically, HLA-G has been proposed to protect trophoblast from maternal natural killer (NK) cell-mediated lysis (see below).

2.4 Role of Trophoblast Lymphocyte Cross-Reactive Antigen

Description of the lymphocyte cross-reactive (TLX) alloantigen system evolved from studies which showed that heterologous antisera produced to individual preparations of purified syncytiotrophoblast microvilli were cytotoxic when tested in complement-dependent assays against a panel of lymphocyte donors McIntyre and Faulk 1982). Mathematical analysis of the cytotoxic reaction patterns revealed three TLX antigen groupings which were independent of the HLA and AB0 designations assigned to the lymphocyte donors (McIntyre et al. 1983). Further studies of the TLX antigen system showed that these alloantigens, in addition to trophoblast and lymphocytes, are also expressed on platelets (Kajino et al. 1987) and are present in seminal plasma (Kajino et al. 1988) the latter being secreted by the seminal vesicle luminal epithelia (Thaler et al. 1989, 1990). Antibodies to TLX antigens were subsequently detected in the blood of a subgroup of women who suffered from repeated pregnancy failures (McIntyre et al. 1986). Experimental manipulation of the isolated human anti-TLX antibodies (discussed below) led to the hypothesis that normal pregnancy represents a balanced idiotype-antiidiotype TLX network, and that failure to establish or maintain such a balanced network can result in pregnancy failures (McIntyre et al. 1989). Immunochemical investigations have implicated the association of a complement component (C3b) with membrane cofactor protein (MCP, or CD46) that are necessary to produce an allotypic antigen that is recognizable by anti-TLX antisera (Roussev et al. 1991). Some investigators have mistakenly referred to MCP as the TLX antigen. This technical discretion is discussed in Roussev et al. (1993).

3 Evasion of the Efferent Arm of the Immune System

Although it is broadly agreed, with the original immunocytochemical observation, that conventional HLA molecules are not expressed on trophoblast (FAULK and TEMPLE 1976), other allotypic molecules can be recognized by the maternal immune system. It is therefore possible that mechanisms designed to regulate the efferent arm of the immune response provide protection from rejection. These modulatory mechanisms could be categorized as being either "specific" or "nonspecific," depending upon whether they function in a distinct antigen-restricted manner or via general nonspecific means.

3.1 Nonspecific Mechanisms

3.1.1 HLA-G

Selective expression of the class IB antigen HLA-G by trophoblast raises the prospect that it may have some biological function in pregnancy. Although no function has been definitively assigned to HLA-G, there is convincing evidence that it provides a degree of protection to cells from lysis by decidual NK-like cells (CHUMBLEY et al. 1994). Transfection of HLA-G into an HLA-A, B, C, negative cell line rendered partial resistance to lysis by decidual large granular lymphocytes (LGL). Curiously, resistance of the target cells to LGL-mediated lysis was dependent upon expression of transfected HLA-G reaching a critical level. This may contribute to the finding that in general the normal trophoblast is resistant to NK-mediated lysis (KING et al. 1989; HEAD 1989) as well as to macrophage-mediated damage (SIONOV et al. 1993). This of course assumes that investigators know what constitutes a normal trophoblast; however, such knowledge is based solely on morphological observations.

Lysis of trophoblast by decidual lymphokine-activated killer cells is possible (KING and LOKE 1993). Lysis by these activated NK-like cells can be suppressed by augmenting class I expression in the trophoblast with γ interferon (KING and LOKE 1993). The caveat to these induction experiments is that the interferon response element has been deleted from the 5' flanking region of HLA-G (SCHMIDT and ORR 1993). Nonetheless, expression of HLA-G may enable trophoblast to evade destruction by the maternal innate immune system, and the degree of expression may be critical to afford this protection.

3.1.2 Complement Regulatory Proteins

Complement components when activated can participate in both humoral and cellular immune responses to eliminate foreign antigens. Regulation of complement activity is an important adaptation for trophoblast which, as a foreign tissue, must evade maternal immunological rejection reactions (reviewed by VANDERPUYE et al.

1992). Indeed, maternal antibodies capable of fixing complement are formed during the course of both normal and abnormal pregnancies (KAJINO et al. 1988). Thus, the presence and unusually high density of membrane-bound complement regulatory proteins on trophoblast is not an unexpected observation.

Three membrane-bound glycoproteins have been described for trophoblast, each of which independently is capable of deactivating maternal complement should it become activated. These are: (a) MCP (CD46) (b) decay-accelerating factor (DAF, or CD55) and (c) membrane attack complex inhibitor (MAC inhibitor, or CD59). We and others have shown that these complement regulatory proteins are expressed on trophoblast in higher concentrations than in either kidney or liver cells (VANDERPUYE et al. 1993; HOLMES et al. 1992).

The two regulatory proteins MCP and DAF function to deactivate both alternative and classical pathway convertases, which are early events in the complement cascade, whereas the MAC inhibitor acts on the final stages of complement activation by inhibiting the assembly of the terminal components, C8 and C9. In spite of the documented presence of these complement regulatory proteins we have been chronically puzzled by the ubiquitous presence of activated complement components on the basement membranes of syncytiotrophoblast and fetal stem vessels of normal human placentae (FAULK and JOHNSON 1977; JOHNSON and FAULK 1978; FAULK et al. 1980). To date we have assumed that they are important in normal pregnancy, for they are increased in abnormal pregnancies (FAULK et al. 1980; SINAH et al. 1984).

3.1.3 Placental Proteins and Hormones

For decades researches have studied proteins and hormones produced by placentae as possible immunosuppressive factors. The driving force of this research has been the assumption that production of such factors by placentae avoids immune detection/rejection, and this has intuitively been thought to be advantageous for survival of the placental graft. Indeed, there is an extensive amount of literature concerning the potential immunosuppressive properties of various specific placental proteins and hormones. Unfortunately, a thorough discussion of the immunomodulating potentials of such factors is beyond the scope of this review. Interested readers are referred to a recent review of this subject (CHARD and GRUDZINSKAS 1992). This review concludes that, with the possible exception of placental protein 14, the specific placental proteins do not possess immunosuppressive properties. Another protein which is associated with growth and possible escape from immunosurveillance in tumor cells in the transferrin receptor (FAULK and GALBEAITH 1979; CRANE et al. 1990; BERCZI et al. 1993). Its role in protection of trophoblast has been discussed in an earlier review of trophoblast antigens (FAULK and HUNT 1988).

3.2 Specific Mechanisms

There is considerable debate as to whether the female immune system recognizes and responds to any fetal trophoblast antigens. Inasmuch as evolution of the immune system is thought to predate viviparous reproduction, it seems reasonable to believe that the maternal immune system has adapted to accept the fetal allograft. Confounding all studies attempting to detect maternal immune responses to trophoblast is the interpretation of negative findings. Depending upon the methods of detection, inability to demonstrate a specific in vitro immune response to trophoblast could be interpreted as meaning that either no immune response was initiated, or that specific down-regulation of a response had occurred. Differentiation between these two distinct possibilities is difficult. In fact, this may explain the often conflicting research reports regarding whether an immune response to trophoblast ensues during human pregnancy. There is evidence to support the concept that cellular immune reactivity to trophoblast is present in women (Yamada et al. 1994; Heyborne et al. 1994). Some of this evidence has been put forward by Chaouat (this volume). The remainder of this review summarizes potential regulation of maternal trophoblast immunity via the humoral immune system.

3.2.1 Idiotype-Antiidiotype Network

Several studies have documented the presence of trophoblast antibodies in the sera of normal pregnant women (Torry et al. 1989, 1991; McCrae et al. 1993; Davies 1985; Davies and Brown 1985; Kajino et al. 1988), although this is not a universal finding (Hole et al. 1987; Johnson et al. 1985). Nonetheless, as it is apparent that trophoblast immunity may occur during pregnancy, regulation of the response may be critical for successful pregnancy. Any putative immune regulatory mechanism hypothesized to act during pregnancy should meet the requirements of specificity and systemic activity. Specificity to assure that immunological acceptance of the fetus does not compromise the mother to other foreign antigens, and systemic to manage the extrauterine exposure to trophoblast antigens that occurs because of deportation of trophoblastic tissues during human pregnancy (O'Sullivan et al. 1982). A mechanism known to act systemically and allow for specific regulation of immune responses is the idiotype-antiidiotype network.

The idiotype of an immunoglobulin is restricted to the antigen-binding region of the antibody. This is the result of variable gene usage and recombinatorial processes used to construct that portion of the immunoglobulin molecule (Bona 1987). Due to the tremendous potential of the immunoglobulin repetroir, the existence of idiotypic determinants on immunoglobulins led to a proposal that antiidiotypes are produced to these determinants, and that such antiidiotypic antibodies serve to regulate the quality and quantity of an immune response (Jerne 1974).

An extensive amount of literature supports the idea that both humoral and cellular immune responses are influenced by the production of antiidiotypic antibodies. Specificity is one of the fundamental aspects of an adaptive immune system. This allows an organism to discriminate between different antigens, and because of idiotypic determinants on the resulting antibodies or T cell receptors, antiidiotype responses allow the organism to regulate independently immune responses to different challenges.

Most studies detailing the production of antiidiotypic antibodies during pregnancy have concentrated on HLA class IA and II specificities (AGRAWAL et al. 1994; BEHAR et al. 1991; HORINI and TERASAKI 1982; REED et al. 1983; SUCIU-FOCA et al. 1983; SINGAL et al. 1984; BONAGURA et al. 1987). Antiidiotypic antibodies to paternally induced DR-reactive maternal antibodies were found to inhibit lymphocytotoxicity in conventional DR typing assays (HORINI and TERASAKI 1982; REED et al. 1983). Such inhibition has been shown to be restricted to typing sera specific for paternal DR antigens. Thus, the antiidiotypes were DR specific, but they recognized cross-reactive idiotypes on cytotoxic DR antibodies. Several studies have shown that reactivity of DR antiidiotype is not restricted to immunoglobulin idiotypes (SUCIU-FOCA et al. 1983; SINGAL et al. 1984; BONAGURA et al. 1987). In these studies DR-specific antiidiotypes were able to bind to autologous maternal lymphocytes primed against paternal lymphocytes or to third party cells that shared DR specificities with the husband. This resulted in a significant reduction in both mixed lymphocyte reactions (SUCIU-FOCA et al. 1983; SINGAL et al. 1984) and cell-mediated cytotoxicity in a DR-restricted manner (BONAGURA et al. 1987).

The biological significance of HLA-DR antiidiotype during pregnancy was postulated in a report which showed that no such antiidiotypes were detected in three of three recurrent aborters, while sera from eight of nine normal parous women contained DR antiidiotype (SINGAL et al. 1984). Since the trophoblast does not express class II antigens, the biological function of DR antiidiotypes in normal pregnancy is unclear.

To date only a limited number of studies have addressed the production and function of trophoblast antiidiotypes during pregnancy (TORRY et al. 1989, 1991; CHAOUAT and LANKAR 1988). The finding of TLX antibodies in the sera of secondary aborters has prompted research into whether normally reproducing women produce TLX antiidiotype to down-regulate their trophoblast immune responses (TORRY et al. 1989).

We have shown that primigravida sera that demonstrated no antipaternal reactivity by conventional cytotoxicity assays were absorbed with immobilized TLX idiotype from a selected secondary aborter they competively displaced the primigravida antiidiotype and demonstrated cytotoxicity against target cells in an HLA-independent manner. In addition, IgG antiidiotype recovered from primigravidae was shown to block in vitro cytotoxicity mediated by secondary aborter sera (TORRY et al. 1989). The ability of an antiidiotype to react with idiotypic determinants from an unrelated source suggests that the antiidiotype recognizes a cross-reactive idiotypic determinant (CRI). These data also suggest that pregnant women normally produce antibodies to trophoblast antigens.

We have used a different approach to characterize the degree of CRI on secondary aborter TLX antibodies which provides a more practical method to screen for TLX antibodies in normal primigravidae and multiparae (Torry et al. 1991). In this approach rabbit antiidiotype was raised to affinity-isolated TLX antibodies from a single secondary aborter. This xenogeneic antiiodiotype detected a CRI in 6 of 11 secondary aborter IgG preparations known to contain demonstrable TLX immunoreactivity. The public idiotype specificity of the rabbit antiidiotype allowed studies to determine whether normal multiparae and primigravidae produce IgG TLX antibodies. A competitive binding assay was developed in which IgG from three of eight multiparous women and one of four primigravid women inhibited the rabbit antiidiotype from binding to its immunizing idiotype.

These data suggest that normally reproducing women produce TLX antibodies. By virtue of the experimental design these studies do not reflect the frequency with which normal women produce trophoblast antibodies but rather provide evidence that trophoblast immunity does occur during normal pregnancy. Notably, none of the multiparae or primigaravidae sera studied demonstrated antipaternal cytotoxicity in conventional assays. Thus, it would have been erroneously concluded that these women had no trophoblast directed immunity if their sera had been studied by using conventional antigen-binding assays.

The biological significance of trophoblast antiidiotype production during human pregnancy remains to be fully explored. However, studies performed in the mouse model of recurrent pregnancy loss support a role for trophoblast antiidiotype in assuring pregnancy success (Chaouat and Lankar 1988). For example, female CBA/J mice mated with DBA/2 males experience a high spontaneous resorption rate that can be prevented by preimmunization of the females with nonpaternal strain (BALB/c) lymphocytes (Kiger et al. 1985; Chavez et al. 1987). In an elegant study to determine whether trophoblast antiidiotype plays a role in protecting the pregnancy in this mating combination, CBA mice were immunized with BALB/c lymphocytes and anti-BALB/c idiotype purified by affinity isolation from BALB/c trophoblast (Chaouat and Lankar 1988). The isolated CBA anti-BALB/c antibodies were injected into naive CBA mice, and the resulting antiidiotype was affinity purified via column chromatography by using immobilized CBA anti-BALB/c idiotype. Such affinity-purified trophoblast antiidiotype was found to prevent the high resorption rate in CBA females when passively administered between days 0 and 6 of pregnancy. Interestingly, no effect was seen after day 8, suggesting that antiidiotype production is important during the initial stages of trophoblast implantation and outgrowth. These data significantly strengthen the possibility that the idiotype-antiidiotype network is a key mechanism by which the trophoblast evades the efferent arm of the maternal immune system.

Clinical manipulation of the trophoblast idiotype-antiidiotype network during human pregnancy may represent an attractive potential in the treatment of immunologically mediated recurrent pregnancy loss. One current treatment regime for recurrent pregnancy loss is the use of intravenously administered pooled IgG

(Coulam et al. 1991). The beneficial use of intravenous immunoglobulin (IvIg) in the treatment of antiphospholipid antibody syndrome has been ascribed to the presence of phospholipid antiidiotypic antibodies in the IvIg (Caccavo et al. 1994). Similarly, the beneficial use of IvIg as an alternative to immunization with leukocytes in the treatment of unexplained recurrent miscarriage is thought to be due to the passive increase in the patient of antiidiotypic antibodies present in the IvIg preparation (Maruyama et al. 1994). More detailed studies are required to characterize the presence and function of trophoblast idiotype-antiidiotype interactions in human pregnancy.

4 Concluding Remarks

The genetic disparity between the embryo and mother during pregnancy is certainly acceptable to and somehow tolerated by the maternal immune system. This may even be necessary for the normal growth and development of the fetoplacental unit. The mechanisms allowing this immune relationship are not well understood but probably involve aversion of both immune recognition and immune destruction of trophoblast. Immunological acceptance of the fetus is probably the culmination of both nonspecific and antigen-driven mechanisms.

Since a central function of the immune system is the recognition of nonself antigens, it is easy to accept that rejection of such antigens can be attained by either nonspecific or specific reactions. Contrary to this, it would appear that immunological acceptance would be best attained by antigen-specific mechanisms. Thus the pregnant woman immunologically recognizes the conceptus and, by as yet unknown means, allows the antigenically disparate graft to survive. This is quite distinct from the possibility that the embryo is devoid of antigenic determinants which allow it to evade maternal immune recognition entirely.

Pivotal to the lack of understanding of the mechanisms by which extraembryonic tissue evades maternal immune reactions is a fundamental lack of knowledge about the antigenic status of trophoblast. Conclusive evidence that a maternal immune response and regulation of that response are required for successful pregnancy will become clearer once discrete allotypic trophoblast antigens are characterized more definitively. The idea that such antigens exist has been based largely on the presence of maternal so called blocking antibodies in eluates of human placentae (Faulk et al. 1978), but the chemistry has not yet been carried out.

In closing, it should be stated that most research on the chemistry of trophoblast antigens has employed biochemical methods designed to identify proteins (e.g., TA1 antigens by Faulk et al. 1978; McIntyre and Faulk 1979a,b, and R80K antigens by Jalali et al. 1993), and only recently have candidate carbohydrate antigens been investigated (Arkwright et al. 1994). Additional studies will help to resolve these areas of investigation.

References

Agrawal S, Sharma RK, Kishore R, Agarwal SS (1994) Development of anti-idiotypic antibodies to HLA antigens during pregnancy. Indian J Med Res 99:42–46

Alizadeh M, Legras C, Semana G, Le Bouteiller P, Genetet B, Fauchet R (1993) Evidence for a polymorphism of HLA-G gene. Hum Immunol 38(3):206–212

Arkwright P, Rademacher T, Boutigon F, Dwek R, Redman C (1994) Suppression of allogeneic reactivity in vitro by the syncytiotrophoblast membrane glycocalyx of the human term placenta is carbohydrate dependent. Glycobiology 4:39–47

Behar E, Carp H, Livneh A, Gazit E (1991) Anti-idiotypic IgM antibodies to anti-HLA class I antibodies in habitual abortion. Am J Reprod Immunol 26(4):143–146

Berczi A, Barabas K, Sizensky JA, Faulk WP (1993) Adriamycin conjugates of human transferrin bind transferrin receptors and kill K562 and HL60 cells. Arch Biochem Biophys 300:356–362

Billingham RE (1964) Transplantation immunity and the maternal-fetal relation. N Engl J Med 270:667–672

Bona C (1987) Regulatory idiotopes. In: Bona C (ed) Modern concepts in immunology, vol 2 Wiley, New York, pp 152–174

Bonagura VR, Ma A, McDowell J, Lewison A, King DW, Suciu-Foca N (1987) Anticlonotypic autoantibodies in pregnancy. Cell Immunol 108:356–365

Boucraut J, Guillaudeux T, Alizadeh M, Boretto J, Chimini G, Malecaze F, Semana G, Fauchet R, Pontarotti P, Le Bouteiller P (1993) HLA-E is the only class I gene that escapes CpG methylation and is transcriptionally active in the trophoblast-derived human cell line JAR. Immunogenetics 38:117–130

Caccavo D, Vaccaro F, Ferri GM, Amoroso A, Bonomo L (1994) Anti-idiotypes against antiphospholipid antibodies are present in normal polyspecific immunoglobulins for therapeutic use. J Autoimmunity 7(4):537–548

Chaouat G, Lankar D (1988) Vaccination against spontaneous abortion in mice preimmunized with an anti-idiotypic antibody. Am J Reprod Immunol Microbiol 16:146–150

Chard T, Grudzinskas JG (1992) Plancental proteins and steriods and the immune relationship between mother and fetus. In: Coulam C, Faulk WP, McIntyre JA (eds) Immunological obstetrics. Norton, New York, pp 282–289

Chavez DJ, McIntyre JA, Collives JA, Faulk WP (1987) Allogeneic matings and immunization have different effects in nulliparous and multiparous mice. J Immunol 139:85–88

Chiang MH, Main EK (1994) Nuclear regulation of HLA class I genes in human trophoblasts. Am J Reprod Immunol 32(3):167–172

Chumbley G, King A, Holmes N, Loke YW (1993) In situ hybridization and northern blot demonstration of HLA-G mRNA in human trophoblast populations by locus-specific oligonucleotide. Hum Immunol 37(1):17–22

Chumbley G, King A, Robertson K, Holmes N, Loke YW (1994) Resistance of HLA-G and HLA-A2 transfectants to lysis by decidual NK cells. Cell immunol 155(2):312–322

Coulam C, Peters A, McIntyre JA, Faulk WP (1991) The use of IVIG for the treatment of recurrent spontaneous abortion. In: Morell A, Nydegger U (eds) Immunotherapy with intravenous immunologulins. Academic, London, pp 395–400

Crane FL, Low H, Sun IL, Morre DJ, Faulk WP (1990) Interaction between oxidoreductase, transferrin receptor and channels in the plasma membrane. In: Sara VR, Hall K, Low H (eds) Growth factors. From genes to clinical applications. Raven, New York, pp 228–239

David-Watine B, Isreal A, Kourilsky P (1990) The regulation and expression of MHC class I genes. Immunol Today 11:286–292

Davies M (1985) The formation of immune complexes in primiparous and multiparous human pregnancies. Immnol Lett 10:199–205

Davies M, Browne CM (1985) Anti-trophoblast antibody responses during normal human pregnancy. J Reprod Immunol 7:285–297

Faulk WP, Galbraith RM (1979) Trophoblast transferrin and transferrin receptors in the host-parasite relationship of human pregnancy. Proc R Soc Lond [Biol] 204:83–97

Faulk WP, Hunt JS (1988) Human trophoblast antigens. In: Rubin JM, Gleicher N (eds) Reproductive immunology. Saunders, Philadelphia, pp 27–47 (Immunology and allergy clinics of North America)

Faulk WP, Johnson PM (1977) Immunological studies of human placentae: identification and distribution of proteins in mature chorionic villi. Clin Exp Immunol 27:365–375

Faulk WP, McIntyre JA (1981) Trophoblast survival. Transplantation 32:1–5

Faulk WP, McIntyre JA (1983) Immunological studies of human trophoblast: markers, subsets and functions. Immunol Rev 75:139–175
Faulk WP, Temple A (1976) Distribution of β_2 microglobulin and HLA in chorionic villi of human placentae. Nature 262:799–802
Faulk WP, Temple A, Lovins RE, Smith (1978) Antigens of human trophoblasts: a working hypothesis for their role in normal and abnormal pregnancies. Proc Natl Acad Sci USA 75:1947–1951
Faulk WP, Galbraith RM, Keane M (1980) Immunological considerations of the feto-placental unit in diabetes. In: Irvine J (ed) Immunology of diabetes. Teviot Scientific, Edinburgh, pp 309–317
Flanagan JR, Murata M, Burke PA, Shirayoshi Y, Appella E, Sharp PA, Ozato K (1991) Negative regulation of the major histocompatibility complex class I promoter in embryonal carcinoma cells. Proc Natl Acad Sci USA 88(8):3145–3149
Giacomini P, Tosi S, Murgia C, Nobili F, Gaetani S, Gambari R, Nicotra MR, Simoni G, Maggi F, Natali PG (1994) First-trimester human trophoblast is class II major histocompatibility complex mRNA+/antigen. Hum Immunol 39(4):281–289
Guillaudeux T, Rodriguez AM, Girr M, Mallet V, Ellis SA, Sargent IL, Fauchet R, Alsat E, Le Bouteiller P (1995) Methylation status and transcriptional expression of the MHC class I loci in human trophoblast cells from term placenta. J Immunol 154(7):3283–3299
Head JR (1989) Can trophoblast be killed by cytotoxic cells? In vitro evidence and in vivo possibilities. Am J Reprod Immunol 20:100-105
Heyborne K, Fu Y-X, Nelson A, Farr A, O' Brein R, Born W (1994) Recognition of trophoblast by gamma/delta T Cells. J Immunol 154:2918–2926
Hole N, Cheng HM, Johnson PM (1987) Antibody reactivity against human trophoblast membrane antigens in the context of normal pregnancy and unexplained recurrent miscarriage? Collogue INSERM 154:213–224
Holmes C, Simpson KL, Okada H et al. (1992) Complement regulatory proteins at the feto-maternal interface during human placental development: distribution of CD59 by comparison with membrane cofactor protein (CD46) and decay accelerating factor (CD55). Eur J Immunol 22:1579–1585
Horini R, Terasaki P (1982) Autoanti-idiotypic antibody against DR antibody. Immunol 5:144–145
Hunt JS, Orr HT (1992) HLA and maternal-fetal recognition. FASEB J 6(6):2344–2348
Hunt JS, Andrews GK, Wood GW (1987) Normal trophoblast resist induction of class I HLA. J Immunol 138:2481–2487
Jalali GR, Rexai A, Underwood JL, Mowbray JF, Allen WR, Surridge S, Marthias S (1995) An 80 kDa syncytiotrophoblast alloantigen bound to maternal alloantibody in term placenta. Am J Reprod Immunol 33:213–220
Jerne NK (1974) Towards a network theory of the immune system. Annu Inst Pasteur Immunol 125c:373–389
Johnson PM, Faulk WP (1978) Immunological studies of human placentae: identification and distribution of proteins in immature chorionic villi. Immunology 34:1027–1035
Johnson PM, Cheng HM, Stevens VC, Matangkasombut P (1985) Antibody reactivity against trophoblast and trophoblast products. J Reprod Immunol 8:347–352
Kajino T, Faulk WP, McIntyre JA (1987) Antigens and human trophoblast: trophoblast-lymphocyte cross-reactive (TLX) antigens on platelets. Am J Reprod Immunol Microbiol 14:70–78
Kajino T, McIntyre JA, Faulk WP, Deng SC, Billington WD (1988) Trophoblast antibodies in normal pregnant and secondary aborting women. J Reprod Immunol 14:267–282
Kiger N, Chaouat G, Kolb JP, Wegmann TG, Guennet JL (1985) Immunogenetic studies of spontaneous abortion in mice. I. Preimmunization of the mother with allogeneic spleen cells. J Immunol 134:2966–2970
King A, Loke YW (1993) Effect of IFN-gamma and IFN-alpha on killing of human trophoblast by decidual LAK cells. J Reprod Immunol 23(1):51–62
King A, Birkby C, Loke YW (1989) Early human decidual cells exhibit NK activity against the K562 cell line but not against first trimester trophoblast. Cell Immunol 118:337–344
Klein J (1990) Antigens and other lymphocyte-activating substances. In: Klein J (ed) Immunology. Blackwell, Cambridge, MA, pp 269–293
Labarrere CA, Faulk WP (1995) Intercellular adhesion molecule-1 (ICAM-1) and HLA-DR antigens are expressed on endovascular cytotrophoblasts in abnormal pregnancies. Am J Reprod Immunol 33:47–53
Le Bouteiller P (1995) Regulation of HLA class I gene expression. In: Kurpisz M, Fernandez N (eds) Immunology of human reproduction. Bios Scientific Publishers, Oxford, pp 205–215

Maruyama T, Makino T, Iwasaki K, Sugi T, Saito S, Umeuchi M, Ozawa N, Matsubayashi H, Nozawa S (1994) The influence of intravenous immunoglobulin treatment on maternal immunity in women with unexplained recurrent miscarriage. Am J Reprod Immunol 31(1):7–18

McCrae KR, DeMichele AM, Pandhi P, Balsai MJ, Samuels P, Graham C, Lala PK, Cines DB (1993) Detection of antitrophoblast antibodies in the sera of patients with anticardiolipin antibodies and fetal loss. Blood 82:2730–2741

McIntyre JA, Faulk WP (1979a) Antigens of human trophoblast: effects of heterologous anti-trophoblast sera on lymphocyte responses in vitro. J Exp Med 149:824–836

McIntyre JA, Faulk WP (1979b) Trophoblast modulation of maternal allogeneic recognition. Proc Natl Acad Sci USA 76:4029–4032

McIntyre JA, Faulk WP (1982) Allotypic trophoblast-lymphocyte cross-reactive (TLX) cell surface antigens. Hum Immunol 4:27–36

McIntyre JA, Faulk WP, Verhulst SJ, Colliver J (1983) Human trophoblast-lymphocyte cross-reactive (TLX) antigens define a new alloantigen system. Science 222:1135–1138

McIntyre JA, Coulam CB, Faulk WP (1989) Recurrent spontaneous abortion. Am J Reprod Immunol 21:100–104

McIntyre JA, Faulk WP, Nichols-Johnson VR, Taylor CG (1986) Immunological testing and immunotherapy in recurrent spontaneous abortion. Obstet Gynecol 67:169–175

O' Sullivan MJ, McIntyre JA, Prior M, Warriner G, Faulk WP (1982) Identification of human trophoblast membrane antigens in maternal blood during pregnancy. Clin Exp Immunol 48:279–287

Razin A, Cedar H (1991) DNA methylation and gene expression. Microbiol Rev 55:451–458

Reed E, Bonagura V Kung P, King DW, Suciu-Foca N (1983) Anti-idiotypic antibodies to HLA DR4 and DR2. Eur J Immunol 131:2890–2894

Roussev RG, Vanderpuye OA, Wagenknecht DR, McIntyre JA (1991) A role for TLX antigens in pregnancy. Acta Eur Fertil 22:181–187

Roussev RG, Vanderpuye OA, McIntyre JA (1993) TLX alloantigens and pregnancy. In: Naz RK (ed) Immunology of reproduction. CRC, New York, pp 169–207

Schmidt CM, Orr HT (1993) Maternal/fetal interactions: the role of the MHC class I molecule HLA-G (Review). Crit Rev Immunol 13(3–4):207–224

Shawar SM, Vyas JM, Rodgers JR, Rich RR (1994) Antigen presentation by major histocompatibility complex class I-B molecules. Annu Rev Immunol 12:839–880

Singal DP, Butler L, Liao SK, Joseph S (1984) The fetus as an allograft: evidence for anti-idiotypic antibodies induced by pregnancy. Am J Reprod Immunol 6:145–151

Sinah D, Wells M, Faulk WP (1984) Immunological studies of human placentae: complement components in pre-eclamptic chorionic villi. Clin Exp Immunol 56:175–184

Sionov RV, Yagel S, Har-nir R, Gailliy (1993) Trophoblasts protect the inner cell mass from macrophage destruction. Biol Reprod 49:588–595

Suciu-Foca N, Reed E, Rohowsky C, Kung P, King DW (1983) Anti-idiotypic antibodies to anti-HLA receptors induced by pregnancy. Proc Natl Acad Sci USA 80:830–834

Thaler CJ, Critser JK, McIntyre JA, Faulk WP (1989) Seminal vesicles: a source of trophoblast lymphocyte cross-reactive antigen. Fertil Steril 52:463–468

Thaler CJ, McIntyre JA, Critser JK, Knapp PM, Coulam CB, Faulk WP (1990) Congential aplasia of seminal vesicles: absence of trophoblast-lymphocyte crossreactive (TLX) antigens from seminal plasma. Fertil Steril 53:948–949

Torry DS, Faulk WP, McIntyre JA (1989) Regulation of immunity to extraembryonic membranes in human pregnancy. Am J Reprod Immunol 21:76–81

Torry DS, Faulk WP, McIntyre JA (1991) Trophoblast immunity in human pregnancy defined by antiidiotype. Am J Reprod Immunol 25:181–184

Van der Ven K, Ober C (1994) HLA-G polymorphisms in African Americans. J Immunol 153(12):5628–5633

Vanderpuye OA, Labarrere CA, McIntyre JA (1992) The complement system in human reproduction. Am J Reprod Immunol 27:145–155

Vanderpuye OA, Labarrere CA, McIntyre JA (1993) Expression of CD59, a human complement system regulatory protein in extraembryonic membranes. Int Arch Allergy Immunol 101:376–384

Yamada H, Polgar K, Hill JA (1994) Cell-mediated immunity to trophoblast antigens in women with recurrent spontaneous abortion. Am J Obstet Gynecol 170(5):1339–1344

Traffic of Leukocytes Through the Maternofetal Placental Interface and Its Possible Consequences

N. PAPADOGIANNAKIS

1 Introduction

If, as is often the case, pregnancy and the survival/acceptance of the semiallogeneic embryo can be referred to as a paradox, we can surely regard the existence of circulating immune cells on the "wrong" side of the fetoplacental barrier, as nothing less than a self-contradiction. The presence and possible functional consequences of fetal cells such as lymphocytes in maternal blood and vice versa is fascinating, provocative, and challenging from a number of biological, ethical, and philosophical aspects. This review summarizes the evidence that such a curious cell traffic does in fact take place in human pregnancy.

The transplacental passage of cell types other than leukocytes is generally accepted. The passage of fetal erythrocytes into the maternal circulation is nowadays a well-established fact and can lead to isoalloimmunization, notably against the rhesus antigen, with potentially life-threatening consequences for the embryo/neonate (JACKSON and SCOTT 1992). Similarly, the presence of fetal platelets in maternal blood has been documented and can be the cause of alloimmune thrombocytopenia (JACKSON and SCOTT 1992). On the other hand, the presence of small amounts of maternal erythrocytes in fetal blood is regularly demonstrated in normal pregnancy (BENIRSCHKE and KAUFMANN 1990). Deportation of trophoblast has been known for at least 100 years to occur in maternal lungs (SCHMORL 1893). Recent studies have convincingly shown circulating syncytiotrophoblast and villous

Karolinska Institute, Department of Pathology, Huddinge University Hospital, 14186 Huddinge, Sweden

cytotrophoblast in the peripheral blood of mothers in normal pregnancy (MUELLER et al. 1990; HAWES et al. 1993). These trophoblast cells may not be totally inert, and in any case they constitute a source of fetal antigenic material in maternal blood and body tissues.

The trafficking of fetal lymphocytes or other populations of leukocytes through the placenta into the maternal organ systems, including blood circulation, remains a controversial issue. Even more so, the concept of maternal leukocyte passage into the fetus under normal conditions is debated and is sometimes rejected in strong and absolute terms (HUNZIKER and WEGMANN 1986; ADINOLFI 1993). Nearly 30 years after the seminal observations of WALKNOWSKA et al. (1969) which effectively began the modern era of transplacental lymphocyte trafficking research, the most important biological questions pertaining to this bidirectional cell traffic remain largely unanswered. Thus the precise frequency and extent of the postulated leukocyte passage are not matters of agreement. The kinetics of the transplacental passage during pregnancy as well as eventual postpartum chimerism are essentially unexplored. Even the exact phenotypic characteristics and origin of the trafficking cells are controversial.

A considerable amount of effort has been invested during recent years in the identification and characterization of circulating fetal cells in maternal blood (SIMPSON and ELIAS 1994; BIANCHI 1995). However, in my opinion, many relevant investigations carry an inherent bias towards the development of test systems for prenatal diagnosis of fetal diseases. Another point of confusion has been the uncritical extrapolation to humans of results obtained in other mammalian models, such as mouse or rat (HUNZIKER and WEGMANN 1986). It is well recognized that placental morphology is highly variable among mammals, probably more so than that of any other organ (HAIG 1993; LEISER and KAUFMANN 1994). Interspecies differences in placenta structure and details of function, in conjunction with differences in the constitution of the immunological apparatus, including lymphocyte homing and recirculation, are probably reflected in species-specific profiles of transplacental lymphocyte trafficking (ANDERSON 1971; HAIG 1993; DE SOUSA 1994). In an elegant article HAIG (1993) has discussed the way in which placental evolution and divergence among lineages may be driven by internal forces in each separate species, presupposing a continuous exchange of cells and/or information between mother and her offspring.

2 Feasibility of Transplacental Cell Trafficking

Maternal and fetal blood circulations are anatomically clearly separate from each other in humans. Further, the prevailing dogma in the literature presumes the existence of an effective immunological barrier at the maternofetal interface, i.e., villous trophoblast (FINN et al. 1976; BEER and SIO 1982; HUNZIKER and WEGMANN 1986). This barrier would prevent the entry of potentially harmful maternal leukocytes into the fetus and safeguard the integrity and survival of trophoblast, avoiding rejection of the fetoplacental unit. The original hypothesis postulated that trophoblast is protected from immune attack through an outer surface layer of "fibrinoid" material, serving as mechanical or electrostatic barrier to maternal lymphocytes (Fox 1978; BENIRCHKE and KAUFMANN 1990). This material, especially concentrated in the intervillous trophoblast, is eventually enriched in highly sulfated mucoproteins, sialic and hyaluronic acid, thereby masking histocompatibility antigens expressed by trophoblast cells. The deposition of immunoglobulins, complement, and immune complexes in these areas strengthened the impression that the fibrinoid material is probably the outcome of local immunological interactions. However, this concept was seriously challenged by many subsequent investigations which failed by electron microscopy to demonstrate any constant separation of maternal and trophoblastic tissues or did not succeed in rendering the trophoblast immunogenic by removing components of the mucoprotein "barrier" (ROBERTSON and WARNER 1974; FOX 1978).

The postulated placental barrier may be functional/biological rather than physical. Thus, the excessive production of potent immunosuppressive substances such as human chorionic gonadotropin, chorionic somatomammotrophin and placental lactogen at the immediate vicinity of the villous syncytiotrophoblast (AMOROSO and PERRY 1975; FOX 1978; MUES et al. 1989) can conceivably counteract the proliferation and effector function of "aggressive" maternal leukocytes with antifetal/paternal specificities, without presupposing an absolute, cell-impermeable barrier. A feasible route of leukocyte transfer is the well-documented fetomaternal and maternofetal bleedings (BENIRSCHKE and KAUFMANN 1990). Although massive, clinically significant, transplacental hemorrhage is uncommon, small amounts of blood pass regularly in both directions in normal pregnancy (DE ALMEIDA and BOWMAN 1994), with unavoidable carrying over of leukocytic populations, probably in very low (but essentially unknown) numbers (BEER and BILLINGHAM 1974). The reasons for these bleedings are often obscure but may involve minute traumata or breaks in the continuity of trophoblast interface (KLINE 1948). The rate of transplacental blood exchange is largely unpredictable, and the amount of blood may not necessarily increase with advancing gestational age (COHEN et al. 1964; COHEN and ZUELZER 1965). Testimony of the intermingling of maternal and fetal circulations are the intervillous thromboses, frequently found in placentae at term and containing an admixture of fetal and maternal blood cell elements (KAPLAN et al. 1982; GILLE et al. 1986).

Direct demonstration of active leukocyte migration through the placenta has not yet been provided but can be predicted, especially towards the end of pregnancy with the gradual attenuation of the trophoblast cell layer. By term most cytotrophoblast has disappeared, and large areas of the syncytiotrophoblast are replaced by the so-called vasculosyncytial membranes, or epithelial plates, which can be as thin as 1–2 μm (BENIRSCHKE and KAUFMANN 1990; BURTON and THAM 1992). These membranes are regarded as specialized obtrusions of segments of fetal capillaries, without nuclei but rich in pinocytic vesicles. The intriguing existence of transtrophoblastic channels or pores, possibly facilitating exchange of smaller molecules has recently been described (BURTON and THAM 1992). Other examples of close proximity between maternal and fetal tissues include the findings that the anchoring villi of the placenta are deprived of surface trophoblast layer, allowing direct contact between maternal decidual and fetal villous stroma (ENDERS 1968).

Thus, a great number of observations suggest that the separation of maternal and fetal tissues is often incomplete, and that the concept of a structural immune "barrier" at the placental interface must be revised.

3 Evidence of Mutual Maternofetal Recognition and Interaction

A plethora of observations derived from in vitro and in vivo studies supports the notion of transplacental leukocyte trafficking. In general these studies involve either demonstration of signs of recognition and sensitization of the maternal immune system of fetal leukocytic antigens, and vice versa, or the documentation of the actual presence of maternal and fetal leukocytes on the opposite side of the placental interface.

Most modern theories, for explaining the invariable success of "nature's allograft" presuppose a dynamic state of immunological equilibrium obtained through the extensive and continuous exchange of immune cells and antigens through the placenta (ANDERSON 1971, 1982; BEER and BILLINGHAM 1974; REDMAN 1986; DAUNTER 1992; HAIG 1993). The teleological argument is persuasive. If, in agreement with the widely held view, the fetoplacental unit resembles an allograft/transplant, it should basically obey the immunological rules of transplantation, in analogy with a solid organ transplant. According to the current "two-way" paradigm (STARZL et al. 1995), graft acceptance is based upon mutual chimerism between graft and recipient, involving migration of immune cells, probably lymphocytes and/or dendritic cells in both directions.

An array of studies have demonstrated the production of maternal antibodies (Abs) with high specificity against fetal or paternal HLA class I or II antigens (AHRONS 1971; ANDERSON 1971; SCHRÖDER 1975a; REDMAN 1986; AANTCZAK 1989; REED et al. 1991). Some of these Abs can develop even during the first pregnancy, excluding maternal sensitization only during labor, but in general the titers of the Abs rise with advancing gestational age and parity (MORIN-PAPUNEN et al. 1984). In most cases the maternal alloantibodies are not harmful for the fetus (AHRONS 1971; BALASCH et al. 1981), probably because of the specialized immunoadsorbent function of the placenta. However, failure may occur, with formation of autoantibodies and passively acquired fetal autoimmune disease. The function of the alloreactive antifetal Abs can be agglutinating, complement inactivating, cytotoxic, protective (NEPPERT et al. 1989), and in some cases unknown. The existence of anti-idiotypic Abs to HLA antigens in pregnancy has also been proposed (REED et al. 1991; AGRAWAL et al. 1994).

Another line of evidence demonstrates suppression of mixed lymphocyte reaction (MLR), mitogen stimulation, or leukocyte migration factor with the addition of maternal or fetal plasma (REDMAN 1986; DAUNTER 1992), again, strongly implicating anti-fetal or anti-maternal alloantibodies or factors. Other investigators have failed to find signs of alloreactivity in pregnancy (ADINOLFI 1993; MANYONDA et al. 1993). These discrepancies may be explained by the observations that sensitization of maternal cells to fetal HLA is intermittent and random within one pregnancy or in successive pregnancies of the same individual (HOFF and PETERSON 1995). It is obvious that the bulk of the antigenic stimulation of the maternal immune system must reside on fetal leukocyte populations, because trophoblast cells, at the placental interface or in maternal blood, in essence lack HLA antigens, with the exception of the oligomorphic HLA-G or other minor antigens, the antigenicity of which has not been clearly documented (OBER and VAN DER VEN, this volume).

There is also evidence for sensitization of the cellular immune system of the mother during pregnancy. In vivo studies have shown a striking hypertrophy of the lymph nodes draining the uterus, pointing to an immunological stimulation of the mother by fetal antigenic material (BEER and BILLINGHAM 1974). Skin grafts exchanged between mother and fetus survive significantly longer than expected, showing maternal reactivity towards transplantation antigens of the offspring. These experiments led to the formulation of the theory of "immunological inertia of viviparity" (ANDERSON 1971), which postulates that the transplacental passage of immunocompetent leukocytes contribute to a suppression of harmful alloreactive responses and to mutual adaptation or accommodation of maternal and fetal immune systems.

In addition to cytotoxic Abs, alloreactive antifetal cytotoxic or killer T cells have been shown in maternal blood during pregnancy (REDMAN 1986). HOFF and PETERSON (1995) recently measured soluble markers of immune activation, such as soluble CD8 antigen, soluble interleukin-2 receptor and β_2-microglobulin and found evidence further supporting a mutual sensitization with activation of either immunosuppressive or immunotrophic networks in pregnancy, requiring transplacental passage of leukocytes.

The fetal immune system similarly shows signs of sensitization towards possibly transplacentally transferred maternal leukocytes. MIYAGAWA (1984) found in cord blood IgM Abs against maternal alloreactive T cells, evidencing mutual recognition of maternal and fetal immune systems. Some fetal responses are directed against maternal antigens not present on fetal cells (HORTON et al. 1976), which necessitates transplacental passage of leukocytes. Furthermore, neonates are sometimes sensitized to infectious agents which do not cross the placenta, again suggesting a transplacental transfer of cellular immunity (CRAMER et al. 1974; THONG et al. 1974; DAUNTER 1992).

A multitude of studies have addressed the presence of fetal cells including leukocytes or lymphocytes in the maternal blood circulation, with varying perspective and final outcome. A smaller number of studies have attempted to demonstrate maternal cells in fetal blood or tissues. Both types of results are detailed below. In general terms the methodology used has been quite variable and is, naturally, becoming increasingly sophisticated. The various methods are discussed in many excellent reviews, for example, by PARKS and HERZENBERG (1982), HOLZGREVE et al. (1992) and SENYEI and WASSMANN (1993).

4 Fetal Leukocytes in Maternal Blood

WALKNOWSKA et al. (1969) were the first to demonstrate fetal lymphoid cells in the blood circulation of pregnant women, using a conventional cytogenetic technique employing the bright fluorescence of Y chromatin as a marker of separating fetal and maternal metaphases. The fetal cells were identified as lymphoid stem cells or lymphocytes, they appeared as early as the 14th week of pregnancy and were responsive to stimulation with phytohemagglutinin (PHA). However, both false-positive and false-negative results were obtained in the prediction of fetal sex. These results were later challenged by JACOBS and SMITH (1969), who found evidence of 46XY cells in the blood of normal, nonpregnant women and by SHARPE (1970) who found practically no transplacental passage of lymphocytes. Similarly, ZIMMERMAN and SCHMICKEL (1971), GOLOB and KUNZE-MUHL (1971), and TAKAHARA et al. (1972) observed only minimal transfer of fetal leukocytes in maternal blood and concluded that the method was inadequate for prenatal determination of sex.

Nevertheless, a substantial number of studies subsequently reproduced in essence the original findings of WALKNOWSKA et al. (1969). Using either conventional cytogenetic methods or various modifications for detection of Y-bodies even in interphase nuclei, numerous groups have reported the presence of significant numbers of fetal lymphocytes or lymphocytelike cells in maternal blood. These include DE GROUCHY and TRÉBUCHET (1971), SCHINDLER et al. (1972), WHANG-PENG et al. (1973), SCHRÖDER (1974, 1975a), SCHRÖDER and DE LA CHAPELLE (1972), SCHRÖDER et al. (1974, 1977), ROGALL and ZINSER (1973), GROSSET et al. (1974), SIEBERS et al. (1975), ZILIACUS et al. (1975a), CIARANFI et al. (1977), KIRSCH-VOLDERS et al. (1980), and WESSMANN et al. (1992). ZILIACUS et al. (1975b) described a case of massive invasion of mother's blood by fetal lymphocytes following an induced abortion. The presence of fetal lymphocytes was recorded as early as the 8th week (WHANG-PENG et al. 1973) or the 10–12th weeks (SCHINDLER et al. 1972) in normal pregnancies. Some studies demonstrate postpartum persistence of fetal cells, i.e., for at least 6 months (WHANG-PENG et al. 1973), 1 year (SCHRÖDER 1974), or 5 years (CIANRAFI et al. 1977). TIILIKAINEN et al. (1974) suggested that masking of paternal HLA antigens on fetal lymphocytes contribute to their persistence in maternal blood after delivery. Different studies gave variable estimates of the proportion of circulating fetal lymphocytes, from 0.02% (ZILIACUS et al. 1975a) up to 3.7% (CIANRAFI et al. 1977).

The immune capacity of fetal lymphocytes in maternal blood has been the issue of some controversy. In many studies fetal cells show good response to PHA

(WALKNOWSKA et al. 1969; DE GROUCHY and TRÉBUCHET 1971; GOLOB and KUNZE-MUHL 1971; SCHRÖDER and DE LA CHAPELLE (1972). SELYPES and LORENCZ (1988) using a unique "air-culture" technique reported large numbers of fetal mitotic cells from maternal whole-blood cultures. In contrast, other studies (SCHRÖDER et al. 1977) have found no mitotic capacity of fetal cells using PHA, pokeweed mitogen, lipopolysaccharide or MLR. THARAPEL et al. (1993) found no fetal metaphases in FACS-separated cells from maternal blood. These findings raised the possibility that the circulating fetal lymphocytes are not of conventional T-cell phenotype, display immature, blastlike (?) characteristics, or are even of B-cell (SCHRÖDER 1975b) or monocytic lineage. The reasons for the observed poor mitogenic response are not clear. SCHRÖDER (1975b) proposed some kind of coating mechanism rendering the fetal cells unresponsive. However, this deviating behavior may be somehow associated with the well-recognized functional immaturity of the fetal/neonatal cellular immune system. A variety of observations (SPLAWSKI et al. 1991), including our own (PAPADOGIANNAKIS et al. 1986; PAPADOGIANNAKIS 1995), suggest that fetal/neonatal immune cells display signs of dysregulation, especially regarding suppressor cell function, requirements for lymphocyte activation, signal transduction, and lymphocyte-monocyte cooperation.

In many of the studies cited above (WALKNOWSKA et al. 1969; SCHRÖDER and DE LA CHAPELLE 1972; CIARANFI et al. 1977; SIEBERS et al. 1975) the number of fetal lymphocytes was not concordant with the amount or the kinetics during pregnancy of the fetomaternal blood leakage, suggesting an active migration or transport of fetal cells in the maternal circulation. HERZENBERG et al. (1979) and IVERSON et al. (1981) isolated fetal cells in maternal blood after enrichment using both Y-chromosome and HLA antigens as markers. They found fetal cells from the 15th week at a frequency of 1:1000–1:5000 in maternal lymphocytes. They characterized the fetal cells as lymphocytelike, mononuclear, and HLA positive. KULOZIK and PAWLOWITZKI (1982) isolated fetal lymphocytes from maternal blood using immunohistochemistry and α-fetoprotein as a marker for fetal cells.

The existence of fetal granulocytes in maternal blood has been indicated or demonstrated in several instances (MOSZKOWSKI et al. 1971; SCHRÖDER and DE LA CHAPELLE 1972; ROGALL and ZINSER 1973; SIEBERS et al. 1975; WESSMANN et al. 1992), as early as the 8th–10th weeks of pregnancy, often in parallel with circulating fetal lymphocytes.

Although many discrepant and conflicting results have been obtained regarding the nature and biological behavior of fetal leukocytes in maternal blood, as delineated above, the concensus has been that the low number of fetal lymphoid cells in maternal blood and the laborious and cumbersome methodology make fetal leukocytes an unattractive candidate target for prenatal diagnosis. An impressive and ever increasing amount of research in recent years has focused on the isolation and amplification of fetal-specific DNA sequences, with the perspective of developing an effective, noninvasive instrument for prenatal diagnosis of a variety of fetal diseases (GEIFMAN-HOLTZMAN et al. 1994; SIMPSON and ELIAS 1994).

The results of these studies were not concordant regarding the frequency or the exact nature of the fetal cells in maternal blood. GÄNSHIRT-ALERT et al. (1990),

Adinolfi et al. (1989), Nakagome et al. (1991) and Hamada et al. (1993) found practically no or only extremely low amounts of fetal DNA in maternal blood. In contrast, Lo et al. (1989, 1990, 1993), Yeoh et al. (1991), Hsieh et al. (1993), Liou et al. (1993), Adkinson et al. (1994), Geifman-Holtzman et al. (1994), Thomas et al. (1995), and Bianchi et al. (1996) found measurable amounts of fetal DNA in mother's blood, with potential applications for accurate prenatal diagnosis. Attempts have been made to employ fetal-specific markers not dependent on the male Y-sequences (Geifman-Holtzman et al. 1994, 1995). It is noteworthy that Bianchi et al. (1996) recorded persistence of fetal DNA for as long as 27 years postpartum. The detected fetal cells were $CD34^+$ or $CD34^+38^+$, mononuclear, and probably of progenitor type.

Some of the above discrepancies may be explained by differences in methodology, for example, prior enrichment protocol, choice of target sequence, and type of polymerase chain reaction method applied (Adkinson et al. 1994). On the other hand, there may well be an unrecognized or hitherto unexplored biological variability in the time of appearance, the amount of fetal cells during different stages of pregnancy (Hamada et al. 1993; Lo et al. 1993; Thomas et al. 1995), and differences between individual pregnancies.

5 Maternal Leukocytes in Fetal Tissues

Relatively few investigations have addressed the presence of maternal lymphocytes or other populations of leukocytes in normal human pregnancy. Desai and Creger (1963) injected atabrine-labeled leukocytes into the maternal circulation before delivery and subsequently detected in six of nine cases the labeled fluorescent mononuclear leukocytes, as well as platelets and granulocytes, in umbilical cord blood. This was the first direct demonstration that normal maternal leukocytes can actually cross the placenta. The estimated number of maternal cells was low, and no information was provided about the kinetics, tissue distribution, or function of the colonizing maternal cells. Although the authors were careful to exclude nonspecific effects of cell labeling, this method is considered relatively unreliable. El-Alfi and Hathout (1969) described an infant with cytogenetic and immunological evidence of maternofetal lymphocyte transfer, probably occurring early in pregnancy. Moszkowski et al. (1971) found cytogenetic evidence for materno-fetal transfusion of polymorphonuclear leukocytes in the cord blood of 24 of 30 healthy babies. Turner et al. (1966) found evidence of materno-fetal leukocyte transfer in only two out of 183 cases; both infants showed serious developmental defects and died shortly after delivery. Schröder (1974) examined a large number of cells with the help of Y-chromosome marker and found maternal leukocytes in the peripheral blood of one of ten newborns. He estimated the proportion of maternal cells to 0.07%, and some maternal mitoses were also observed. In contrast, other studies (Taylor and Polani 1965; Turner et al. 1966; Olding 1972) have failed to detect any mitogenically active, PHA-responsive maternal lymphocytes in neonatal blood following normal deliveries. OLDING (1972) discussed the possibility of a very rare passage of maternal cells with rapid elimination from the systemic circulation of the fetus, or differences in the immunological reactivity between maternal and fetal lymphocytes. SHARPE (1970) and ANDERSON and FERGUSON-SMITH (1971) similarly found no convincing female (maternal) karyotypes in the cord blood of normal newborns. Recently HARD et al. (1991) searched the lymph nodes of three normal newborns and two fetuses for maternal DNA sequences, using highly specific polymorphic probes and came up with negative results.

A number of studies have firmly established that transplacental passage of maternal lymphoid cells with subsequent engraftment in the fetus is a frequent phenomenon when the fetal immune system is gravely debilitated, for example, in cases of severe combined immunodeficiency (SCID; POLLACK et al. 1982) and diverse abnormalities of the thymus (KADOWAKI et al. 1965; LISCHNER et al. 1967; GITHENS et al. 1969).

The amounts of maternal lymphocytes are variable (SOTTINI et al. 1995) and the cells may persist in the blood circulation of infants for long periods of time, at least 6 months (BORZY et al. 1984). In most cases the identified maternal cells are of T cell lineage, but engraftment of B cells can also occur (GEHA and REINHERZ 1983). Although anatomically intact, the maternal lymphocytes appear in general anergic, showing reduced or no response to mitogen stimulation as well as inadequate effector functions (O'REILLY et al. 1989; SOTTINI et al. 1995). There is great variability in the clinical picture following engraftment of maternal lymphocytes in SCID (ALAIN et al. 1993). However, in most instances only a mild, transient graft versus host disease (GvHD) is evident (GITHENS et al. 1969; POLLACK et al. 1982; BORZY et al. 1984; BARRETT et al. 1988). VAIDYA et al. (1991) described the case of an infant with SCID in which the engrafted maternal T cells had an apparently protective-suppressive effect on the otherwise lethal GvHD from the simultaneous engraftment of donor T lymphocytes.

The reasons for the apparent inactivity and special biological profile of maternal lymphocytes that cross the placenta in SCID patients remain obscure. It is equally unclear whether the passage of maternal cells is secondary to the immune defect state, or whether it contributes to the development of the immune abnormality. WAHN et al. (1991) described a fascinating case of a SCID infant with transient, clonal expansion of maternally derived $CD3^+CD8^+$ γ/δ^+ T lymphocytes. The child showed signs of only mild GvHD and no malignancy. The authors raised the intriguing question of whether the engrafted maternal T cells might possess individual attributes allowing them to cross the placenta. In a recent interesting report SOTTINI et al. (1995) found high numbers of engrafted maternal T cells in a SCID patient. The maternal cells were, in accordance with previous results, unresponsive to PHA and to the combination of OKT3 and interleukin-2, but they showed good proliferative response to superantigens. Furthermore, the transplacentally acquired maternal T cells expressed a random set of T cell receptor variable segments but displayed an extremely restricted V-D-J junctional diversity, indicating that the maternal cells may be in some way positively selected.

Transplacental passage of maternal leukemic cells has been recorded in some instances (CRAMBLETT et al. 1958; DIAMANDOPOULOS and HERTIG 1963; RIGBY et al. 1964; OSADA et al. 1990), but it appears to be a very rare event, and the fetus remains mostly disease-free even in the presence of numerous leukemic cells in the intervillous space (Fox 1978; BENIRSCHKE and KAUFMANN 1990).

Further support for the notion of transplacental migration of maternal lymphocytes comes from studies of placentae with villitis of unknown etiology (VUE). VUE is a common placental lesion and is observed in many, or most, normal placentae at term (LABARRERE and FAULK 1995). VUE is characterized by focal infiltration of the villous stroma by mononuclear inflammatory cells. Recent studies using immunocytochemistry (ALTEMANI 1992; LABARRERE and FAULK 1995) or in situ hybridization with X and Y chromosome probes (REDLINE and PATTERSON 1993) demonstrate unequivocally that the majority of the invading cells are maternally derived mature T cells or monocytes. These findings are a strong indication that maternal immune cells are able to cross the trophoblastic barrier. The precise mechanism of placental transport has not been elucidated, but the patchy distribution of VUE lesions suggests multiple, independent, probably continuous episodes of maternal cell migration (REDLINE and PATTERSON 1993).

Thus, the collected data clearly demonstrate the capacity of maternal leukocytes to pass through the trophoblastic "barrier", at least under certain (pathological?) conditions. The paucity of demonstrable maternal, mitotically active lymphocytes in normal pregnancy can be interpreted in several ways, not mutually exclusive: by low sensitivity of the detection method, by a rapid elimination mechanism in fetal blood (BILLINGTON 1992), by special kinetics of recirculation or engraftment of the transported cells, and by the actual absence of a normally operating maternofetal transfer mechanism. Our results (PAPADOGIANNAKIS et al. 1990) suggest another plausible mechanism: the strong, nonspecific suppressor activity residing in fetal/neonatal lymphocytes. The suppressive effect is mediated largely by prostaglandins (PG), mainly PGE_2, which are potent inhibitors of immune cell functions, such as proliferation, lymphokine production, cytotoxicity, and antibody production. The fetal environment is probably enriched in PG, which largely escape catabolism because of the inactivation of fetal lungs (FERREIRA and VANE 1967). We have shown that PHA-stimulated fetal lymphocytes are more resistant to the antiproliferative effect of PGE_2, than lymphocytes from their mothers or other adults. Thus, it is feasible that the heavily PG-suppressed maternal cells are hardly detectable in the fetal circulation, whereas the relatively unharmed fetal lymphocytes remain immunologically competent and can eventually recruit additional antimaternal mechanisms, such as cytotoxic cells and Abs (MIYAGAWA 1984). However, definite conclusions on the fate of the placenta-passing maternal cells in normal situations must await further research focusing on the distribution and recirculation of maternal cells and maternal DNA in blood as well peripheral lymphoid tissues of the fetus.

6 Possible Consequences of Bidirectional Traffic of Leukocytes Through the Placenta

The evidence detailed above provides a convincing, albeit incomplete, picture of fetal and maternal lymphoid cells frequently transgressing the placento-trophoblastic "barrier". The provocative long-term (up to 27 years!) persistence of fetal cells in the maternal circulation (BIANCHI et al. 1996) suggests that pregnancy may constitute a valuable, hitherto neglected model for the study of spontaneous chimerism in humans. Future research must concentrate on the investigation of possible leukocyte chimerism in the peripheral lymphoid tissues (MASSEYEFF et al. 1983; HARD et al. 1991; SHIMAMURA et al. 1994). At any given time the majority, perhaps more than 80%, of the total lymphocyte numbers in the body are found not in blood but in peripheral lymphoid organs, such as lymph nodes, spleen, bone marrow, and liver (DAUNTER 1992; BUTCHER and PICKER 1996).

The continuous, low-grade leakage of lymphoid cells through the placental interface results in direct and repeated encounter between maternal and fetal immune systems. This is in agreement with the modern concept of solid organ transplantation (STARZL et al. 1995) and probably contributes to a reciprocal acceptance and the nonrejection of the fetoplacental unit (ANDERSON 1982; KNOBLOCH and MILLER 1988; HAIG 1993). The best documented sequel of feto-maternal leukocyte transfer is the rich production of various anti-HLA Abs by the mother (ANTCZAK 1989). However, the characterization and clinical significance of these Abs remain incomplete. BEER and BILLINGHAM (1974) suggested that fetal lymphocytes in maternal blood contribute to the generation of sensitized maternal effector cells.

Most investigators agree that the low numbers of fetal leukocytes in maternal circulation are not amenable to accurate, cost-effective prenatal diagnosis of fetal inherited diseases (SIMPSON and ELIAS 1994; BIANCHI 1995). However, reservation may be appropriate until the precise nature of placenta-crossing mononuclear cells (lymphoblastoid? monocytoid? dendritic?) is fully revealed.

The most obvious consequence of transfer of immunocompetent maternal cells in the fetus would be GvHD. This is well documented in rodents and is described as runting disease (BEER and BILLINGHAM 1974). In humans GvHD is manifest in some newborns with SCID but is generally of mild severity (POLLACK et al. 1982). BASSUKAS (1992) hypothesized that erythema toxicum neonatorum, a common and transient skin disease of the newborn, may be a limited acute GvHD by transferred maternal lymphocytes. We have proposed a mechanism which may prevent or counteract maternal GvHD under physiological conditions, i.e., the strong suppressor activity of fetal/neonatal lymphocytes mediated by PG (PAPADOGIANNAKIS et al. 1990).

It is unclear whether maternal lymphocytes in the fetus contribute to the pathogenesis of SCID (HANSEN et al. 1977; POLLACK et al. 1982; HAMILTON et al. 1988). On the other hand, the migrating maternal cells are certainly a major component and a probable etiological factor in VUE, a common condition with potentially harmful effects for the fetus (LABARRERE and FAULK 1995). The association of transferred maternal cells with other complications of pregnancy, such as recurrent spontaneous abortion is debatable (OSSA et al. 1994) and may be mediated by GvHD-like mechanism engaging idiotypic recognition networks in both mother and fetus.

The continuous exposure of fetal immune system to low numbers of immunocompetent maternal lymphocytes may be associated with the state of neonatal tolerance. Recent investigations (LAFFERTY 1995; RIDGE et al. 1996) have emphasized the crucial role of second signals in the acquisition of tolerance and in graft rejection. In other words, the low-grade sensitization of fetal immune system by transplacentally acquired maternal leukocytes in the presence of functionally inadequate, or down-regulated, dendritic cells (HUNT et al. 1994) or monocytes (PAPADOGIANNAKIS 1995), unable to provide the appropriate second signals, may turnout to be tolerogenic. This is a fascinating scenario, but more research is needed before its validity is established in humans.

The transfer of sensitized maternal leukocytes into the fetus might otherwise contribute to the shaping of the immunological repertoire of the fetus/neonate. There is evidence indicating that prenatal sensitization of the fetus to specific antigens can occur during normal pregnancy (CRAMER et al. 1974)

Finally, the existence and possible persistence of immunocompetent maternal lymphocytes, with GvHD potential, in umbilical cord blood, even in low numbers (PETIT et al. 1995) may have serious clinical implications for cord blood transplantation, which has been initiated in recent years.

References

Adinolfi M (1993) The maternal-fetal interaction: some controversies and solutions. Exp Clin Immunogenet 10:103–117

Adinolfi M, Camporese C, Carr T (1989) Gene amplification to detect fetal nucleated cells in pregnant women. Lancet ii:328–329

Adkison LR, Andrews RH, Vowell NL, Koontz WL (1994) Improved detection of fetal cells from maternal blood with polymerase chain reaction. Am J Obstet Gynecol 170:952–955

Agrawal S, Sharma RK, Kishore R, Agarwal SS (1994) Development of anti-idiotypic antibodies to HLA antigens during pregnancy. Indian J Med Res 99:42–46

Ahrons S (1971) HL-A antibodies: influence on the human foetus. Tissue Antigens 1:129–136

Alain G, Carrier C, Beaumier L, Bernard J, Lemay M, Lavoie A (1993) In utero acute graft-versus-host disease in a neonate with severe combined immunodeficiency. J Am Acad Dermatol 29:862–865

Altemani AM (1992) Immunohistochemical study of the inflammatory infiltrate in villitis of unknown etiology. A qualitative and quantitative analysis. Pathol Res Pract 188:303–330

Amoroso EC, Perry JS (1975) The existence during gestation of an immunological buffer zone at the interface between maternal and fetal tissues. Philos Trans R Soc Lond B Biol Sci 271:343–361

Anderson JM (1971) Transplantation – nature's success. Lancet ii:1077–1082

Anderson JM (1982) The effects of transplacental cell (antigen) traffic. J Reprod Fertil [Suppl] 31:161–173

Anderson JM, Ferguson-Smith MA (1971) Nature's transplant. BMJ 2:166–167

Antczak DF (1989) Maternal antibody responses in pregnancy. Curr Opin Immunol 1:1135–1140

Balasch J, Ercilla G, Vanrell JA, Vives J (1981) Effects of HLA antibodies on pregnancy. Obstet Gynecol 57:444–446

Barrett MJ, Buckley RH, Schiff SE, Kidd PC, Ward FE (1988) Accelerated development of immunity following transplantation of maternal marrow stem cells into infants with severe combined immunodeficiency and transplacentally acquired lymphoid chimerism. Clin Exp Immunol 72:118–123

Bassukas ID (1992) Is erythema toxicum neonatorum a mild self-limited acute cutaneous graft-versus-host-reaction from maternal-to-fetal lymphocyte transfer? Med Hypotheses 38:334–338

Beer AE, Billingham RE (1974) The embryo as a transplant. Sci Am 230:36–46

Beer AE, Sio JO (1982) Placenta as an immunological barrier. Biol Reprod 26:15–27

Benirschke K, Kaufmann P (1990) Pathology of the human placenta. Springer, Berlin Heidelberg New York

Bianchi DW (1995) Prenatal diagnosis by analysis of fetal cells in maternal blood. J Pediatr 127:847–856

Bianchi DW, Zickwolf GK, Weil GJ, Sylvester S, DeMaria MA (1996) Male fetal progenitor cells persist in maternal blood for as long as 27 years postpartum. Proc Natl Acad Sci USA 93:705–708

Billington WD (1992) The normal fetomaternal immune relationship. Baillieres Clin Obstet Gynecol 6:413–438

Borzy MS, Magenis E, Tomar D (1984) Bone marrow transplantation for severe combined immune deficiency in an infant with chimerism due to intrauterine-derived maternal lymphocytes: donor engraftment documented by chromosomal marker studies. Am J Med Genet 18:527–553

Burton GJ, Tham SW (1992) Formation of vasculo-syncytial membranes in the human placenta. J Dev Physiol 18:43–47

Butcher EC, Picker LJ (1996) Lymphocyte homing and homeostasis. Science 272:60–66

Ciaranfi A, Curchod A, Odartchenko N (1977) Survie de lymphocytes foetaux dans le sang maternel post-partum (in French). Schweiz Med Wochenschr 107:134–138

Cohen F, Zuelzer WW (1965) The transplacental passage of maternal erythrocytes into the fetus. Am J Obstet Gynecol 93:566–569

Cohen F, Zuelzer WW, Gustafson DC, Evans MM (1964) Transplacental bleeding from the fetus. Blood 23:621–646

Cramblett HG, Friedman JL, Najjar S (1958) Leukemia in an infant born of a mother with leukemia. N Engl J Med 259:727–729

Cramer DV, Kunz HW, Gill TJ III (1974) Immunologic sensitization prior to birth. Am J Obstet Gynecol 120:431–439

Daunter B (1992) Immunology of pregnancy: towards a unifying hypothesis. Eur J Obstet Gynecol Reprod Biol 43:81–95

De Almeida V, Bowman JM (1994) Massive fetomaternal hemorrhage: Manitoba experience. Obstet Gynecol 83:323–328

De Grouchy J, Trébuchet C (1971) Transfusion foeto-maternelle de lymphocytes sanguins et détection du sexe du foetus (in French). Ann Genet 14:133–137

de Sousa M (1994) Lymphocyte traffic and positioning in vivo: an expanded role for the ECM, the VLA proteins and the cytokines. Pathol Res Pract 190:840–850

Desai RG, Creger WP (1963) Maternofetal passage of leukocytes and platelets in man. Blood 21:665–673

Diamandopoulos GTH, Hertig AT (1963) Transmission of leukemia and allied diseases from mother to fetus. Obstet Gynecol 21:150–154

El-Alfi OS, Hathout H (1969) Maternofetal transfusion: immunologic and cytogenetic evidence. Am J Obstet Gynecol 103:599–600

Enders A (1968) Fine structure of anchoring villi of the human placenta. Am J Anat 122:419–451

Ferreira SH, Vane JR (1967) Prostaglandins. Their disappearance from and release into the circulation. Nature 216:868–873

Finn R, Davis JC, Hill CA, Hipkin LJ, Hervey M (1976) The placenta as an immunological barrier. BMJ 2:527

Fox H (1978) Pathology of the placenta. Saunders, Philadelphia

Gänshirt-Ahlert D, Pohlschmidt M, Gal A, Miny P, Horst J, Holzgreve W (1990) Ratio of fetal to maternal DNA is less than 1 in 5000 at different gestational ages in maternal blood. Clin Genet 38:38–43

Geha RS, Reinherz E (1983) Identification of circulating maternal T and B lymphocytes in uncomplicated severe combined immunodeficiency by HLA typing of subpopulations of T cells separated by the fluorescence activated cell sorter and of Epstein Barr virus derived B cell lines. J Immunol 130:2493–2495

Geifman-Holtzman O, Blatman RN, Bianchi DW (1994) Prenatal genetic diagnosis by isolation and analysis of fetal cells circulating in maternal blood. Semin Perinatol 18:366–375

Geifman-Holtzman O, Holtzman EJ, Vadnais TJ, Philips VE, Capeless EL, Bianchi DW (1995) Detection of fetal HLA-DQ-alpha sequences in maternal blood – a gender-independent technique of fetal cell identification. Prenat Diagn 15:261–268

Gille J, Schwerd W, von. Criegern T (1986) Zusammensetzung intervillöser Thromben aus maternem und fetalen (in German). Blut Z Geburtshilfe Perinat 190:133–136

Githens JH, Muschenheim F, Fulginiti VA, Robinson A, Kay HEM (1969) Thymic alymphoplasia with XX/XY lymphoid chimerism secondary to probable maternal-fetal transfusion. J Pediatr 75:87–94

Golob E, Kunze-Muhl E (1971) Feto-maternal crossing of lymphocytes and its eventual significance in prenatal sex diagnosis (in German). Z Geburtshilfe Perinatol 175:132–138

Grosset L, Barrelet V, Odartchenko N (1974) Antenatal fetal sex determination from maternal blood during early pregnancy. Am J Obstet Gynecol 120:60–63

Haig D (1993) Genetic conflict in human pregnancy. Q Rev Biol 68:495–532

Hamada H, Arinami T, Kubo T, Hamaguchi H, Iwasaki H (1993) Fetal nucleated cells in maternal peripheral blood: frequency and relationship to gestational age. Hum Genet 91:427–432

Hamilton MS, Becker J, Hamilton BL (1988) Maternally-induced graft-vs-host disease to minor antigens as a possible etiology of an acquired immunodeficiency syndrome in mice. Cancer Detect Prev 12:205–210

Hansen JA, Good RA, Dupont B (1977) HLA-D compatibility between parent and child. Increased occurrences in severe combined immunodeficiency and other hematopoietic diseases. Transplantation 23:366–374

Hard RC Jr, Slosberg AM, Salzberg AM (1991) Use of polymorphic DNA probes to test the lymph nodes of infants and fetuses for spontaneous chimerism. Arch Pathol Lab Med 115:891–894

Hawes CS, Suskin HA, Petropoulos A, Latham SE, Mueller UW (1994) A morphologic study of trophoblast isolated from peripheral blood of pregnant women. Am J Obstet Gynecol 170:1297–1300

Herzenberg LA, Bianchi DW, Schröder J, Cann HM, Iverson GM (1979) Fetal cells in the blood of pregnant women: detection and enrichment by fluorescence-activated cell sorting. Proc Natl Acad Sci USA 76:1453–1455

Hoff C, Peterson RDA (1995) Associations between maternal and fetal serum levels of immune activation markers and fetal growth. Am J Hum Biol 7:453–458

Holzgreve W, Garritsen HP, Gänshirt-Ahlert D (1992) Fetal cells in the maternal circulation. J Reprod Med 37:410–418

Horton JE, Oppenheim JJ, Chan SP, Baker JJ (1976) Relationship of transformation of newborn human lymphocytes by dental plaque antigen to the degree of maternal periodontal disease. Cell Immunol 21:153–160

Hsieh T-T, Pao CC, Hor JJ, Kao S-M (1993) Presence of fetal cells in maternal circulation after delivery. Hum Genet 92:294–295

Hunt DWC, Huppertz H-I, Jiang H-J, Petty RE (1994) Studies of human cord blood dendritic cells: evidence for functional immaturity. Blood 84:4333–4343

Hunziker RD, Wegmann TG (1986) Placental immunoregulation. CRC Crit Rev Immunol 6:245–285

Iverson GM, Bianchi DW, Cann HM, Herzenberg LA (1981) Detection and isolation of fetal cells from maternal blood using the fluorescence-activated cell sorter (FACS). Prenat Diagn 1:61–73

Jacobs PA, Smith PG (1969) Practical and theoretical implications of fetal/maternal lymphocyte transfer. Lancet ii:745

Jackson GM, Scott JR (1992) Alloimmune conditions and pregnancy. Baillieres Clin Obstet Gynecol 3:541–563

Kadowaki J-I, Zuelzer WW, Brough AJ, Thompson R, Woolley PV Jr, Gruber D (1965) XX/XY lymphoid chimerism in congenital immunological deficiency syndrome with thymic alymphoplasia. Lancet ii:1152–1155

Kaplan C, Blanc WA, Elias J (1982) Identification of erythrocytes in intervillous thrombi: a study using immunoperoxidase identification of hemoglobins. Hum Pathol 13:554–556

Kirsch-Volders M, Lissens-van Assche E, Susanne C (1980) Increase in the amount of fetal lymphocytes in maternal blood during pregnancy. J Med Genet 17:267–272

Kline BS (1948) Microscopic observations of the placental barrier in transplacental erythrocytic anemia (erythroblastosis fetalis) and in normal pregnancy. Am J Obstet Gynecol 56:226–237

Knobloch V, Miller I (1988) The development of immunological relationship between mother and fetus under physiological and pathological conditions. Allergy Immunol 34:219–231

Kulozik A, Pawlowitzki H (1982) Fetal cells in the maternal circulation: detection by direct AFP-immunofluorescence. Hum Genet 62:221–224

Labarrere C, Faulk WP (1995) Maternal cells in chorionic villi from placentae of normal and abnormal human pregnancies. Am J Reprod Immunol 33:54–59

Lafferty KJ (1995) Role of second signals in the induction of T cells and graft rejection. Immunologist 5–6:256–258

Leiser R, Kaufmann P (1994) Placental structure: in a comparative aspect. Exp Clin Endocrinol 102:122–134

Liou J-D, Pao CC, Hor J-J, Kao S-M (1993) Fetal cells in the maternal circulation during first trimester in pregnancies. Hum Genet 92:309–311

Lischner HW, Punett HH, DiGeorge AM (1967) Lymphocytes in congenital absence of the thymus. Nature 214:580–582

Lo Y-MD, Wainscoat JS, Gillmer MDG, Patel P, Sampietro M, Fleming KA (1989) Prenatal sex determination by DNA amplification from maternal peripheral blood. Lancet ii:1363–1365

Lo Y-MD, Patel P, Sampietro M, Gillmer MDG, Fleming KA, Wainscoat JS (1990) Detection of single-copy fetal DNA sequence from maternal blood. Lancet 335:1463–1464

Lo Y-MD, Patel P, Baigent CN, Gillmer MDG, Chamberlain P, Travi M, Sampietro M, Wainscoat JS, Fleming KA (1993) Prenatal sex determination from maternal peripheral blood using the polymerase chain reaction. Hum Genet 90:483–488

Manyonda IT, Pereira RS, Pearce JM, Sharrock CE (1993) Limiting dilution analysis of the allo-MHC anti-paternal cytotoxic T cell response. I. Normal primigravid and multiparous pregnancies. Clin Exp Immunol 93:126–131

Masseyef R, Soubiran P, Philip PJM, Aynaud N (1983) In: Edelman P, Sureau C (eds) Immunologie de la reproduction humaine. Boz, Paris, pp 93–96

Miyagawa Y (1984) Further characterization of IgM antibodies against maternal alloreactive T cells produced by cloned Epstein Barr virus transformed cord B cells. J Immunol 133:1270–1277

Morin-Papunen L, Tiilikainen A, Hartikainen-Sorri AL (1984) Maternal HLA immunization during pregnancy: presence of anti-HLA antibodies in half of multigravidous women. Med Biol 62:323–325

Moszkowski EF, Eby B, Shocket C, Govila V (1971) Cytogenetic evidence for materno-fetal transfusion of polymorphonuclears. J Reprod Med 6:26–28

Mueller UW, Hawes CS, Wright AE, Petropoulos A, DeBoni E, Firgaira FA, Morley AA, Turner DR, Jones WR (1990) Isolation of fetal trophoblast cells from peripheral blood of pregnant women. Lancet 336:197–200

Mues B, Langer D, Zwadlo G, Sorg C (1989) Phenotypic characterization of macrophages in human term placenta. Immunology 67:303–307

Nakagome Y, Seki S, Nagafuchi S, Nakahori Y, Sato K (1991) Absence of fetal cells in maternal circulation at a level of 1 in 25000. Am J Med Genet 40:596–508

Neppert J, Mueller-Eckhardt G, Neumeyer H, Malchus R, Kiefel V, Gerhard I, Kuhn V, Westphal E, Harpprecht J (1989) Pregnancy maintaining antibodies: workshop report (Giessen, 1988). J Reprod Immunol 15:156–167

Olding L (1972) The possibility of materno-foetal transfer of lymphocytes in man. Acta Pediatr Scand 61:73–75

O'Reilly RJ, Keever CA, Small TN, Broschtein J (1989) The use of HLA-non-identical T-cell depleted marrow transplants for correction of severe combined immunodeficiency disease. Immunodefic Rev 1:273–281

Osada S, Horibe K, Oiwa K, Yoshida J, Iwamura H, Matsuoka H, Adachi K, Ohno R, Ueda R (1990) A case of infantile acute monocytic leukemia caused by vertical transmission of the mother's leukemic cells. Cancer 65:1146–1149

Ossa JE, Cadavid AP, Maldonado JG (1994) Is the immune system necessary for placental reproduction? A hypothesis on the mechanisms of alloimmunotherapy in recurrent spontaneous abortion. Med Hypotheses 42:193–197

Papadogiannakis N (1995) (–)-Indolactam induced mitogenesis in human fetal/neonatal and adult T cells: lower response of neonatal cells and possible regulatory role of monocytes in protein kinase C mediated pathways. Cell Immunol 162: 288–294

Papadogiannakis N, Johnsen SA, Olding LB (1986) Monocyte regulated hyporesponsiveness of human cord blood lymphocytes to OKT3 monoclonal antibody induced mitogenesis. Scand J Immunol 23:91–99

Papadogiannakis N, Johnsen SA, Olding LB (1990) Suppressor cell activity in human cord blood. In: Chaouat G (ed) Immunology of the fetus. CRC, Roca Baton, pp 215–227

Parks DR, Herzenberg LA (1982) Fetal cells from maternal blood: their selection and prospects for use in prenatal diagnosis. Methods Cell Biol 26:277–295

Petit T, Gluckman E, Carosella E, Brossard Y, Brison O, Socié G (1995) A highly sensitive polymerase chain reaction method reveals the ubiquitous presence of maternal cells in human umbilical cord blood. Exp Hematol 23:1601–1605

Pollack MS, Kirkpatrick D, Kapoor N, Dupont B, O'Reilly RJ (1982) Identification by HLA typing of intrauterine derived maternal T cells in four patients with severe combined immunodeficiency. N Engl J Med 307:662–666

Redline RW, Patterson P (1993) Villitis of unknown etiology is associated with major infiltration of fetal tissue by maternal inflammatory cells. Am J Pathol 143:473–479

Redman CW (1986) Immunology of the placenta. Clin Obstet Gynecol 13:469–499

Reed E, Beer AE, Hutcherson H, West King D, Suciu-Foca N (1991) The alloantibody response of pregnant women and its suppression by soluble HLA antigens and anti-idiotypic antibodies. J Reprod Immunol 20:115–128

Ridge JP, Ephraim JF, Matzinger P (1996) Neonatal tolerance revisited: turning on newborn T cells with dendritic cells. Science 271:1723–1726

Rigby PG, Hanson TA, Smith RS (1964) Passage of leukemic cells across the placenta. N Engl J Med 271:124–127

Robertson WB, Warner B (1974) The ultrastructure of the human placental bed. J Pathol 112:203–211

Rogall H, Zinser HK (1973) Prenatal sex determination through demonstration of the Y-chromatin in blood leukocytes of pregnant women (in German). Geburtshilfe Frauenheilkd 33:277–281

Schindler A-M, Graf E, Martin-du-Pan R (1972) Prenatal diagnosis of fetal lymphocytes in the maternal blood. Obstet Gynecol 40:340–346

Schmorl G (1893) Pathologisch-anatomische Untersuchungen über puerperal Eklampsie (in German). Vogel, Leipzig

Schröder J (1974) Passage of leukocytes from mother to fetus. Scand J Immunol 3:369–373

Schröder J (1975a) Transplacental passage of blood cells. J Med Genet 12:230–242

Schröder J (1975b) Are fetal cells in maternal blood mainly B lymphocytes? Scand J Immunol 4:279–285

Schröder J, de la Chapelle A (1972) Fetal lymphocytes in the maternal blood. Blood 39:153–162

Schröder J, Tiilikainen A, de la Chapelle A (1974) Fetal leukocytes in the maternal circulation after delivery. I. Cytological aspects. Transplantation 17:346–354

Schröder J, Schröder E, Cann HM (1977) Fetal cells in maternal blood. Lack of response of fetal cells in maternal blood to mitogens and mixed leukocyte culture. Hum Genet 38:91–97

Selypes A, Lorencz R (1988) A noninvasive method for determination of the sex and karyotype of the fetus from the maternal blood. Hum Genet 79:357–359

Senyei AE, Wassman ER (1993) Fetal cells in the maternal circulation. Technical considerations for practical application to prenatal diagnosis. Obstet Gynecol Clin North Am 20:583–598

Sharpe HBA (1970) Human foetal maternal barrier. Nature 226:453–454

Shimamura M, Ohta S, Suzuki R, Yamazaki K. (1994) Transmission of maternal blood cells to the fetus during pregnancy: detection in mouse neonatal spleen by immunofluoerescence flow cytometry and polymerase chain reaction. Blood 83:926–930

Siebers JW, Knauf I, Hilemanns HG, Vogel W (1975) Antenatal sex determination in blood from pregnant women. Humangenetik 28:273–280

Simpson JL, Elias S ed (1994) Fetal cells in maternal blood. Prospects for noninvasive prenatal diagnosis. Ann N Y Acad Sci 731:1–262

Sottini A, Quiros-Roldan E, Notarangelo L, Malagoli A, Primi D, Imberti L (1995) Engrafted maternal T cells in a severe combined immunodeficiency patient express T cell receptor variable beta segments characterized by a restricted V-D-J junctional diversity. Blood 85:2105–2113

Splawski JB, Jelinek DF, Lipsky PE (1991) Delineation of the functional capacity of human neonatal lymphocytes. J Clin Invest 87:545–553

Starzl TE, Demetris AJ, Murase N, Trucco M, Thomson AW, Rao AS (1995) The changing immunology of organ transplantation. Hosp Pract 60:31–42

Takahara H, Kadotani T, Kusumi I, Makino S (1972) Some critical aspects on prenatal diagnosis of sex in leukocyte cultures from pregnant women. Proc Jpn Acad 48:603–607

Taylor AI, Polani PE (1965) XX/XY mosaicism in man. Lancet i:1226

Tharapel AT, Jaswaney VL, Dockter ME, Wachtel SS, Chandler RW, Simpson JL, Shulman LP, Meyers CM, Elias S (1993) Inability to detect fetal metaphases in flow-sorted lymphocyte cultures based on maternal-fetal HLA differences. Fetal Diagn Ther 8:95–101

Thomas MR, Tutschek B, Frost A, Rodeck CH, Yazdani N, Craft I, Williamson R (1995) The time of appearance and disappearance of fetal DNA from the maternal circulation. Prenat Diagn 15:641–64

Thong YH, Hurtado RC, Rola-Pleszczynski M, Hensen SA, Vincent MM, Micheletti SA, Bellanti JA (1974) Transplacental transmission of cell mediated immunity. Lancet i:1286–1287

Tiilikainen A, Schröder J, de la Chapelle A (1974) Fetal leukocytes in the maternal circulation after delivery. II. Masking of HL-A antigens. Transplantation 17:355–360

Turner JH, Wald N, Quinlivan WLG (1966) Cytogenetic evidence concerning possible transplacental transfer of leukocytes in pregnant women. Am J Obstet Gynecol 95:831–833

Vaidya S, Mamlok R, Daeschner CW, Williams J, Ruth J, Goldblum RM (1991) Suppression of graft-versus-host reaction in severe combined immunodeficiency with maternal-fetal engraftment. Am J Pediatr Hematol Oncol 13:172–175

Wahn V, Yokota S, Meyer KL, Janssen JWG, Hansen-Hagge TE, Knobloch C, Koletzko S, Stein H, Friedrich W, Bartram CR (1991) Expansion of a maternally derived monoclonal T cell population with CD3+/CD8+/T cell receptor-γ/δ+ phenotype in a child with severe combined immunodeficiency. J Immunol 147:2934–2941

Walknowska J, Conte FA, Grumbach MM (1969) Practical and theoretical implications of fetal/maternal lymphocyte transfer. Lancet i:1119–1122

Wessmann M, Ylinen K, Knuutila S (1992) Fetal granulocytes in maternal venous blood detected by in situ hybridization. Prenat Diagn 12:993–1000

Whang-Peng J, Leikin S, Lee HE, Sites J (1973) The transplacental passage of fetal leukocytes into the maternal blood. Proc Soc Exp Biol Med 142:50–53

Yeoh SC, Sargent IL, Redman CWG, Wordsworth BP, Thein SL (1991) Detection of fetal cells in maternal blood. Prenat Diagn 11:117–123

Ziliacus R, de la Chapelle A, Schröder J, Tiilikainen A, Kohne E, Kleihauer E (1975a) Transplacental passage of foetal blood cells. Scand J Hematol 15:333–338

Ziliacus R, de la Chapelle A, Schröder J, Tiilikainen A (1975b) Massive invasion of fetal lymphocytes into the mother's blood at induced abortion. Scand J Immunol 4:601–605

Zimmerman A, Schmickel R (1971) Fluorescent bodies in maternal circulation. Lancet i:1305

Suppressive Cellular and Molecular Activities in Maternofetal Immune Interactions; Suppressor Cell Activity, Prostaglandins, and Alpha-Fetoproteins

L.B. OLDING[1], N. PAPADOGIANNAKIS[1], B. BARBIERI[1], and R.A. MURGITA[2]

1 Introduction

Pregnancy has been termed an immunological "paradox" because the fetoplacental unit – although genetically and antigenically alien to its mother – is usually accepted by her as a "semi-allograft". Several models have been proposed to explain this apparent paradox. BILLINGHAM's (1964) concept of the fetoplacental unit as a semi-allograft is still valid form a purely genetic point of view, but otherwise has some shortcomings. First, in contrast to a grafted organ, a fetal "graft's" blood circulation is structurally separated from that of the mother by a barrier in humans consisting of trophoblastic cells, fetal capillary endothelium, and basal membranes with mesenchymal cells in between (see REDLINE, this volume). Second, trophoblastic cells invade the endometrium like a cancer and at least partly clog the maternal spiral arteries in the decidua (HUSTIN and SCHAAPS 1987; R.W. REDLINE, this

[1]The Karolinska Institute, Department of Immunology, Microbiology, Pathology and Infectious Diseases, Division of Pathology, Huddinge University Hospital, 141 86 Huddinge, Sweden
[2]Department of Microbiology and Immunology, McGill University, Montreal, Quebec, Canada O3A 2P4

volume), thereby at least partly hindering circulating maternal immune cells from reaching the intervillous space and the syncytiotrophoblastic membrane in the beginning of gestation. Third, and most important, is the overwhelming amount of evidence that classical major histocompatibility complex (MHC) class I and II antigens are not expressed on the villous syncytiotrophoblast (see, for example, GALBRAITH et al. 1981; FAULK et al. 1982), and only a unique MHC class I antigen, HLA-G, is expressed on the extravillous invasive trophoblast at the placental site in the decidua (for an overview, see Ober and van der Ven, and Arch and Clark, this volume). Besides, it is unclear whether this unique oligomorphic HLA antigen is functional (regulating the natural killer (NK) cells and the NK-like large granular lymphocytes (LGLs) in the decidua?) or merely a non-functional evolutionary relic.

Accordingly, the concept of pregnancy as an ordinary organ transplant is, from an immunological point of view, limp. It seems, instead, to be a unique relationship designed and modified under the pressure of an array of evolutionary events. However, many basic questions remain concerning the success of fetal implantation and its maintenance until term. In this context, we briefly review possible suppressor cells and suppressor factors of importance for immune interactions between the pregnant woman and the fetoplacental unit and for the maintenance of pregnancy. With respect to suppressor substances, we focus on the role of prostaglandins and α-fetoproteins and their possible interactions with cytokines. First, the immunocompetence of the pregnant women is briefly discussed (The ontogeny of immunocompetence of the fetus is extensively reviewed by M. ADINOLFI in this volume.)

2 Immunocompetence of the Pregnant Woman

There is a general consensus that women are not generally immunocompromised during normal pregnancy. Most researchers agree that the immunomodulation necessary for implantation of the blastocyst and for the ensuing maintenance of gestation takes place locally at the blastocyst implantation site in the decidua, at the syncytiotrophoblast cover of the chorionic villi, and at the endovascular trophoblast replacing endothelial cells in maternal spiral arteries. However, in general, there is evidence to suggest that pregnant women have depressed cell-mediated immunity and increased humoral immunity. This is consistent with the concept that pregnancy is biased towards the production of TH_2 cytokines which promote B-cells development and at the same time down regulate TH_1-derived interleukin-2 (IL-2), interferon-γ (IFN-γ), and tumor necrosis factor (TNF), which are considered deleterious for pregnancy (WEGMANN et al. 1993, LIN et al. 1993). This paradigm would further help explain why autoimmune diseases mediated primarily by T cells undergo temporary remission during pregnancy (DA SILVA and SPECTOR 1992), while those involving excessive autoantibody production tend to be exacerbated (EL-ROEIY and SHOENFELD 1985). TH1 cytokines would promote NK cell reactivity which could be detrimental to the fetus. However, NK-cell activity is reported to be diminished in the blood of pregnant women and in the fetus and newborn (LUFT and REMINGTON 1984; LEE et al. 1987; BALEY and SCHACTER 1985).

Ideally, maternal immunosuppression should be sufficient to prevent unwarranted antifetal responses while at the same time functioning in a selective enough manner to leave other protective features of the immune system intact. This optimal situation is not completely attained as pregnancy can result in increased susceptibility to infectious diseases (MORELL 1995; FRIED and DUFFY 1996). Thus, pregnancy tends to increase susceptibility to infections by viruses such as hepatitis virus (KHUOROO et al. 1981), Epstein-Barr virus (EBV; SAKAMOTO et al. 1982), and herpes simplex virus (HSV; BROWN et al. 1985). In addition, decreased immune reactivity to viral antigens e.g., cytomegalovirus (CMV), is evident in vitro (GEHRZ et al. 1981). Those changes can presumably be attributed to a decreased number of circulating cells and a reduced NK-cell activity throughout pregnancy. On the other hand, pregnancy-induced alterations to the immune system can also result in beneficial effects on some disease processes including certain cancers and autoimmune diseases. Pregnant women have an altered susceptibility to cancer. For example, breast cancer is less common in parous than nulliparous women (BERAL 1983; JACOBSON et al. 1989) and Kaposi's sarcoma has been noted to regress during pregnancy (LUNARDL-ISKANDAR et al. 1995). PERSELLIN (1977) has reported improvement or remission of rheumatoid arthritis (RA) in 74% of 274 individual pregnancies.

By and large, the total number of circulating lymphocytes in pregnant women does not seem to differ from that in nonpregnant women. However, temporary variations may arise, for example, a decreased T/B cell ratio during the first 20 weeks of gestation (STRELKAUSKAS et al. 1975, 1978). Some results conflict as to the number of T-cell subtypes present during pregnancy; for example, JACOBY and OLDSTONE (1983) using monoclonal OKT antibodies as markers found a relatively slight increase in helper (CD_4^+) cells in pregnant compared with nonpregnant women (48.5% vs 41%), whereas CASTILLA et al. (1989) reported a slight decrease in those cells during pregnancy. Values for T killer/suppressor (CD_8^+) cells seem to be virtually unchanged (JACOBY and OLDSTONE 1983). The reactivity of pregnant and nonpregnant womens' lymphocytes to alloantigens in a one-way mixed lymphocyte reaction (MLR) seems to be comparable (CARR et al. 1974; OLDING et al. 1977).

A dramatic reduction in the numbers and activity of committed B lymphocyte precursors in the bone marrow of normal pregnant mice has recently been reported (MEDINA et al. 1993; MEDINA and KINCADE 1994). There is as yet no information available on humans regarding the effects of pregnancy of B-cell lymphopoiesis. However, there has been an increase in the number of reports describing the synthesis of lymphohematopoietic cytokines during pregnancy (POLLARD 1991; WEGMANN 1993).

Complement bound to and activated by antigen–antibody complexes constitutes a potential risk for antibody-dependent cell mediated cytotoxicity reactions directed against placental tissues, particularly villous and extravillous trophoblasts.

It is therefore of interest that several complement regulatory proteins have been detected on the trophoblast; these are membrane cofactor protein (CD 46; PURCELL et al. 1990), decay accelerating factor (CD 55), and inhibitor of the membrane attack complex (CD 59; HSI et al. 1991; HOLMES et al. 1992). These proteins might contribute to the relative resistance of trophoblastic cells to antibody- and complement-mediated lysis (TEDESCO et al. 1993).

3 Suppressor Cells

The concept of suppressor T lymphocytes that downregulate humoral and cellular immune response mechanisms originated from experiments by GERSHON and KONDO (1971) in the context of so-called infectious tolerance. Thereafter, an abundance of reports on that theme surfaced which were highly controversial among immunologists. It is beyond the scope of this chapter to review the abundant literature on this topic. Extensive reviews have been published (PARASKEVAS 1984; KLEIN 1986; BLOOM et al. 1992; GREEN and WEBB 1993).

The suppressor T cell was until recently believed to belong exclusively to the CD_8^+ phenotype, and thus, to be phenotypically indistinguishable from the cytotoxic T cell. In addition, based on many experimental investigations, a very complicated "cascade" was proposed which is specifically triggered by antigen-specific I–J restricted CD_4^+ "suppression-inducer" cells, followed by CD_8^+ anti-idiotypic-specific cells and concluded by CD_8^+ antigen-specific effector cells that exert suppression not restricted by MHC antigens. Three soluble factors, an antigen-specific factor (T suppressor F_1), an anti-idiotypic factor (T-suppressor F_2) and a nonspecific factor (T suppressor F_3), connected with the various cells are involved in the cascade (reviewed by KLEIN 1986; BLOOM et al. 1992).

Subsequently, a more simplified, functional model was suggested based on the dominating kinds of cytokines produced by various T lymphocytes of *both* the CD_4^+ (reviewed by JANEWAY et al. 1988; MOSMANN and COFFMAN 1989) and CD_8^+ (BLOOM et al. 1992) type which recognize antigens or T-cell receptor idiotypes together with MHC antigens. Similar to the case of CD_4^+ cells for which two subtypes were recently described (TH_1 and TH_2), two subtypes of CD_8^+ cells (type 1 and type 2) have been suggested. In this model, both TH_1 an CD_8^+ type 1 cells suppress B-cell function and induce delayed-type hypersensitivity (DTH) and cytotoxic T lymphocyte activity, where TH_2 cells and CD_8^+ type 2 cells both serve as B helper cells (BLOOM et al. 1992).

In addition, many immunosuppressor cells which are nonspecific in their induction conditions and effector activity have been described. For example, they might be induced by various mitogens, autologous cells, hormones, or α-fetoproteins, or they might arise spontaneously without any obvious induction (reviewed by MURGITA et al. 1981; PARASKEVAS 1984).

3.1 Suppressor Cell Activity in Cord Blood

We found that peripheral blood mononuclear leukocytes (PBMLs) derived from cord blood of human neonates harbor a strong nonspecific suppressor cell activity in vitro. This was found by coculturing PBMLs from mothers who had recently given birth with PBMLs from the cord blood of their male newborn babies in the ratio 1:1 and by stimulating the cocultures with phytohemagglutinine (PHA; OLDING and OLDSTONE 1974; OLDING et al. 1974). The use of the XY chromosome as a marker for dividing male newborns cells and the XX chromosome to identify the mother's cells, along with a fluorescent chromosome assay, enabled us to demonstrate that 88%–100% of the dividing cells were fetal and only 0%–12% were of maternal origin. We also showed that the strong suppression or abrogation of the division of maternal PBMLs in the presence of PBMLs from the newborn was not caused by significant variations in the reactivity to PHA between maternal and neonatal PBMLs. Neither the gender differences of these cells nor genetic factors were influential; new born females' PBMLs suppressed the reactivity of cells from various unrelated male adults to an equal degree, whereas PBMLs from unrelated adult males and females cocultured with PHA did not suppress one another, nor did those from unrelated newborn males and females (OLDING et al. 1974).

Similarly, allogeneic stimulation of maternal and newborns' PBMLs by a two-way MLR, presumably reflecting allogeneic stimulation in vivo, incited the same strong suppression of maternal cell mitogenesis (90%–100%) that emerged after 6 days in culture (OLDING et al. 1977). The suppression was not linked to any measurable cytotoxicity (OLDING et al. 1974). Furthermore, the suppressive activity of cord PBMLs seemed to be an exclusive function of T lymphocytes (OLDING and OLDSTONE 1976; OLDSTONE et al. 1977). Such suppression was abrogated by irradiation (with 6000 rads) and even turned into a strong stimulatory effect on maternal lymphocytes (mitotic index 7.2). This observation tallied with experiments in mice (WALLIS et al. 1976; SKOWRON-CENRZAK and PTAK 1976). The strong suppressor activity was not restricted to the perinatal period, but emerged as early as the 8th week of gestation among lymphoid cells in the fetal liver and lingered until 11 months after birth (UNANDER and OLDING 1981).

PBMLs from the human neonate strongly inhibit the synthesis of immunoglobulin (Ig) by adult B cells in pokeweed mitogen (PWM-) induced B-cell differentiation assays. For example, the Ig synthesis by maternal PBMLs stimulated by PWM after 8 days in culture gradually decreases as the amount of added (non-antigen-stimulated) neonatal PBMLs increases; in contrast, the amount of Ig synthesized rises, as increasing amounts of autologous PBMLs are added (OLDSTONE et al. 1977; JACOBY and OLDSTONE 1983). Similar results which show the importance of T suppressor cells from newborns in the regulation of adult B-cell differentiation have been reported and reviewed (ANDERSSON et al. 1981; MIYAWAKI et al. 1981; UNANDER et al. 1982).

3.2 T-cell Subsets in Cord Blood Responsible for Immunosuppression

The mode of characterizing functional suppressor T cells has changed over the last twenty years. MORETTA et al. (1977) introduced the use of Fc receptors for IgG (Fc γ) and IgM (Fc μ) to delineate suppressor and helper T cells, respectively. Later, monoclonal antibodies to various clusters of differentiation (CD) antigens on cell surfaces were produced, and subsequently a method to delineate functional subsets of CD_4^+ T cells was introduced based on their production of various cytokines (JANEWAY et al. 1988; MOSMANN and COFFMAN 1989).

The use of Fc γ and Fc μ markers to differentiate between different lymphocytes of the newborn gave conflicting results. OLDSTONE et al. (1977) showed that the neonatal suppressor cell was a Tγ cell, whereas HAYWARD and LYDYARD (1978) indicated that a Tμ cell was suppressive. Ensuing investigations by DURANDY et al. (1979) pointed to the presence of *both* Tγ and Tμ suppressor cell populations in the newborn's blood, with different modes of action: the Tμ cells exerted a significant but transient suppression, whereas the effect of Tγ cells occurred later and was more long-lasting. The reason for this is obscure but might be explained by the fact that the expression of Fc receptors changes during the maturation process of T cells (PICHLER and BRODER 1981).

There has been some controversy as to the CD phenotype of the neonatal T suppressor cell, but the majority of authors have reported a CD_4^+ and CD_8^- phenotype. This was borne out in both negative and positive selection experiments. With negative selection by a monoclonal OKT_8^+ antibody and complement, JACOBY and OLDSTONE (1983) removed CD_8^+ cells from cord blood and found that the CD_8^- cord PBMLs (i.e., enriched for CD_4^+) suppressed the IgG synthesis of adult PWM-induced PBMLs in a dose-dependent manner (by up to 86%). In contrast, no suppression was noticed when cord blood deprived of CD_4^+ cells was used. Basically the same results were obtained by YACHIE et al. (1981), whereas some reports have indicated that cord CD_8^+ cells are the suppressor T cells (HAYWARD and MERILL 1981; DURANDY et al. 1985). A dichotomy in the suppressor cell activity in cord blood was reported by ANDERSSON et al. (1983), who found that the cord suppressor cell activity exerted on PWM-induced Ig secretion belonged to the CD_8^+ phenotype, whereas both cord CD_8^+ and CD_4^+ T cells suppressed EBV-induced B-cell secretion of Ig. In our experiments, cord blood lymphocytes were mixed with maternal cells in a 1:1 ratio in a two-way MLR supported by PHA. The results indicated that the fetal/neonatal suppressor cell was mainly of the CD_4^+/CD_8^- phenotype. Whereas the depletion of the CD_4^+ cells from cord T cells either by panning or by complement-mediated lysis totally abrogated the suppression of maternal lymphocytes, the depletion of cord CD_8^+ cells caused only an occasional, small reduction in suppression (PAPADOGIANNAKIS et al. 1985a). Accordingly, some additional suppressive effect of CD_8^+, presumably based on cooperation between cord CD_4^+ and CD_8^+ cells, could not be excluded.

A "suppressor–inducer" effect of neonatal CD_4^+ cells on maternal CD_8^+ cells, as suggested by THOMAS et al. (1981) and RICH et al. (1986) seems unlikely. For example, removal of maternal CD_8^+ cells by using a monoclonal antibody and complement did not abrogate the suppression exerted by neonatal CD_4^+ cells on maternal B-cell function, nor did irradiation (1200 rads), which is known to inhibit the radiosensitive suppressor fraction of T cells (JACOBY and OLDSTONE 1983). We achieved similar results in a two-way proliferation MLR assay of neonatal and maternal PBMLs from which maternal CD_8^+ cells had been removed (PAPADOGIANNAKIS et al. 1985b). Similar results have also been reported by CHENG et al. (1985).

Hence, a logical conclusion is that the nonspecific suppression of adult lymphocytes by fetal/neonatal cells is basically a direct function of the neonatal CD_4^+ subfraction and that the maternal/adult target cell also is a CD_4^+ cell. Interestingly, some evidence indicates that mitogen-activated suppressor CD_4^+ cells from human newborns, but not autologous conventional CD_8^+ suppressor cells, can directly suppress the IgG secretion of B cells from adults (BLAESE et al. 1982; JACOBY and OLDSTONE 1983), presumably at the plasma cell level (BLAESE et al. 1982). Neither monocytes nor macrophages seem to be involved in this kind of suppression, in contrast to their participation in prostaglandin (PG)-mediated suppression (see below).

A CD_4^+ T cell – instead of the "traditional" CD_8^+ suppressor T cell – as a suppressor cell in the cord blood might seem paradoxical. However, a sound explanation lies in the current concept of two functional subsets of CD_4^+ cells with different kinds of predominant cytokine production either mediating cell-mediated delayed-type hypersensitivity and suppressing B cell function (TH_1 cells) or promoting B-cell development suppressing DTH (TH_2 cells; BLOOM et al. 1992; see above). Also suggested is the possibility that the CD_4^+ function might be diverted towards TH_2 functions during pregnancy (WEGMANN et al. 1993), considering that TH_1 cytokines IL-2, TNF-α, and IFNγ could be deleterious for the fetus. For example, TNF-α could damage trophoblastic cells directly, or, like IL-2 and IFN-γ, activate NK cells and the NK-like LGLs to destructive lymphokine-activated killer cells in the decidua.

This hypothesis is supported by clinical observations of a weakening of cell-mediated immunity, i.e., TH_1 cell function, in normal pregnant women and a simultaneous increase in antibody-mediated immunity (i.e., TH_2 function). Women with systemic lupus erythematosus, which is mainly an antibody-mediated disease, often encounter an aggravation of their symptoms during gestation (DA SILVA and SPECTOR 1992), whereas pregnant women with RA, in whom immunity is predominantly-mediated rather than humoral, experience an improvement of their symptoms (see above). The potential risk of TH_1 cell activity is further emphasized by the presence of TNF-α mRNA in syncytiotrophoblasts, in endovascular trophoblasts within maternal spiral arteries (CHEN et al. 1991), and in NK cells and macrophages occupying the decidua (JOKHI et al. 1994) and by the presence of IFN-γ in syncytiotrophoblasts (BULMER et al. 1990). Investigations by us and by others of the suppressor activity resides in fetal/neonatal lymphocytes have been detailed in reviews by JACOBY et al. (1984) and PAPADOGIANNAKIS et al. (1990). Recent investigations of the cytokines in the placenta and decidua have been extensively reviewed by LOKE and KING (1995).

4 Soluble Suppressor Factors

4.1 Prostaglandins

In mammalian cells, arachidonic acid (AA) can enzymatically and, to some extent, non-enzymatically be metabolized to several biologically active derivatives. These derivatives are divided into three major classes according to the enzyme that catalyzes the initial step of AA metabolism: (1) prostaglandin H (PGH) synthase, which produces PGH. PGH is then metabolized to other prostaglandins (PGs) and thromboxanes (TXs); (2) lipoxygenases, which produce leucotrienes, hydroxy derivatives and lipoxins; and (3) cytochrome p-450 which produces hydroxy derivatives and epoxide-containing derivatives.

The principal step in the formation of the AA-derived eicosanoids – the collective name for metabolites of 20-carbon fatty acids, from the Greek word *eicosi*, meaning twenty – is the calcium-dependent release of free AA from the cell membrane phospholipid pool (Smith and Marnett 1991; Reilly and Fitzgerald 1993). Several factors can induce the liberation of AA (reviewed by Herschman 1994). Such factors can be inflammatory (Vane 1987), immunological (Goodwin 1989; Bray 1987), mechanical, or hormonal, and function by activating phospholipase A_2 (PLA_2) which degrades the cell membrane phospholipids into arachidonic acid and diacyl glycerol moieties. Phospholipase C may also release AA by liberating a diglyceride from phosphatidylinositol-4,5-diphosphate, which is then hydrolyzed by another lipase to yield AA (Reilly and Fitzgerald 1993).

Although AA has an almost unique function as a precursor for eicosanoids, it should be emphasized that in most cells, AA, like other fatty acids, undergoes β-oxidation even if other common fuels are available (Barbieri et al. 1994). However, the extent to which AA is used in the β-oxidation reaction varies with the cell type (Barbieri et al. 1995).

Details of the mechanism of release of arachidonate esterified to the glycerol moiety of phospholipids are beyond the scope of this discussion. The relevant point is that it has not yet been established whether PGs and leucotrienes are produced from the same or different phospholipid pools.

The PGs are composed of a 20-carbon fatty acid containing a cyclopentane ring, the so-called hypothetical prostanoic acid. PGs fall into three subclasses; PG_1, PG_2, and PG_3. The PG_2 class is the most abundant in man and the only one for which AA is the precursor. Following its release, the AA is metabolized by PGH synthase (Rollins and Smith 1980; Smith et al. 1983). This enzyme, which exhibits both cyclooxygenase and peroxidase activity produces the endoperoxides PGG_2 and PGH_2. The cyclooxygenation is inhibited by aspirin, indomethacin, and several other nonsteroidal anti-inflammatory drugs (Meade et al. 1993; Vane 1994; Laneuville et al. 1994). PGH_2, a labile intermediate, can be converted into stable PGs, such as PGE_2, PGD_2, and $PGF_{2\alpha}$, by their respective synthase enzymes. In addition, PGH_2 can be metabolized to TXA_2 by TX synthase and to PGI_2 by prostacyclin synthase.

It is generally believed that the rate-limiting step in PG synthesis is AA release from the phospholipid pool. This theory assumes that AA is converted to PGH_2 by the constitutively expressed enzyme PGH synthase 1, proposed to be present in excess (HERSCHMAN 1994). However, another subtype of the isozyme, PGH synthase 2, (LYSZ and NEEDLEMAN 1982; MEADE et al. 1993) is inducible by, for example, growth factors, tumor promotors, endotoxins, and other substances known to elevate PG production by cells.

Regulation of PGH synthase 2 expression is presumably critical for the production of PGs in cells expressing both isozymes or only PGH synthase 2 (RAZ et al. 1989; VARFOLMEYER and MEVKH 1993; HERSCHMAN 1994). Hence, it seems as if PG production is limited by steps beyond the AA liberation level, so that, despite a massive release of AA, an ensuing excess in PG production with potential harmful effects can be avoided.

A rapid regulation of cell function by PGs is achieved by maintaining a low basal level of PGs in tissues and rapidly inactivating them when formed. Thus, typical PG-mediated regulation requires that (a) PG is synthesized at a speed exceeding the inactivation rate and (b) PG must occupy a sufficient number of specific receptors in order to induce regulatory signals in the cell. Moreover, the PG synthesized must exit the cell to reach the actual receptors on the target cell and also enter a cell for oxidative degradation. Most PGs in the blood circulation are rapidly degraded due to their instability or by PG dehydrogenase enzymes preferentially located in the lungs and liver. Although PGs are deprotonated at physiological pH and diffuse poorly across membranes they have been assumed to exit cells in which they are produced by simple diffusion across the membranes. There does not seem to be clear evidence for active or carrier-mediated transport of PG in the literature. However, the existence of a PG-transporting protein has been reported (KANAI et al. 1995).

The kind and amount of eicosanoids produced depend on the tissue or cell. In the context of this chapter we should mention that the main immunoregulatory PG, PGE_2, is produced mainly by monocytes and macrophages, and *not* by lymphocytes. Most authors agree (reviewed by GOLDYNE 1989) that lymphocytes regardless of phenotype do *not* produce PGE_2 or any other AA metabolite. This proposal was confirmed in repeated in vitro experiments (B. BARBIERI, unpublished work). Furthermore, lymphocytes apparently do not express PGH synthase type 1 or 2, and reports claiming AA metabolism in lymphocytes can probably be attributed to insufficient removal of monocytes. In experiments performed with $5–10 \times 10^6$ lymphocytes, the presence of monocytes even in an amount which is only 2% of the total cell number might produce a significant amount of PGE_2 (GOLDYNE 1989). Any contamination by monocytes is even more critical if the cells are stimulated, which would promote expression of PGH synthase 2.

4.1.1 Prostaglandins in Pregnancy

AA metabolites are essential in many respects during pregnancy. For example, PGE_2 is important in softening the cervix uteri by increasing the collagenase activity and making the cervix "ripe" for parturition (reviewed by CALDER 1994). PGE_2 and $PGF_{2\alpha}$ are essential for the initiation of parturition in cooperation with progesterone and estrogen in a complicated and still not fully understood way (reviewed by MAGGI et al. 1994). However, recent investigations suggest that PGs enhance the estrogen-induced expression of oxytocin receptors in the myometrium following sensitization by progesterone (NEULEN and BRECKWOLDT 1994). It is well known that $PGF_{2\alpha}$ provokes abortion by inducing contractions of the uterus myometrium. Also well known is that PGE_2, and possibly PGI_2, combined with a low oxygen tension in fetal blood prohibits preterm closure of the ductus arteriosus (reviewed by GERSONY 1986).

The placenta with the fetal membranes and the decidua are major producers of AA metabolites. This is evident from many investigations using various techniques such as perfusion whole cell homogenates, microsome cell fractions, culture of dissociated cells, and perifusion of cell cultures. The eicosanoids have been measured by radio-thin layer chromatography, gas chromatography–masspectrometry, radioimmunoassay and immunochemistry. Conversion of exogenous AA to PGF_2 was found to occur in homogenized tissues from the chorioamnion, villous placenta, placenta arteries, and myometrium, and to $PGF_{2\alpha}$ in the chorioamnion, villous placenta, placental vessels, and myometrium, and to thromboxane B_2 in the villous placenta, placental vessels and myometrium (CHRISTENSEN and GRÉEN 1983; DIMOV et al. 1983). Similar results were obtained by MTICHELL (1986). Cultured human trophoblastic cells produce PGs, mainly PGE_2 (KELLY et al. 1995; SHIMONOVITZ et al. 1995). Dissociated human decidua cells at term yield PGs and more $PGF_{2\alpha}$ than PGE_2, and bone-marrow-derived ($CD45^+$) cells in the decidua produce more PGs than the decidua cells (NORWITZ et al. 1991). Furthermore, enzymes associated with PG synthesis have been found in the placenta and decidua according to several reports: phospholipase A_2 (ANDERSEN et al. 1994) and PGH synthase (cyclooxygenase) have been found in the decidua, extravillous trophoblast, and villous syncytiotrophoblast (DIVERS et al. 1995), PGH synthase 1 and 2 in the human amnion (TEIXEIRA et al. 1994), PGH synthase 1 mRNA in the human amnion, decidua, and chorionic villi (FREED et al. 1995), and PG dehydrogenase in the trophoblastic cells (CHEUNG et al. 1992).

4.1.2 Prostaglandin-Mediated Immunosuppression

PGE, and specifically PGE_2, has turned out to be the main suppressor of cellular and humoral immune response among various PGs tested (A, E_1, E_2, $F_{1\alpha}$, $F_{2\alpha}$, I_2). This major immunosuppressive effect is apparent in a multitude of functional processes (GOODWIN and WEBB 1980; BRAY 1980; PAPADOGIANNAKIS et al. 1990).

We found that PBMLs from mothers who had recently given birth were strongly suppressed in vitro by enriched PBMLs from cord blood of their own (male or female) babies or of alien babies by means of a soluble and dialyzable factor of less than 500 dalton (OLDING et al. 1977). This result was borne out by experiments in a Marbrook-Diener double chamber system in which PHA-stimulated PBMLs from a mother and her baby were cultured for 60 to 72 h on each side of a dialysis filter. Maternal cell proliferation was suppressed, although only 40%–71% as measured by the uptake of ^{3}H-labeled thymidine. In contrast, a two-way MLR supported by PHA showed a strong predominance of dividing cells from newborns (88%–100%; see above). The addition of indomethacin (2.8 or 28 μM), which blocks the PGH synthase (see above) and thereby blocks the first step in PG synthesis from AA, not only abrogated suppression of the maternal PHA-induced PBML proliferation by 100% but even reverted suppression to a significant stimulation of this maternal PBML response (JOHNSEN et al. 1982). Similar results were obtained by using eicosatetraynoic acid (3.3 or 33 μM), an acetylenic AA analogue that competes with AA but lacks the ability to be metabolized (AHERN and DOWNING 1970).

When indomethacin (2.8 or 28 μM) was added to a two-way MLR of maternal and neonatal PBMLs (tested by fluorescent chromosome markers – see above) the suppression decreased significantly (from 58%–92% to 15%–31%; JOHNSEN et al. 1982). Our experiments confirmed PGE_2 as a major immunosuppressive factor which is bound to fetal and neonatal PBMLs. Fetal/neonatal and maternal/adult PBMLs – and presumably only monocytes (see above) – convert ^{14}C-labeled AA in vitro mainly to PGE, and preferentially to PGE_2, but also to small amounts of $PGF_{2\alpha}$ and thromboxane B_2 according to gas chromatography–mass spectrometry (JOHNSEN et al. 1983).

PBMLs from adults are 100 times more sensitive to PGE_2 than cells from newborns. After testing several concentrations of PGE_2, it was found that 1.4×10^{-8} M PGE_2 yielded as much suppression in adults as 1.4×10^{-6} M did in newborns' PBMLs. However, there was a dichotomy in the effect of PGE_2: smaller amounts (1.4×10^{-9} M in adults and 1.4×10^{-7} M in newborns) reversed the suppressive effect to one of slight stimulation (JOHNSEN et al. 1982). Enriched T cells from mothers and newborns (deprived of monocytes by nylon wool or plastic adherence) cocultured with PHA displayed a similar suppressive pattern as PBMLs (PAPADOGIANNAKIS et al. 1985b). The suppression was largely reduced by various PG synthase inhibitors. However, various subtypes (phenotypes) of the newborns' T cells displayed different sensitivities. Whereas cord CD_4^+ CD_8^- T cells (i.e., conventional T helper cells) were virtually insensitive to PGE_2, the CD_8^+ CD_4^- T cells (i.e., conventional T suppressor cells) were significantly suppressed by four of five PGE_2 doses (1.4×10^{-5} through 1.4×10^{-9} M) (PAPADOGIANNAKIS et al, 1985a). In contrast, both CD_4^+ and CD_8^+ T cells from the mother were strongly suppressed by the same doses of PGE_2 sensitivity of the cells.

The mechanism(s) by which PGE_2 suppresses the proliferation of mitogen-induced PBMLs from adults has been studied in several ways. The impact of PGs on immune cells seems to be mainly mediated by binding of the PGs to specific high-affinity cell surface receptors (RAO 1988; PLAUT 1987). Such receptors have been described and partly characterized on PBMLs, lymphocytes, monocytes, and thymocytes (Samuelsson et al. 1978; Goodwin et al. 1979; Eriksen et al. 1985; Dailey et al. 1988; Brown and Phipps 1995). The PG receptor has recently been purified and cloned (Narumiya 1994). The receptor proteins are linked via G proteins to effectors such as adenylate cyclase (AC) and phospholipase C (Narumiya 1994). Accumulation of activated AC generates cAMP from ATP. The effect of PG on cell function is subsequent to the action of cAMP itself and involves binding to cAMP-specific protein kinases and phosphorylation of various substrate proteins. cAMP displays various suppressive effects on immune functions such as the proliferation of T and B cells, killer T cell (T_K), killer cell (K) and NK cell cytotoxicity, antibody production by B cells, and secretion of some cytokines and growth factors (reviewed by Goodwin 1989; Plaut 1987). This can be caused, for example, by inhibition of an antigen- or mitogen-induced rise in intracytoplasmic Ca^{2+} (Papadogiannakis et al. 1989a).

We found that enriched PBMLs from both cord blood and blood from mothers who had recently given birth displayed specific high affinity binding (dissociation constant of 6.5×10^{-9} *M*; Johnsen and Olding 1983) and that the maternal cells bound about three times more PGE_2 molecules than the cord cells. Thus, the relative resistance of neonatal lymphoid cells to the antiproliferative effect of PGE_2 could be explained by a lower density of specific PGE_2 binding sites on these cells than on maternal cells. However, because PBMLs (including both lymphocytes and monocytes) were used, the density of binding sites exclusively on lymphocytes could not be determined in this investigation.

Next, the kinetics of cAMP production in fetal/neonatal and maternal/adult cells was investigated. Cord PBMLs showed an overall lower rate of AC activity than maternal PBMLs in response to PGE_2 and other autacoids, such as isoproterenol and histamine, and to receptor-independent stimulation by forskolin (Papadogiannakis et al. 1989b). However, cord PBMLs also displayed a significantly lower rate of degradation of cAMP by cAMP-phosphodiesterase. The net accumulation of PGE_2-induced cAMP was similar in cord and maternal PBMLs. However, PHA-stimulated cord cells were much less sensitive to the antiproliferative effect of cAMP-raising agents, such as the receptor-independent forskolin and dibutyryl cAMP (a synthetic cAMP analogue), than PHA-activated maternal cells (Papadogiannakis et al. 1989b). These results suggest that cord lymphocytes are genuinely less susceptibile to the effect of cAMP itself than maternal/adult cells. Although the reasons for this remain unclear, they presumably involve steps following the generation of cAMP, i.e., functions and kinetics of cAMP kinases, as discussed above.

When the monoclonal anti-CD^3 antibody OKT3 (linked to the T-cell receptor for antigen) was used as a mitogen instead of PHA in our cocultures with chromosome markers, the proliferation of maternal cells was still significantly suppressed, but less than in the PHA-supplemented cultures (Papadogiannakis and Johnsen 1988). In cultures of separate cord PBMLs and T cells stimulated by OKT3 or by the calcium ionophore A23187 (which promotes cell proliferation by raising the intracellular concentration of Ca^{2+}), cord cells were as sensitive to the immunosuppressive effect of PGE_2 as the maternal cells (Papadogiannakis and

JOHNSEN 1987). Furthermore, cord cells exhibited a lower mitogenic response to OKT3 (PAPADOGIANNAKIS et al. 1986a) and this could be largely explained by the existence or function of an excessively PG-producing autologous monocyte population (PAPADOGIANNAKIS et al. 1986b). Moreover, the suppression in OKT3-induced cocultures appeared to be insensitive to the action of PG synthase inhibitors such as indomethacin.

4.2 α-Fetoproteins

In the remainder of this chapter we confine our remarks to an updated analysis of the immunoregulatory properties of AFP. Where possible we will emphasize what we consider to be the important parallels between experimentally determined in vitro and in vivo patterns of AFP-mediated regulatory effects on lymphoid cell growth and function and the altered immune responsiveness of pregnant females and the newborn who have normally elevated serum AFP levels.

AFP, an embryo-specific glycoprotein synthesized primarily by the yolk sac and liver, is the first α-globulin to appear in mammalian sera during ontogenic development and remains a dominant serum protein throughout embryonic life. In early murine ontogeny AFP is mostly transcribed in the yolk sac and fetal liver, representing approximately 10% and 15%, respectively, of the total mRNA in these tissues. The onset of AFP expression occurs on day 10 of gestation in the mouse and is detectable by the 4th week of gestation in the human. The concentration of AFP in human fetal serum peaks at levels of 2–4 mg/ml at 12–16 weeks of gestation. Synthesis then remains constant until the 32nd week, thereafter declining until terms when the levels are approximately 0.1 mg/ml. Postnatally, AFP rapidly disappears from the serum and the trace amount that is characteristically found in the adult, about 1–10 ng/ml, is reached by 4–5 weeks of age. The AFP in maternal serum increases during pregnancy over the very low normal adult value up to a range of 100–500 ng/ml depending on the gestational stage. The highest levels are reached in the third trimester. Maternal AFP is thought to be entirely derived from the fetus (ADINOLFI 1979).

The effects of AFP on the immune system have been extensively studied (reviewed by DEUTCH 1991). The results of numerous investigations show that AFP can exert strong regulatory influences on lymphoid cell growth and function. The first direct evidence that AFP suppresses certain types of immune responses was obtained in the murine system (MURGITA and TOMASI 1975; reviewed by MURGITA and WIGZELL 1981). Fetal-derived AFP, purified to homogeneity, was found to exert a potent noncytotoxic inhibitory effect on primary and secondary antibody responses to T-cell-dependent, but not T-cell-independent (MURGITA and WIGZELL 1976) antibody responses. IgA was most sensitive to suppression by AFP, IgG was intermediate, and IgM was least susceptible to inhibition by AFP (MURGITA and TOMASI 1975).

It has been hypothesized that in normal physiology AFP protects the developing embryo from an immune attack by the mother by entering the maternal circulation and selectively suppressing the immune system during the stages of gestation when the fetus is potentially vulnerable. An earlier study in the murine system (MURGITA 1976) has shown that certain immune functions are inhibited during pregnancy and that these temporary changes in immune reactivity could, at least in part, be attributed to immunoregulatory AFP molecules in the maternal circulation. Notably, the pattern of AFP-mediated immunosuppression in this pregnancy study was the same as that reported in the initial studies describing the inhibitory effects of purified fetal AFP on in vitro immune responses by normal mouse spleen cells (MURGITA and TOMASI 1975). Similar findings were subsequently reported by TODER et al. (1979). That AFP is able to suppress cytokine-activated NK cells (COHEN et al. 1986) is consistent with the results of LUFT and REMINGTON (1984) which show that pregnancy is associated with an impaired ability to augment NK activity. Downregulation of NK cells by AFP may also help prevent fetal loss as a consequence of overproduction of NK-derived TNF-α and IFN-γ (TRANGRI et al. 1994). Support for this concept comes from studies employing transgenic mice which express human AFP (YAMASHITA et al. 1993). The transgenic mice had a diminished ability to eliminate an infection with a facultative intracellular pathogen due to an AFP-mediated inhibition of IFN-γ and TNF in NK cells and macrophages (YAMASHITA et al. 1994).

There are a number of reports that AFP purified from human cord blood or hepatoma serum can suppress human lymphocyte reactions in vitro (YACHNIN 1976; ALPERT et al. 1978; MURGITA et al. 1978a). YACHNIN and LESTER (1976) showed that human fetal-derived AFP was one to three times more suppressive than was AFP isolated from human hepatoma fluids. Three molecular variants of human AFP were detected electrophoretically in fetal- and hepatoma-derived AFP preparations. The immunosuppressive potency of AFP isolated from a given source could be correlated with the proportion of a certain electronegative species contained in it (LESTER et al. 1978). VAN OERS et al. (1989) directly examined the functional significance of microheterogeneity of AFP by quantitatively isolating each isomeric form (VAN OERS et al. 1990). All of the immunosuppressive activity of AFP was localized to a single molecular variant which represented only 6% of the total composition of fetal (mouse) AFP. CHAKRABORTY and MANDAL (1993) have shown in a cross-species study that the antiproliferative effect of human fetal AFP is not only limited to human lymphocytes, but also extends to lymphocytes of mice, hamsters, and rats.

The degree of selectivity in the immunoregulatory effects of AFP was further emphasized in a series of studies designed to test the impact of AFP on T-cell proliferation toward defined sets of histocompatibility antigens in primary and secondary allogeneic MLRs; (PECK et al. 1978). These studies showed that T-cell proliferation involving MHC class II region differences was almost completely eliminated in the presence of AFP. This included proliferative reaction against isolated class II region incompatibilities, reactions against class II plus class I region differences as well as reactions against whole MHC haplotype histoincompatibilities. In contrast, no detectable inhibition of T-cell proliferation in MLRs against isolated class I alloantigens was observed. On the contrary, alloantigenic lymphocyte-activating systems where class II association was not required were often substantially augmented in the presence of AFP. Thus, AFP could be shown to exert its suppressive activity on allogeneic MLRs through a selective interference with class II region T-cell triggering systems.

There are several convergent lines of evidence indicating that AFP might be capable of exerting an ameliorating effect on certain autoimmune diseases. A primary target for AFP-mediated immunosuppression is the MHC class II restricted CD_4^+ T cell (PECK et al. 1978; HOOPER and EVANS 1989). MHC class II molecules play an essential role in immune activation events in autoimmunity (NEPORN and ERLICH 1991), and there is strong evidence for the participation of CD_4^+ T cells in the pathogenesis of many autoimmune diseases (WRAITH et al. 1989), including RA (WENDLING et al. 1992), myasthenia gravis (PROTTI et al. 1993), experimental allergic encephalomyelitis (ZAMVIL and STEINMAN 1990), multiple sclerosis (HOHLFELD et al. 1995), and insulin-dependent diabetes (KATZ et al. 1995).

The autologous mixed lympocyte reaction (AMLR; BATTISTO and PONZIO 1981; WEKSLER et al. 1983) consists of a proliferative response by CD_4^+ T cells to self class II MHC-encoded gene products (GLIMCHER et al. 1981). Both mouse (HOOPER and MURGITA 1981) and human AFP (O'NEILL et al. 1982; HOOPER et al. 1989) were shown to exert strong suppressive effects on AMLR. On the basis of these findings, a role for endogenous fetal AFP in the regulation of autosensitization was proposed . Internal regulation of the immune system occurs through self recognition which constitutes the most basic form of autoimmunity. Since self-recognizing lymphocytes are normal components of the immune system (SMITH and STEINBERG 1983), it is likely that regulatory mechanisms have evolved to control these beneficial expressions of physiological autoimmunity in order to avert possible conversions to disease-provoking autodestructive events.

Self-recognizing lymphocytes can produce overt autocytolytic reactions in vivo when normal control mechanisms are circumvented (COHEN and WEKERLE 1973; ROSENKRANTZ et al. 1985). It is possible that immature T cells on the verge of becoming immunologically reactive would be at particular risk for expression of aggressive forms of autoreactivity. Indeed, there is evidence that the mechanisms for generating thymic and/or peripheral tolerance are inefficient during the perinatal period (BONOMO et al. 1994). Although negative selection of self-reactive T cells (capable of recognizing self antigens expressed in the thymus) clearly takes place in the thymus (KAPPLER et al. 1987) there is evidence of thymic exit of potentially autoreactive T cells (BYRNE et al. 1994). The migration of self-reactive T cells to the periphery may be increased during the perinatal period; T cells bearing autoreactive T-cell receptors can be readily found in secondary lymphoid tissues of neonatal but not of adult animals (SCHNEIDER et al. 1989). These findings indicate a need for the strict control of autoreactivity in ontogeny. There is accumulating data in support of the contention that endogenous levels of AFP in the circulation of the fetus and newborn play a key role in keeping fetal/neonatal autoreactive T cells in check (SAKAGUCHI and SAKAGUCHI 1990).

The regular association of pregnancy with immunization against fetal-specific products (HAMILTON 1983; BRENT et al. 1983) coupled with the heightened potential for maternal T-cell autoreactivity (HOSKIN et al. 1985) led to an examination of syngeneically mated mice for evidence of cellular immune responses specific for fetal autoantigens. The result of this investigation (HOSKIN and MURGITA 1989) demonstrated the existence of a specific maternal antifetal lymphoproliferative response. Splenic CD_4^+ T cells obtained from primiparous CBA/J mice pregnant by syngeneic matings proliferate in response to coculture with class II positive fetal cells whereas CD_4^+ T cells from age-matched virgin female controls failed to react in this system. Fetal AFP was shown to suppress this specific form of maternal antifetal T-cell reactivity.

The in vitro studies described briefly above strongly indicate that autoreactive CD_4^+ T cells are preferential targets for AFP-mediated immunosuppression. A primary function of AFP may therefore be to protect the developing fetus from exposure to autoaggressive self-reactive T cells. As pointed out earlier, fetal-derived AFP is elevated in the maternal circulation, one consequence of which is the selective inhibition of the maternal immume system (MURGITA 1976; TODER et al. 1979). Maternal AFP levels may also play a role in the remissions of certain autoimmune diseases, experienced by a high percentage of pregnant women. This is supported by in vivo studies which show that administration of AFP can ameliorate experimental allergic encephalomyelitis (ABRAMSKY et al. 1982), and myasthenia gravis (BRENNER et al. 1984; ABRAMSKY and BRENNER 1983; BUSCHMAN et al. 1987). This concept has been strengthened by studies on experimental antigen-induced arthritis in transgenic mice expressing human AFP (OGATA et al. 1995). In these studies a transgenic mouse, designated TG-3, maintains a constant serum level of AFP which corresponds to the maternal mouse serum AFP level during pregnancy. Definite arthritis was observed in 21% of the transgenic mice and in 56% of control mice. The results show that endogenously synthesized human AFP can function in vivo to significantly reduce the incidence of experimental autoimmune disease.

There is evidence for more than one mechanism of action for AFP-mediated immunoregulatory effects on the immune system. Cell surface receptors for AFP have been identified on malignant cells (VILLACAMPA et al.1984) as well as on normal lymphoid cells, particularly on activated T cells (TORRES et al. 1989) and monocytes (SUZUKI et al. 1992; ESTEBAN et al. 1993). These latter findings coupled with the linkage of AFP-induced suppression with class II determinants provides at least an initial insight into observations by three independent laboratories that AFP causes a selective downregulation of class II molecules of monocytes (LU et al. 1984; CRAINIE et al. 1989; LAAN-PÜTSEP et al. 1991). Altered expression of class II molecules may involve coreceptor-mediated endocytosis or interference with cytokine-induced expression of monocyte and macrophage differentiation markers. It has been demonstrated that purified human AFP downregulates human monocytic cell TNF-α and Il-1B production and gene expression (WANG and ALPERT 1995). In any event, efficient AFP-mediated inhibition of class II expression on lymphoid cells would have an obvious impact on induction and progression of autoimmue reactions (NEPORN and ERLICH 1991) and could help to explain the delay in immunoresponsiveness in the newborn which has been attributed to a deficit in class II-bearing macrophages (LU et al. 1979).

Other studies have linked at least some aspects of AFP-mediated immunoregulation to an interference at the macrophage level (OLINESCU et al 1978; VETVICKA et al. 1988; PECK et al. 1982).

A number of studies have demonstrated in both the murine (MURGITA et al. 1977) and human (ALPERT et al. 1978) system that AFP suppresses certain T-cell-dependent immune response through its ability to activate populations of inhibitory cells. Like naturally occurring suppressor T cells in the newborn, AFP-induced inhibitory T cells in adult spleens belong to the CD_4^+ CD_8^- subset of T lymphocytes (MURGITA et al. 1978b; MURGITA et al. 1981). A second population of AFP-induced inhibitory cells was identified in the spleen of pregnant mice which lacked many of the conventional cell surface markers normally associated with mature lymphocytes (HOSKIN et al. 1983). A panel of monoclonal antibodies were raised against the pregnancy-associated "null" suppressor cells (HOSKIN et al. 1989). Administration of such antibodies to pregnant mice resulted in embryo resorption (GRONVIK et al. 1987). A more thorough analysis in pregnant mice of the inhibitory cell type in spleen lacking mature lymphocyte markers revealed that most of the regulatory cells are of an immature T-cell lineage carrying the CD_3^+ CD_4^- CD_8^- $CD45R^+$ phenotype (BROOKES-KAISER et al. 1992). These double negative regulatory T cells from spleens of pregnant animals are very similar to a suppressor cell population identified in human blood which downregulates autoreactive T-cell responses to self class II autologous MLR (KAWANO et al. 1990).

In addition to altering the expression of the MHC class II on lymphoid cells and inducing populations of regulatory suppressor cells, there is evidence that AFP can act as an embryonic cytokine through its ability to control the growth of cells either directly (HOSKIN et al. 1985; VAN OERS et al. 1989), or indirectly by acting synergistically or antagonistically with other cytokines to regulate cell growth (NUNEZ 1994). The idea that AFP may regulate growth of distinct cell types is consistent with its frequent association with rapidly dividing cell populations in normal, restorative, and malignant conditions.

Finally, a comment on some reports in the literature claiming that the immunoregulatory effects ascribed in numerous detailed investigations to intrinsic properties of highly purified and defined AFP molecules are not inherent features of the molecule itself, but can instead be attributed to putative low molecular weight active factors transported to target sites by AFP which acts as an inert carrier protein. While accumulated evidence in support of a direct immunoregulatory role for AFP is, as briefly reviewed here, preponderate, assertions to the contrary should be addressed and clarified.

Many proteins in plasma bind ligands, including albumin and AFP, but most are not considered to function as transport proteins. Of the limited number of transport proteins in plasma, the albumin family of molecules belongs to a category having low affinities and generally low specificities for ligands (HERVÉ et al. 1994). These characteristics are associated with restrictive binding where the carrier functions as a clearance protein to neutralize and remove excess ligand which might otherwise accumulate to toxic levels. For instance, a detoxification function for AFP has been proposed (ATTARDI and RUOSLAHTI 1976) as a result of its estrophilic properties. In this capacity AFP may protect fetal tissues by binding and clearing potentially harmful levels of circulating maternal estrogens. Those who have invoked the idea that an active ligand linked to AFP accounts for functional activity must assume that a permissive form of ligand binding is operating in this system. Permissive complex formation where ligand activity and distribution to target tissue is unlimited is associated with high affinity binding (HERVÉ et al. 1994).

Careful evaluation and comparison of studies by groups which have assigned to AFP a passive role as a protective carrier of a putative immunoregulatory moiety reveals a lack of consensus as to the nature of the active factor. For example, one group who earlier on had reported that AFP isolated from mouse amniotic fluid (MAF) must first bind estrogen before obtaining the capacity to elicit immunosuppressive activity (KELLER et al. 1976) have more recently ascribed all of the inhibitory activity in MAF to a transforming growth factor β2 (TGF-β2)-like factor bound in an active form to neutral AFP carrier molecules (ALTMAN et al. 1990). Another report on studies with human amniotic fluid (LANGE and SEARLE 1994) differs significantly from the earlier investigation mentioned above in that immunosuppressive activity was incompletely neutralized by anti-TGF-β2 antibodies and reversed by a combination of this antibody and anti-TGF-β1 antibody. As human-amniotic-fluid-mediated suppression was not abolished by the combined anti-TGF-β1 and -β2 antibody treatment, this study implied the existence of one or more additional inhibitory components in amniotic fluid, which are not neutralizable by anti-TGF-β antibodies.

Reports by DEUTCH (1991) and KHAIR-EL-DIN et al. (1995) maintain that the binding of nonesterified fatty acids, particularly arachidonic and docosahexaenoic acids, confers immunosuppressive activity to AFP. These studies, which focus on certain hormones, fatty acids, and peptide growth factors as essential active ligands, have failed to take into account a body of work which demonstrates that AFP isolated from tumor sources where these ligands would not be available to interact with it is inhibitory (LESTER et al. 1977; MURGITA et al. 1978a). Moreover, YACHNIN et al. (1980a,b) have performed very careful studies on purified human AFP designed to exclude any ligand-binding role for a variety of known factors including fatty acids as elements contributing to the immunosuppressive action of AFP. Any attempt to precisely identify an active immunoregulator factor(s) in unfractionated amniotic fluid is problematic in that this material represents a complex mixture of several factors capable of exerting both positive and negative regulatory influences on the immune system (MURGITA and WIGZELL 1981; JYONOUCHI et al. 1987; BUSBY et al. 1988). It has been emphasized before (VAN OERS et al. 1989) that it is quite likely that immunoregulatory AFP molecules act in conjuction with other active factors present in amniotic fluid as well as in maternal, fetal/newborn and tumor sera from which AFP can be isolated. Finally, it has recently been shown that recombinant AFP produced in either procaryotic or eucaryotic expression systems retain full biological activity when compared with the natural protein (SEMENIUK et al. 1995; BOISMENU et al. 1996). In these studies it was possible to perform functional comparisons between recombinant and natural fetal-derived AFP in carefully controlled in vitro environments where the potential contribution of putative exogenous active factors could be eliminated.

Thus, the extreme view that AFP serves only as an inert carrier for active immunoregulatory factors, the identity of which individual studies cannot agree on, is essentially untenable.

5 Conclusions

It is obvious from several investigations including our own, as briefly reviewed in this chapter, that a significant immunomodulatory potency resides in cells and soluble factors at the maternal–fetal interface and in human feta/neonatal lymphoid cells. These cells and factors are preferentially able to strongly and non-specifically suppress both proliferation and Ig synthesis of lymphoid cells from pregnant women and other adults. Some different patterns of the immunomodulation can be distinguished:

1. A primarily prostaglandin- or AFP-independent suppression, involving fetal/neonatal suupressor T cells and maternal target T cells both of the same CD_4^+ CD_8^- (T helper cell) phenotype. The mechanism of suppression is unclear. However, the current concept of two subtypes of CD_4^+ lymphocytes, TH_1 and TH_2, producing suppressive and stimulatory cytokines, respectively, offers the hypothesis that TH_1 suppressive cytokines such as TNF-α, IFN-γ, and IL-2 dominate in interactions between fetal/neonatal CD_4^+ cells and maternal CD_4^+ cells. Except for immune cells, cells at the maternal–fetal interface in the placenta can produce various cytokines. For example, TNF-α is secreted by villous syncytio- and cytotrophoblasts (King et al. 1995). Secretion of IFN-γ by trophoblastic cells has been reported (Tao and Cao 1993). IL-2, a potent activator of NK cells, has been found in normal trophoblastic cells by some investigators (Boehm et al. 1989; Soubiran et al. 1987); this observation, however, has been questioned by others (Haynes et al. 1993; Kelly et al. 1995; King et al. 1995).
2. A strong antiproliferative immunosuppression of maternal immune cells can obviously be exerted by PGs, and especially by PGE_2. The suppression is dose-dependent and to some extent dependent on the kind and strength of the mitogenic stimulus. The suppression is apparently linked to differences in density of PGE_2 binding sites on lymphoid cells derived from the mother and from her fetus/newborn, and to a lower sensitivity of the fetal/neonatal lymphocytes to cAMP and its suppressive effect on cell proliferation. Maternal T cells recognizing alloantigens on the trophoblast and simultaneously exposed to PGE_2 in the placenta or decidua might become suppressed in their proliferation and, accordingly, in the generation of specific antibody and cell-mediated immunity in the lymphoid organs.

3. PGs, and particularly PGE_2 might serve as immunomodulatory agents, "fine tuning" the immune response as suggested by Bray (1980, 1987). We believe that this effect of PGs is important in maternal–fetal interactions. The net effect might be suppressive or stimulatory. Interactions between cytokines and PGs derived from the placenta or decidua have been investigated. IL-1 produced in human trophoblast cultures increases the trophoblast-derived PGE levels by 500% (Shimonovitz et al. 1995). In addition, PGE_2 decreases the release of IL-1 by means of a feedback mechanism (Scales et al. 1989). TGF-β1 synthesized in the villous and extravillous trophoblast as indicated by the presence of TGF-β mRNA (King et al. 1995) inhibits the IL-1 induced enhancement of PGE release from the trophoblast (Shimonovitz et al. 1995). TNF-α production by syncytiotrophoblasts and endovascular trophoblasts (Chen et al. 1991), and by cytotrophoblasts (King et al. 1995) NK, and T cells in the decidua is suppressed by PGE_2 (Scales et al. 1989). We suggest that PGs, by these mechanisms, divert immune reactions towards TH_2 and away from TH_1 responses in pregnancy according to the theory of Wegmann et al. (1993).
   Presumably, the various kinds of immunoregulation, as suggested above, concur in vivo to complicated interactions. PGs are attractive candidates for local immuno-regulators in the placenta because they are produced by various tissues in the placenta and are rapidly degraded in the systemic circulation of the mother or even by PG-dehydrogenase present in the villous trophoblast (Cheung et al. 1992).
   In this context, the ability of PGs (like AFP) to modulate the expression of MHC antigens should be considered. Downregulation of the expression of Ia antigens (corresponding to MHC class II antigens in humans) on mouse macrophages by PGE_2 was originally reported by Snyder et al. (1982). It is well established that HLA-D antigens are absent on human trophoblasts. However, HLA-D mRNA (but not the antigen) has recently been demonstrated on human first trimester cytotrophoblasts (Giacomini et al. 1994). The question is whether the HLA-D antigens are posttranscriptionally downregulated by PGs in a (presumably) PG-rich environment at the maternal–fetal interface in the placenta.
   Furthermore, a PG-mediated immunosuppressive effect like the one described by us could selectively inactivate maternal immunocompetent cells in the fetal circulation (see N. Papadogiannakis, this volume). We speculate that cord blood lymphoid cells and their precursors, when used to reconstitute the bone marrow of heavily irradiated cancer patients, should be able to evade rejection by locally suppressing the patients' immune cells.
4. Exemption of the fetus from premature immune attack depends in part on the cumulative action of specific and nonspecific immunoregulatory factors. One of the contributing regulatory factors is AFP. Since AFP is a major α-globulin component of fetal and newborn sera, and since the serum levels of AFP in pregnant females is normally elevated, it must be considered an important regulatory agent which helps maintain the maternal–fetal immunological relationship. It does so by suppressing unwarranted maternal antifetal autoreac-

tions. AFP is capable of exerting a direct antiproliferating effect on autoreactive T cells and can also efficiently induce populations of natural suppressor cells. Recent studies employing recombinant AFP have established that immunoregulatory activity is intrinsic to the molecule itself.

Acknowledgements. The authors wish to thank Mrs Phyllis Minick and Mrs Maj-Len Holm for their help in preparing the manuscript.

References

Abramsky O, Brenner T (1983) A role of alpha-fetoprotein in autoimmune disease. Ann N Y Acad Sci 183:108–116
Abramsky O, Brenner T, Mizrachi O, Soffer D (1982) Alpha-fetoprotein suppresses experimental allergic encephalomyelitis. J Neuroimmunol 2:1–7
Adinolfi M (1979) Human alpha-fetoprotein 1956–1978. Adv Hum Genet 9:165–228
Ahern DG, Downing DT (1970) Inhibition of prostaglandin biosynthesis by eicosa 5, 8, 11, 14 tetraynoic acid. Biochim Biophys Acta 210:456–461
Alpert E, Dienstag JL, Sepersky S, Littman B, Rocklin R (1978) Immunosuppressive characteristics of human AFP: Effect on tests of cell-mediated immunity and induction of human suppressor cells. Immunol Comm 7:163–185
Altman DJ, Schneider SL, Thompson DA, Cheng HL, Tomasi TB (1990) A transforming growth factor B2 (TGF-B2)-like immunosuppressive factor in amniotic fluid and localization of TGF-B2 mRNA in the pregnant uterus. J Exp Med 172:1391–1401
Andersen S, Sjursen W, Laegreid A, Austgulen R, Johansen B (1994) Immunohistological detection of non-pancreatic phospholipase A_2 (type II) in human placenta and its possible involvement in normal parturition at term. Prostaglandins Leukot Essent Fatty Acids 51:19–26
Andersson U, Bird AG, Britton S, Palacios R (1981) Humoral and cellular immunity in humans studied at the cell level from birth to two years of age. Immunol Rev 57:5–38
Andersson U, Britton S, deLey M, Bird G (1983) Evidence for the ontogenic precendence of suppressor T cell functions in the human neonate. Eur J Immunol 13:6–16
Attardi B, Ruoslahti E (1976) Fetoneonatal oestradiol-binding protein in mouse brain cytosol is alpha-fetoprotein. Nature 263:685–689
Baley JE, Schacter BZ (1985) Mechanisms of diminshed natural killer cell activity in pregnant women and neonates. J Immunol 134:3042–3048
Barbieri B, Papadogiannakis N, Eneroth P, Hansson C, Roepstorff P, Olding LB (1994) Identification of a substance, previously shown to enhance mitogenesis of human lymphocytes, as the acetamide of p-aminobenzoic acid. Biochim Biophys Acta 1214:309–316
Barbieri B, Papadogiannakis N, Eneroth P, Olding LB (1995) Arachidonic acid is preferred acetyl donor among fatty acids in the acetylation of p-aminobenzoic acid by human lymphoid cells. Biochim Biophys Acta 1257:157–166
Battisto JR, Ponzio NM (1981) Autologous and syngeneic mixed lymphocyte reactions and their immunological significance. Prog Allergy 28:160–192
Beral V (1983) Parity and susceptibility to cancer. In: Evered D and Whelan J (eds) Fetal antigens and cancer. (Ciba Foundation Symposium 96.) Pitman, London, pp 182–203
Billingham RE (1964) Transplantation immunity and the maternal-fetal relation. N Engl J Med 270:667–672
Blaese RM, Pike S, Tosato G (1982) Suppressor T-cell function in man: suppression of immunoglobulin production by the direct action of immunoregulatory T cells on the B cell in four separate, distinct systems. Clin Immunol Immunopath 23(2):162–171
Bloom BR, Salgame P, Diamond B (1992) Revisiting and revising suppressor T cells. Immunol Today 13:131–136

Boehm KD, Kelley MF, Ilan J (1989) The interleukin 2 gene is expressed in the syncytio-trophoblast of the human placenta. Proc Natl Acad Sci USA 86:656–660

Boismenu R, Semeniuk D, Murgita RA (1997) Purification and characterization of human and mouse recombinant alpha-fetoproteins expressed in Escherichia coli. Protein Expr Purif (in press)

Bonomo A, Kehn PJ, Shevach EM (1994) Premature escape of double positive thymocytes to the periphery of young mice. Possible role for autoimmunity. J Immunol 152:1509–1514

Bray MA (1980) Prostaglandins: fine tuning of the immune system? Immunol Today 1:65–69

Bray M (1987) Prostaglandins and leukotrienes: fine tuning of the imune response. ISI Atlas Sci Pharmacol 1:101–106

Brenner T, Zielinski A, Argo A, Abramsky O (1984) Prevention of experimental myasthenia gravis in rats by fetal alpha-fetoprotein-rich fractions. Tumour Biol 5:263–274

Brent L, Hunt R, Hutchinson IV, Medawar PB, Palmer L, Welsh L (1983) Host recognition of fetal antigens: do they induce specified antibodies? In: Evered D, Whelan J (eds) Fetal antigens and cancer. (Ciba Foundation Symposium 96.) Pitman, London, pp 125–145

Brookes-Kaiser JC, Murgita RA, Hoskin DW (1992) Pregnancy-associated suppressor cells in mice: functional characteristics of T cells with natural suppressor activity. J Reprod Immunol 21:103–125

Brown DM, Phipps RP (1995) Characterization of prostaglandin E2 receptors on normal and malignant B lymphocytes. Adv Prostaglandin Thromboxane Leukot Res 23:299–301

Brown ZA, Vontver LA, Benedetti J, Critchlow CW, Hickoc DE, Selz CJ, Berry S, Corey L (1985) Genetical herpes in pregnancy: risk factors associated with recurrences and asymtomatic viral shedding. Am J Obstet Gynecol 153:24–30

Bulmer JN, Morrison L, Johnson PM, Meager A (1990) Immunochemical localization of interferons in human placental tissue in normal, ectopic, and molar pregnancy. Am J Reprod Immunol 22:109–116

Busby WH, Klapper DG, Clemmons DR (1988) Purification of a 31,000-dalton insulin-like growth factor binding protein from human amniotic fluid. J Biol Chem 263:14203–14210

Buschman E, van Oers NSC, Katz M, Murgita RA (1987) Experimental myasthenia gravis induced in mice by passive transfer of human myasthenic immunoglobulin. J Neuroimmunol 13:315–330

Byrne JA, Stankovic AK, Cooper MD (1994) A novel subpopulation of primed T cells in the human fetus. J Immunol 152:3098–3106

Calder AA (1994) Prostaglandins and biological control of cervical function. Aust N Z J Obstet Gynaecol 34:347–351

Carr M, Stites DP, Fudenberg H (1974) Cellular immune aspects of the human fetal–maternal relationship. III. Mixed lymphocyte reactivity between related maternal and cord blood lymphocytes. Cell Immunol 11:332–341

Castilla JA, Rueda R, Vargas ML, Gonzalez-Gomez F, Garcia-Olivares E (1989) Decreased levels of circulating CD_4^+ T lymphocytes during normal pregnancy. J Reprod Immunol 15:103–111

Chakraborty M, Mandal C (1993) Immunosuppressive effect of human alpha-fetoprotein: a cross species study. Immunol Invest 22:329–339

Chen H-L, Yang Y, Hu X-L, Yelavarthi K, Fishback JL, Hunt JS (1991) Tumor necrosis factor alpha mRNA and protein are present in human placental and uterine cells at early and late stages of gestation. Am J Pathol 139:327–335

Cheng H, Sehon AH, Delespesse G (1985) Human cord blood suppressor T lymphocytes. I. Phenotype and target of the inducer and suppressor cell factor. Am J Reprod Immunol Microbiol 9:93–99

Cheung PY, Walton JC, Tai HH, Riley SC, Challis JR (1992) Localization of 15-hydroxy prostaglandin dehydrogenase in human fetal membranes, decidua, and placenta during pregnancy. Gynecol Obstet Invest 33:142–146

Christensen NJ, Gréen K (1983) Bioconversion of arachidonic acid in human pregnant reproductive tissues. Biochem Med 30:162–180

Cohen IR, Wekerle H (1973) Regulation of autosensitization. J Exp Med 137:224–232

Cohen BL, Orn A, Gronvik K-O, Gindlund M, Wigzell H, Murgita RA (1986) Natural killer cell activity stimulated in vitro and in vivo by interferon and interleukin-2. Scand J Immunol 23:211–223

Crainie M, Semeluk A, Lee KC, Wegmann T (1989) Regulation of constitutive and lymphokine-induced Ia expression by murine alpha-fetoprotein. Cell Immunol 118:41–52

Dailey MO, Schreurs J, Schulman H (1988) Hormone receptors on cloned T lymphocytes. Increased responsiveness to histamine, prostaglandins and β-adrenergic agents as a late stage event in T cell activation. J Immunol 140:2931–2936

Da Silva JA, Spector TD (1992) The role of pregnancy in the course and aetiology of rheumatoid arthritis (review). Clin Rheumatol 11:189–194

Deutch HF (1991) Chemistry and biology of alpha-fetoprotein. Adv Cancer Res 56:253–309

Dimov V, Christensen NJ, Gréen K (1983) Analysis of prostaglandins formed from endogenous and exogenous arachidonic acid in homogenates of human reproductive tissues. Biochim Biophys Acta 754:38–43
Divers MJ, Lilford RJ, Miller D, Bulmer JN (1995) Cyclo-oxygenase distribution in human placenta and decidua does not change with labour after term or preterm delivery. Gynecol Obstet Invest 39:157–161
Durandy A, Fischer A, Griscelli C (1979) Active suppression of B lymphocyte interaction by two different newborn T lymphocyte subsets. J Immunol 123:2644–2650
Durandy A, Brami C, Griscelli C (1985) The effects of indomethacin administration during pregnancy on women's and newborns' T-suppressor lymphocyte activity and on HLA class II expression by newborn's lymphocytes. Am J Reprod Immunol Microbiol 8:94–100
El-Roeiy A, Shoenfeld Y (1985) Autoimmunity and pregnancy. Am J Reprod Immunol Microbiol 9:25–32
Eriksen EF, Richelsen B, Beck-Neilsen H, Melsen F, Kraemmer-Neilsen H, Mosekilde L (1985) Prostaglandin E2 receptors on human peripheral blood monocytes Scand J Immunol 21:167–172
Esteban C, Trojan J, Macho A, Mishal Z, Lafarge-Forgoyssinet C, Uriel J (1993) Activation of an alpha-fetoprotein/receptor pathway in human normal and malignant peripheral blood mononuclear cells. Leukemia 7:1807–1816
Faulk WP, Hsi BL, McIntyre JA, Yeh CJG, Mucchielli A (1982) Antigens of the human extra-embryonic membranes. J Reprod Fertil 31 (Suppl):181–189
Freed KA, Aitken MA, Brennecke SP, Rice GE (1995) Prostaglandin G/H synthase-1 messenger RNA relative abundance in human amnion, choriodecidua and placenta before, during and after spontaneous onset of labour at term. Gynecol Obstet Invest 39:73–78
Fried M, Duffy PE (1996) Adherence of plasmodium falciparum to chrondroitin sulfate A in the human placenta. Science 272:1502–1504
Galbraith RM, Wener P, Kanton RR, Galbraith GM (1981) Studies on the interaction between human transferrin and specific receptors on the trophoblast membrane. Placenta 3 (Suppl):49–59
Gehrz RC, Christianson WR, Linner KM, Conroy MM, McCue SA, Balfour HH (1981) Cytomegalovirus-specific humoral and cellular immune responses in human pregnancy. J Infect Dis 143:391–395
Gershon RK, Kondo K (1971) Infectious immunological tolerance. Immunology 21:903–910
Gersony WM (1986) Patent ductus arteriosus in the neonate. Pediatr Clin North Am 33:545–560
Giacomini P, Tosi S, Murgia C, Nobili F, Gaetani S, Gambari R, Nicotra MR, Simoni G, Maggi F, Natali PG (1994) First-trimester human trophoblast is class II major histocompatibility complex mRNA$^+$/antigen$^-$. Hum Immunol 39:281–289
Glimcher LH, Longo DL, Green I, Schwartz RH (1981) Murine syngeneic mixed lymphocyte response. I. Target antigens are self Ia molecules. J Exp Med 154:1652–1670
Goldyne ME (1989) Eicosanoid metabolism by lymphocytes: do all human nucleated cells generate eicosanoids? Pharmacol Res 21:241–245
Goodwin JS (1989) Immunomodulation by eicosanoids and anti-inflammatory drugs. Curr Opin Immunol 2:264–268
Goodwin JS, Webb DR (1980) Regulation of the immune response to prostaglandins. Clin Immunol Immunopath 15:106–122
Goodwin JS, Wiik A, Lewis M, Bankhurst AD, Williams RC Jr (1979) High-affinity binding sites for prostaglandin E on human lymphocytes. Cell Immunol 43:150–159
Green DR, Webb DR (1993) Saying the S' word in public. Immunol Today 14:523–526
Gronvik K-O, Hoskin DW, Murgita RA (1987) Monoclonal antibodies against murine neonatal and pregnancy-associated natural suppressor cells induce resoprtion of the fetus. Scan J Immunol 25:533-540
Hamilton MS (1983) Maternal immune responses to oncofetal antigens. J Reprod Immunol 5:249–264
Haynes MK, Jackson LG, Tuan RS, Shepley KJ, Smith BJ (1993) Cytokine production in first trimester chorionic villi: detection of mRNAs and protein products in situ. Cell Immunol 151:300–308
Hayward AR, Lydyard PM (1978) Suppression of B cell differentiation by newborn T lymphocytes with a Fc receptor for IgM. Clin Exp Immunol 34:374–384
Hayward AR, Merill D (1981) Requirement for OKT8$^+$ suppressor cell proliferation for suppression by human newborn T cells. Clin Exp Immunol 45:408–415
Herschman HR (1994) Regulation of prostaglandin synthase-1 and prostaglandin synthase-2. Cancer and Metastasis Rev 13:241–256
Hervé F, Urien S, Duché JC, Tillement J-P (1994) Drug binding in plasma. A summary of recent trends in the study of drug or hormone binding. Clin Pharmacokinet 26:44–58

Hohlfeld R, Londei M, Marsacesi L, Salvetti M (1995) T-cell autoimmunity in multiple sclerosis. Immunol Today 16:259–261

Holmes CH, Simpson KL, Okada H, Okada N, Wainwright SD, Purcell DFJ, Honlihan JM (1992) Complement regulatory proteins at the feto-maternal interface during human placental development: distribution of CD 59 by comparison with membrane co-factor protein (CD 46) and decay accelerating factor (CD 55). Eur J Immunol 22:1479–1585

Hooper DC, Evans RG (1989) Anti-proliferative action of murine alpha-fetoprotein on activated T-lymphocytes. J Reprod Immunol 16:83–96

Hooper DC, Murgita RA (1981) Regulation of murine T-cell responses to autologous antigens by alpha-fetoprotein. Cell Immunol 63:417–425

Hooper DC, O'Neill G, Gronvik K-O, Gold P, Murgita RA (1989) Human AFP inhibits cell proliferation and NK-like cytotoxic activity generated in autologous, but not in allogeneic mixed lymphocyte reactions. In: Mizejewski GJ, Jacobsen J (eds) Biological activities of alpha-fetoprotein, vol II. CRC, Boca Raton, pp 183–197

Hoskin DW, Murgita RA (1989) Specific maternal anti-fetal lymphoproliferative responses and their regulation by natural immunosuppressive factors. Clin Exp Immunol 76:262–267

Hoskin D, Hooper DC, Murgita RA (1983) Naturally occurring non-T suppressor cells in pregnant and neonatal mice: some functional and phenotypic characteristics. Am J Reprod Immunol 3: 72–77

Hoskin DW, Hamel S, Hooper DC, Murgita RA (1985) In vitro activation of bone marrow-derived T and non-T cell subsets by alpha-fetroprotein. Cell Immunol 96:163–174

Hoskin DW, Gronvik K-O, Hooper DC, Reilly BD, Murgita RA (1989) Altered immune response patterns in murine syngeneic pregnancy: presence of natural null suppressor cells in maternal spleen identifiable by monoclonal antibodies Cell Immunol 120:42–60

Hsi B-L, Hunt JS, Atkinson JP (1991) Differential expression of complement regulatory protein on subpopulations of human trophoblast cells. J Reprod Immunol 19:209–223

Hustin J, Schaaps JP (1987) Echocardiographic and anatomic studies of the maternotrophoblastic border during the first trimester of pregnancy. Am J Obstet Gynecol 157:162–168

Jacobson HI, Thompson WD, Janerich DT (1989) Multiple births and maternal risk of breast cancer. J Epidemiol 129:865–869

Jacoby DR, Oldstone MBA (1983) Delineation of suppressor and helper activity within the OKT 4-defined T lymphocyte subset in human newborns. J Immunol 131:1765–1770

Jacoby DR, Olding LB, Oldstone MBA (1984) Immunologic regulation of fetal–maternal balance. In: Dixon FJ, Kunkel HG (eds) Advanced immunology. Academic, New York, pp 157–208

Janeway CA Jr, Carding S, Jones B, Murray J, Portoles P, Rasmussen R, Rojo J, Saizawa K, West J, Bottomly K (1988) CD_4^+ T cells: specificity and function. Immunol Rev 101:39–80

Johnsen S-A, Olding LB (1983) Differences in binding sites for prostaglandin E2 on mononuclear leukocytes from human newborns and from their mothers. Scand J Immunol 17:389–394

Johnsen S-A, Olding LB, Westberg NG, Wilhelmsson L (1982) Strong suppression by mononuclear leukocytes from human newborns on maternal leukocytes: mediation by prostaglandins. Clin Immunol Immunopathol 23:606–615

Johnsen S-A, Olding LB, Green K (1983) Conversion of arachidonic acid in human maternal and neonatal mononuclear leukocytes. Immunol Lett 6:213–218

Jokhi PP, King A, Sharkey AM, Smith SK, Loke YW (1994) Screening for cytokine mRNAs in purified human decidual lymphocyte populations by the reverse-transcriptase polymerase chain reaction (RT-PCR). J Immunol 153:4427–4435

Jyonouchi H, Voss RM, Good RA (1987) IL-1-like activities present in murine amniotic fluid. A significantly larger amount of IL-1-like activity is present in amniotic fluid of autoimmune NZB mice. J Immunol 138:3300–3307

Kanai N, Lu R, Satriano JA, Bao Y, Wolkoff AW, Schuster VL (1995) Identification and characterization of a prostaglandin transporter. Science 268:866–869

Kappler JW, Roehm N, Marrack P (1987) T cell tolerance by clonal elimination in the thymus. Cell 49:273–280

Katz JD, Benoist C, Mathis D (1995) T helper cell subsets in insulin-dependent diabetes. Science 268:1185–1188

Kawano Y, Noma T, Yata J (1990) Identification of a cord blood T cell subset of $CD3^+$ 4^- $45R^+$ suppressing interleukin 2 production in the autologous mixed lymphocyte reaction and the mode of action of exogenous IL-2 in the induction of IL-2 production. Cell Immunol 131:27–40

Keller RH, Calvanico NJ, Tomani TB (1976) Immunosuppressive properties of AFP: role of estrogens. In: Fishman WH, Sell S (eds) Onco developmental gene expression. Academic, New York, pp 287–295
Kelly RW, Carr GG, Elliott CL, Tulppala M, Critchley HOD (1995) Prostaglandin and cytokine release by trophoblastic villi. Hum Reprod 10:3289–3292
Khair-El-Din TA, Sicher C, Vazquez MA, Wright WJ, Lu CY (1995) Docosahexaenoic acid, a major constituent of fetal serum and fish oil diets, inhibits IFN-γ-induced Ia-expression by murine macrophages in vitro. J Immunol 154:1296–1306
Khuroo MS, Teli MR, Skidmore S, Sofi MA, Khuroo MI (1981) Incidence and severity of viral hepatitis in pregnancy. Am J Med 70:252–255
King A, Jokhi PP, Smith S, Sharkey A, Loke YW (1995) Screening for cytokine mRNA expression in purified human villous and extravillous trophoblast populations using the reverse-transcriptase polymerase chain reaction (RT-PCR). Cytokine 7:364–371
Klein J (1986) Natural history of major histocompatibility complex. Wiley, New York pp 423–608
Laan-Pütsep K, Wigzell H, Cotran P, Gidlund M (1991) Human alpha-fetoprotein (AFP) causes a selective down regulation of monocyte MHC class II molecules without altering other induced or noninduced monocyte markers or functions in monocytoid cell lines. Cell Immunol 133:506–518
Laneuville O, Breuer Dk, DeWitt DL, Hla T, Funk CD, Smith WL (1994) Differential inhibition of human prostaglandin endoperoxide H synthase-1 and -2 by nonsteroidal anti-inflammatory drugs. J Pharmacol Exp Ther 271:927–934
Lange AK, Searle RF (1994) The immunomodulatory activity of human amniotic fluid can be correlated with transforming growth factor-beta 1 (TGF-β1) AND β2 activity. Clin Exp Immunol 97:158–163
Lee H, Gregory CD, Rees GB, Scott IV, Golding PR (1987) Cytotoxic activity and phenotypic analysis of natural killer cells in early normal human pregnancy. J Reprod Immunol 12:35–47
Lester EP, Miller JB, Yachnin S (1977) A postsynthetic modification of human alpha-fetoprotein controls its immunosuppressive potency. Proc Natl Acad Sci USA 74:3988–3992
Lester EP, Miller JB, Yachnin S (1978) Human alpha-fetoprotein: immunosuppressive activity and microheterogeneity. Immunol Comm 7:137–161
Lin H, Mosmann TR, Guilbert L, Tuntipopipat S, Wegmann TG (1993) Synthesis of T helper 2-type cytokines at the maternal–fetal interface. J Immunol 151:4562–4573
Loke YW, King A (1995) Human implantation cell biology and immunology. Cambridge University Press, Cambridge
Lu CY, Calmai EG, Unanue ER (1979) A defect in antigen presenting functions of macrophages from neonatal mice. Nature 282:327–329
Lu CY, Changelian PS, Unanue ER (1984) Alpha-fetoprotein inhibits macrophages expression of Ia antigens. J Immunol 132:1722–1727
Luft BJ, Remington JS (1984) Effect of pregnancy on augmentation of natural killer cell activity by Corynebacterium parvum and Toxoplasma gondii. J. Immunol 132:2375–2380
Lunardl-Iskandar Y, Bryant Jl, Zeman RA, Lam VH, Samanlego F, Besnler JM, Hermans P, Thlerry AR, Gill P, Gallo RC (1995) Tumorigenesis and metastasis of neoplastic Kaposi's sarcoma all live in immunodeficient mice blocked by a human pregnancy hormone. Nature 375:64–68
Lysz TW, Needleman P (1982) Evidence for two distinct forms of fatty acid cyclooxygenase in brain. J Neurochem 38:1111–1117
Maggi M, Baldi E, Susini T (1994) Hormonal and local regulation of uterine activity during parturition, part II. The prostaglandin and adrenergic systems (review). J Endocrinol Invest 17:757–770
Meade EA, Smith WL, DeWitt DL (1993) Differential inhibition of prostaglandin endoperoxide synthase (cyclooxygenase) isozymes by aspirin and other non-steroidal anti-inflammatory drugs J Biol Chem 268:6610–6614
Medina KL, Kincade PW (1994) Pregnancy-related steroids are potential negative regulators of B lymphopoiesis. Proc Natl Acad Sci USA 91:5382–5386
Medina KL, Smithson G, Kincade PW (1993) Suppression of B lymphopoeisis during normal pregnancy. J Exp Med 178:1507–1515
Mitchell MD (1986) Pathways of arachidonic acid metabolism with specific application to the fetus and mother. Semin Perinatol 10:242–254
Miyawaki T, Moriya N, Nagaoki T, Taniguchi N (1981) Suppressor activity of T lymphocytes from infants assessed by co-culture with unfractionated adult lymphocytes in the pokeweed mitogen system. J Immunol 123:1092–1096
Morell (1995) Zeroing in on how hormones affect the immune system. Science 269:773–775

Moretta L, Webb S, Grossi CE, Lyolyard PM, Cooper MD (1977) Functional analysis of two human T-cell subpopulations: help and suppression of B cell responses by T cells bearing receptors for IgM or IgG. J Exp Med 146:184–200
Mosmann TR, Coffman RL (1989) TH1 and TH2 cells: different patterns of lymphokine secretion lead to different functional properties (review). Annu Rev Immunol 7:145–173
Murgita RA (1976) The immunosuppressive role of alpha-fetoprotein during pregnancy Scand J Immunol 5:1003–1014
Murgita RA, Tomasi TB (1975) Suppression of the immune response by alpha-fetoprotein. I. The effect of mouse alpha-fetaprotein on the primary and secondary antibody response. J Exp Med 141:269–286
Murgita RA, Wigzell H (1976) The effects of mouse alpha-fetoprotein on T cell-dependent and T cell-independent immune responses in vitro. Scan J Immunol 5:1215–1220
Murgita RA Wigzell H (1981) Regulation of immune functions in the fetus and newborn. Prog Allergy 29:54–133
Murgita RA, Goidl EA, Kontiainen S, Wigzell H (1977) Alpha-fetoprotein induces the formation of suppressor cells in vitro. Nature 267:257–259
Murgita RA, Anderson LC, Sherman MS, Bennich H, Wigzell H (1978a) Effects of human alpha-fetoprotein on human B and T lymphocyte proliferation in vitro. Clin Exp Immunol 33: 347–356
Murgita RA, Goidl EA, Kontiainen S, Beverly PCL, Wigzell H (1978b) Adult murine T cells activated in vitro by alpha-fetoprotein and naturally occurring T cells in newborn mice: identify in function and cell surface differentiation antigens. Proc Natl Acad Sci USA 75:2897–2901
Murgita RA, Hooper DC, Stegagno M, Delovitch TL, Wigzell H (1981) Characterization of murine newborn inhibitory T lymphocytes: functional and phenotypic comparison with an adult T cell subset activated in vitro by alpha-fetoprotein. Eur J Immunol 11:957–964
Narumiya S (1994) Prostanoid receptors: structure, function and distribution. Ann NY Acad Sci 744:126–138
Neporn GT, Erlich H (1991) MHC class II molecules and autoimmunity. Annu Rev Immunol 9: 493–525
Neulen J, Breckwoldt M (1994) Placental progesterone, prostaglandins and mechanisms leading to initiation of parturition in the human. Exp Clin Endorcrinol 102(3):195–202
Norwitz ER, Starkey PM, Lopez Bernal A, Turnbull AC (1991) Identification by flow cytometry of the prostaglandin-producing cell populations of term human decidua. J Endocrinol 131:327–334
Nunez EA (1994) Biological role of alpha-fetoprotein in the endocrinological field: data and hypothesis. Tumor Biol 15:63–72
Ogata A, Yamahita T, Koyama Y, Sakai M, Nishi S (1995) Suppression of experimental antigen-induced arthritis in transgenic mice producing human alpha-fetoprotein. Biochem Biophys Res Comm 213:1322–1327
Olding LB, Oldstone MBA (1974) Lymphocytes from human newborns abrogate mitoses of their mothers' lymphocytes. Nature 249:161–162
Olding LB, Oldstone MBA (1976) Thymus-derived peripheral lymphocytes from human newborns inhibit division of their mother's lymphocytes. J. Immunol 116:682–686
Olding LB, Benirschke K, Oldstone MBA (1974) Inhibition of mitosis of lymphocyte from human adults by lymphocytes from human newborns. Clin Immunol Immunopath 3:79–89
Olding LB, Murgita RA, Wigzell H (1977) Mitogen-stimulated lymphoid cells from human newborns suppress the proliferation of maternal lymphocytes across a cell-impermeable membrane. J Immunol 119:1109–1114
Oldstone MBA, Tishon A, Moretta L (1977) Active thymus-derived suppressor lymphocytes in human cord blood. Nature 269:333–335
Olinescu A, Laky M, Popescu DE, Dumitrescu A, Ganca D (1978) The effect of alpha-fetoprotein on the immune response. Scand J Immunol 8:397–401
O'Neill G, Tsega E, Gold P, Murgita RA (1982) Regulation of human lymphocyte activation by alpha-fetoprotein. Evidence for selective suppression of Ia-associated T cell proliferation in vitro. Oncodevelop Biol Med 3:135–150
Papadogiannakis N, Johnsen S-A (1987) Mitogenic action of phorbol ester TPA and calcium ionophore A 23187 on human cord and maternal/adult peripheral lymphocytes: regulation by prostaglandin E_2. clin Exp Immunol 70:173–181
Papadogiannakis N, Johnsen S-A (1988) Distinct mitogens reveal different mechanisms of suppressor activity in human cord blood. J Clin Lab Immunol 26:37–41

Papadogiannakis N, Johnsen S-A, Olding LB (1985a) Human fetal/neonatal suppressor activity: relation between OKT phenotypes and sensitivity to prostaglandin E_2 in maternal and neonatal lymphocytes. Am J Reprod Immunol Microbiol 9:105–110
Papadogiannakis N, Johnsen S-A, Olding LB (1985b) Strong prostaglandin associated suppression of the proliferation of human maternal lymphocytes by neonatal lymphocytes linked to T versus T cell interactions and differential PGE_2 sensitivity. Clin Exp Immunol 61:125–134
Papadogiannakis N, Johnsen S-A, Olding LB (1986a) Monocyte regulated hyporesponsiveness of human cord blood lymphocytes to OKT3 monoclonal antibody induced mitogenesis. Scand J Immunol 23:91–99
Papadogiannakis N, Johnsen S-A, Olding LB (1986b) A prostaglandin mediated suppressive activity of cord as compared to maternal or other adult adherent cells in OKT3 antibody induced mitogenesis. Cell Immunol 101:51–61
Papadogiannakis N, Nordström TE, Andersson LC, Wolff CHJ (1989a) cAMP inhibits the OKT3-induced increase in cytoplasmic free calcium in the Jurkat T cell line: the degree of inhibition correlates inversely with the amount of CD3 ligand used. Eur J Immunol 19:1953–1956
Papadogiannakis N, Johnsen S-A, Rosberg S, Andersson RG, Olding LB (1989b)Differential sensitivity to cAMP among human cord and maternal/adult peripheral lymphocytes disclose differences between PHA- and OKT3-induced activation pathways. Immunology 68:378–383
Papadogiannakis N, Johnsen S-A, Olding LB (1990) Suppressor activity in human cord blood. In: Chaouat G (ed) The immunology of the fetus. CRC, Florida, pp 215–227
Paraskevas F (1984) Pathways of T-cell suppression. Crit Rev Immunol 5:95–148
Peck AB, Murgita RA, Wigzell H (1978) Cellular and genetic restriction in the immunoregulatory activity of alpha-fetoprotein. I. Selective inhibition of anti-Ia-associated proliferative reactions. J Exp Med 147:667–683
Peck AB, Murgita RA, Wigzell H (1982) Cellular and genetic restrictions in the immunoregulatory activity of alpha-fetoprotein. III. Role of the MLC-stimulating cell population in alpha-fetoprotein-induced suppression of T cell-mediated cytotoxicity. J Immunol 128:1134–1140
Persellin RH (1977) The effect of pregnancy on rheumatoid arthritis. Bull Rheum Dis 27:922–927
Pichler WJ, Broder S (1981) In vitro functions of human T cell expressing Fc-IgG or Fc-IgM receptors. Immunol Rev 56:163–197
Plaut M (1987) Lymphocyte hormone receptors. Annu Rev Immunol 5:621–669
Pollard JW (1991) Lymphohematopoietic cytokines in the female reproductive tract. Curr Opin Immunol 3:772–777
Protti MP, Manfredi AA, Horton RM, Bellone M, Conti-Tronconi BM (1993) Myasthenia gravis: recognition of a human antigen at the molecular level. Immunol Today 14:363–368
Purcell DFJ, McKenzie IFC, Lublin DM, Johnson PM, Atkinson JP, Oglesby TJ, Deacon NJ (1990) The human cell surface glycoproteins HuLy-m5, membrane cofactor protein (MCP) of the complement system, and trophoblast–leucocyte common (TLX) antigen are CD 46. Immunology 70:155–161
Rao CV (1988) Receptors for various prostaglandins. In: Curtis-Prior PB (ed) Biology and chemistry of prostaglandins and related eicosanoids. Churchill Livingstone, Edinbourgh, pp 171–178
Raz A, Wyche A, Needleman P (1989) Temporal and pharmacological division of fibroblast cyclooxygenase expression into transcriptional and translational phases. Proc Natl Acad Sci USA 86:1657–1661
Reilly M, Fitzgerald GA (1993) Cellular activation by thromboxane A_2 and other eicosanoids. Eur Heart J 14 (Suppl K):88–93
Rich PR, El Masry MN, Fox EJ (1986) Human suppressor T cells: induction, differentiation, and regulatory functions. Hum Immunol 17:369–387
Rollins TE, Smith WL (1980) Subcellular localization of prostaglandin-forming cycloogygenase in Swiss mouse 3T3 fibroblasts by electron microscopic immunocytochemistry. J Biol Chem 255:4872–4875
Rosenkrantz K, Dupont B, Flomenberg N (1985) Generation and regulation of autocytotoxicity in mixed lymphocyte cultures: evidence for active suppression of autocytotoxic cells. Proc Natl Acad Sci USA 82:4508–4512
Sakaguchi S, Sakaguchi N (1990) Thymus and autoimmunity: capacity of the normal thymus to produce pathogenic self-reactive T cells and conditions required for their induction of autoimmune disease. J Exp Med 172:537–545
Sakamoto K, Greally J, Gilfillan RF, Sexton J, Barnabei V, Yetz J, Bechtold T, Seeley JK, O'Dwyer E, Purtilo DT (1982) Epstein-Barr virus in normal pregnant women. Am J Reprod Immunol 2:217–221
Samuelsson B, Goldyne M, Granström E, Hamberg M, Hammarström S, Malmsten C (1978) Prostaglandins and thromboxanes. Annu Rev Biochem 47:997–1029

Scales WE, Chensue SW, Otterness I, Kunkel SL (1989) Regulation of monokine gene expression: prostaglandin E_2 suppresses tumor necrosis factor but not interleukin-1a or b-mRNA and cell-associated bioactivity. J. Leukoc Biol 45:416–421

Schneider R, Lees RK, Pedrazzini T, Zinkernagel RM, Hengartner H, MacDonald HR (1989) Postnatal disappearance of self reactive (VB6$^+$) cells from the thymus of MLs^2 mice. J Exp Med 169:2149–2151

Semeniuk DJ, Boismenu R, Tam J, Weissenhofer W, Murgita RA (1995) Evidence that immunosuppression is an intrinsic property of the alpha-fetoprotein molecule. In: Atassi MS, Bixler GS (eds) Immunobiology of proteins and peptides VIII. Plenum, New York, pp 255–269

Shimonovitz S, Yagel S, Anteby E, Finci-Yeheskel Z, Adashi EY, Mayer M, Hurwitz A (1995) Interleukin-1 stimulates prostaglandin E production by human torphoblast cells from first and third trimesters. J Clin Endocrinol Metab 80:1641–1646

Skowron-Cenrzak A, Ptak W (1976) Suppression of local graft–versus–host reactions by mouse fetal and newborn spleen cells. Eur J Immunol 6:451–452

Smith WL, Marnett LJ (1991) Prostaglandin endoperoxide synthase: structure and catalysis. Biochim Biophys Acta 1083:1–17

Smith HR, Steinberg AD (1983) Autoimmunity – a perspective. Annu Rev Immunol 1:175–210

Smith WL, DeWitt Dl, Allen ML (1983) Bimodal distribution of the prostaglandin I_2 synthase antigen in smooth muscle cells. J Biol Chem 258:5922–5926

Snyder DS, Beller DI, Unanue ER (1982) Prostaglandins modulate macrophage Ia expression. Nature 299:163–165

Soubiran P, Zapitelli J-P, Schaffer L (1987) IL-2 like material is present in human placenta and amnion. J Reprod Immunol 12:225–234

Strelkauskas AJ, Wilson BS, Dray S, Dodsom M (1975) Inversion of levels of human T and B cells in early pregnancy. Nature 258:331–332

Strelkauskas AJ, Davies IJ, Dray S (1978) Longitudinal studies showing alterations in the levels and functional response of T and B lymphocytes in human pregnancy. Clin Exp Immunol 32:531–539

Suzuki Y, Zeng CQY, Alpert E (1992) Isolation and partial characterization of a specific alpha-fetoprotein receptor on human monocytes. J Clin Invest 90:1530–1536

Tao Y-X, Cao Y-Q (1993) Modulation of interferon secretion by concanavalin A and interleukin-2 in first trimester placenta explants in vitro. J Reprod Immunol 24:201–212

Tedesco F, Narchi G, Radillo O, Meri S, Fervone S, Betterle C (1993) Susceptibility of human trophoblast to killing by human complement and the role of the complement regulatory proteins. J Immunol 151:1562–1570

Teixeira FJ, Zakar T, Hirst JJ, Guo f, Sadowsky DW, Machin G, Demianczuk N, Resch B, Olson DM (1994) Prostaglandin endoperoxide-H synthase (PGHS) activity and immunoreactive PGHS-1 and PGHS-2 levels in human amnion throughout gestation, at term, and during labor. J Clin endocrinol Metab 78:1396–1402

Thomas Y, Rogozinski L, Irigoyen O, Freedman SM, Kung PC, Goldstein G, Chess L (1981) Functional analysis of human T cell subsets defined by monoclonal antibodies. IV. Induction of suppressor cells within the OKT 3$^+$ population. J Exp Med 154:459–467

Toder V, Blank M, Nebel L (1979) Immunosuppressive effect of alpha-fetoprotein at different stages of pregnancy in mice Dev Comp Immunol 3:537–542

Torres JM, Laborda J, Naval J, Darracq N, Mishal Z, Uriel J (1989) Expression of alpha-fetoprotein receptors by human T lymphocytes during blastogenic transformation. Mol Immunol 26:851–857

Trangri S, Wegmann TG, Lin H, Raghupathy R (1994) Maternal anti-placental reactivity in natural immunologically mediated fetal resorptions. J Immunol 152:4903–4911

Unander MA, Olding LB (1981) Ontogeny and postnatal persistence of a strong suppressor activity in man. J Immunol 127:1182–1186

Unander AM, Smith CI, Hammarström L (1982) Evidence for a spontaneous activity and a weak helper function in cord blood lymphocytes. Int Arch Allergy Appl Immunol 69:245–251

Vane JR (1987) Anti-inflammatory drugs and the arachidonic acid cascade. In: Garaci E, Paoletti R, Santoro MG (eds) Prostaglandins and cancer research. Springer, Berlin Heidelberg New York, pp 12–25

Vane JR (1994) Towards a better aspirin. Nature 367:215–216

van Oers NSC, Cohen BL, Murgita RA (1989) Isolation and characterization of a distinct immunoregulatory isoform of alpha-fetoprotein produced by the normal fetus. J Exp Med 170:811–825

van Oers NSC, Boismenu R, Cohen BL, Murgita RA (1990) Analytical and preparative scale separation of molecular variants of alpha-fetoprotein by amnion-exchange chromatography on Monobead^{TM} resins. J Chromatogr A 525:59–69

Varfolomeyev SD, Mevkh AT (1993) Prostaglandin H synthase as a limiting enzyme of prostaglandin syntheses: substrate-induced inactivation as a new kind of enzyme activity regulation. Biotechnol Appl Biochem 17:291–304
Vetvicka V, Holub M, Kovarum H, Siman P, Kovaru F (1988) Alpha-fetoprotein and phagocytosis in athymic nude mice. Immunol Lett 19:95–98
Villacampa MJ, More R, Naval J, Failly-Crepin C, Lampreave F, Uriel J (1984) Alpha-fetoprotein receptors in human breast cancer cell line. Biochem Biophys Res Commun 122:1322–1327
Wallis WJ, Goldberg EH, Krco CJ, Williams RC (1976) Suppression of stimulation in mixed lymphocyte reaction by newborn splenic lymphocytes. Fed Proc 35:734
Wang W, Alpert E (1995) Down regulation of phorbol 12-myristate 13-acetate-induced tumor necrosis factor-alpha and interleukin 1B production and gene expression in human monocytic cells by human alpha-fetoprotein. Hepatology 22:921–928
Wegmann TG (1993) Lymphohematopoietic cytokines in the placenta: their role in reproduction. In: Chaouat G (ed) Immunology of pregnancy. CRC, Boca Raton, pp 143–150
Wegmann TG, Lin H, Guibert L, Mosmann TR (1993) Bidirectional cytokine interactions in the maternal–fetal relationship: is successful pregnancy a TH_2 phenomenon? Immunol Today 14:353–356
Weksler ME, Moody CE, Kozak RW (1983) The autologous mixed lymphocyte reaction. Adv Immunol 31:271–312
Wendling D, Racadot E, Morel-Fourrier B, Wijdenes J (1992) Treatment of rheumatoid arthritis with anti-CD4 monoclonal antibody. Open study of 25 patients with the B-F5 clone. Clin Rheumatol 11:542–547
Wraith DC, McDevitt HO, Steinman L, Acha-Orbea H (1989) T cell recognition as the target for immune intervention in autoimmune disease. Cell 57:709–715
Yachie A. Miyawaki T, Nagaoki T, Yokoi T, Mukai M, Uwadana N, Taniguchi N (1981) Regulation of B cell differentiation by T cell subsets defined with monoclonal OKT 4 and OKT 8 antibodies in human cord blood. J Immunol 127:1314–1317
Yachnin S (1976) Demonstration of the inhibitory effect of human alpha-fetoprotein on in vitro transformation of human lymphocytes. Proc Natl Acad Sci USA 73:2857–2861
Yachnin S, Lester E (1976) Inhibition of human lymphocyte transformation by human alpha-fetoprotein (HAFP): comparison of fetal and hepatoma HAFP and kinetic studies of in vitro immunosuppression. Clin Exp Imunol 26:484–490
Yachnin S, Soltani K, Lester EP (1980a) Further studies on the mechanism of suppression of human lymphocyte transformation by human alpha-fetoprotein. J Allergy Clin Immunol 65:127–135
Yachnin S, Getz GS, Lusk L, Hsu RC (1980b) Lipid interactions with human alpha-fetoprotein (AFP). A study of the role of such interactions in the ability of human AFP to suppress lymphocyte transformation. Oncodev Biol Med 1:273–285
Yamashita T, Kasai N, Miyoshi I, Sasaki N, Maki K, Sakai M, Nishi S, Namioka S (1993) High level expression of human alpha-fetoprotein in transgenic mice. Biochem Biophys Res Comm 191:715–720
Yamashita T, Nakane A, Watanabe T, Miyoshi F, Kasai N (1994) Evidence that alpha-fetoprotein suppresses the immunological function in transgenic mice. Biochem Biophys Res Comm 201:1154–1159
Zamvil SS, Steinman L (1990) The T lymphocyte in experimental allergic encephalomyelitis. Annu Rev Immunol 8:579–621

The Immunopathology of Recurrent Abortion

A.M. Unander[1,2]

1 Introduction

Medawar's thoughts about the similarities between the fetus and a graft (Medawar 1953) have preoccupied many investigators searching for an explanation for the success of "nature's transplant." In spite of their continous efforts over five decades to solve this question, the mechanisms that are responsible for the non-rejection of the fetus are still unclear. Many of these studies have focused on the differences in immunological reactions between couples with normal fertility and couples with recurrent miscarriages.

Habitual abortion is defined as the occurrence of three or more consecutive pregnancies that have resulted in miscarriages. The risk for a new abortion is increased with the number of previous miscarriages experienced by the same woman, being 20% after two, 40% after three, and at least 54% after four or more previous miscarriages (Parazzini et al. 1988). In accordance with these findings, an

[1]National Board of Health and Welfare, Lilla Bommen 1, S-411 04 Göteborg, Sweden
[2]Department of Obstetrics and Gynecology, Sahlgrenska University Hospital, University of Göteborg, Göteborg, Sweden

international multicenter study showed that the probability of a live birth was reduced by 23% for each additional abortion beyond three (DAYA, and GUNBY 1994). Thus the inclusion of women with two miscarriages in studies of women with recurrent abortion may influence the results: the strict definition of recurrent/habitual abortion should therefore be followed, something which has not always been done so far.

2 Background: The Fetus as an Allograft

During the 1970s, graft survival was found to be significantly prolonged in kidney transplant patients who had received blood transfusions before the transplantations (OPELZ et al. 1973). The prolongation of graft survival depends mainly on the presence of white cells in the transfused blood (PROUD et al. 1979). The transfused allograft recipients develop specific suppressor cells and IgG antibodies that can block their own reactions in one-way mixed lymphocyte culture (MLC) (SINGAL and JOSEPH 1982). These blocking antibodies are directed against recognition sites on T lymphocytes and are associated with prolonged graft survival (SINGAL and JOSEPH 1982). Blocking factors in renal allograft recipients have been thoroughly reviewed (BURLINGHAM 1988).

The concept of the fetus as an antigenically foreign semi-allogeneic allograft led to the idea that the events of abortion might bear similarities to those of rejection, although nobody has ever shown that a true rejection occurs in abortion. If this concept were true, the events following the receipt of blood transfusions containing leukocytes would diminish the risk both of abortion and of rejection of a kidney transplant. The theoretical background to support this notion was provided when it was shown that trophoblast and human leukocytes bear serologically cross-reactive antigens (FAULK et al. 1978; HAMILTON et al. 1980). Based on these findings, a hypothesis was proposed for the maintenance of pregnancy (FAULK et al. 1978) according to which one of these trophoblast antigens can induce a cytotoxic immune response, which might lead to rejection of the placenta, whereas another trophoblast antigen stimulates the B cells to produce antibody that may block the cytotoxic response and thereby protect against abortion.

Many coworking mechanisms have been suggested to explain nonrejection of the fetus, such as a modification of the mother's immune reactivity by hormones and other substances, immunological inertness of the fetus, production of antifetal antibodies during pregnancy, and fetal and maternal suppressor cells, including the underlying cytokine production. The immunopathologic mechanisms suggested to explain recurrent abortion follow the same lines.

3 Possible Mechanisms for the Maintenance of Pregnancy

3.1 Modification of the Mother's Immune Reactivity by Hormones or Other Substances

In animal experiments, both estrogens and progesterone prolong graft survival in the uterine endometrium of a presensitized host. The prolongation of graft survival is maximal when estrogen treatment has been followed by progesterone, a sequence of events that lead to an endometrial reaction of the decidual type, which is present at the time of implantation (Kirby et al. 1966). However, the rejection of grafts in the uterine endometrium of a presensitized host can only be delayed, not abolished by these hormones (Beer and Billingham 1974). Thus these sex hormones alone cannot be responsible for nonrejection of normal pregnancy, and a lack of these hormones cannot be a common explanation for recurrent miscarriage.

Previous ideas that lack of human chorionic gonadotrophin (hCG) could explain repeated miscarriages were tested in a controlled multicenter study in which habitually aborting women received hCG treatment during new pregnancies. This study failed to confirm previous promising data advocating the use of hCG in habitual abortion (Harrison 1992).

Several different proteins that are produced during pregnancy are immunosuppressive in vitro, and many are also immunosuppressive in animal experiments. This is true of alpha fetoprotein (AFP), which is present in amniotic fluid and fetal and maternal serum during pregnancy (Rocklin et al. 1979), and also for early pregnancy factor (EPF), which can be demonstrated during the first two trimesters of human pregnancy (Noonan et al. 1979). Several other proteins that are produced by the placenta remain obscure as far as their function and origin are concerned (Klopper 1980).

3.2 Maternal and Fetal Suppressor Cells

Maternal suppressor cells are found in the regional lymph nodes draining the uterus of allopregnant mice and also in the endometrium of both mice (Clark et al. 1984, 1987) and humans (Daya et al. 1989).

Fetal suppressor T cells have been demonstrated in cord blood (Olding and Oldstone 1974). Such suppressor cells have been found in fetuses from 8 weeks of gestation and persist until around 1 year after birth (Unander and Olding 1981). Their suppression is largely mediated by prostaglandins (Olding et al. 1982.)

3.3 Fetal HLA Antigens, Cytotoxic cells, and Natural Killer Cells

Cytotoxic T cell reactions may be induced by placental and embryo cells (Youtananukorn et al. 1974; Toder et al. 1982; Daya et al. 1989). Human maternal cell-mediated immune reactions to placental antigens develop in pregnancy and increase gradually during the course of pregnancy (Youtananukorn et al. 1974; Taylor et al. 1976). Thus a cytotoxic response of the mother towards the fetus has been shown to be part of the normal course of events during pregnancy. However, conflicting data have since been presented. One recent study has shown that no fertile controls, but many women with recurrent abortion exhibit in vitro evidence of T cell immunity to trophoblast antigen leading to production of embryotoxic factors (Yamada et al. 1994).

It has been claimed that immunologic recognition is a necessary prerequisite for a successful implantation (Clarke and Kirby 1966). T cells are present and capable of recognizing nonself, which furnishes possibilities for blastocyst protection at implantation (Faulk and McIntyre 1981). In mice, the blastocyst is immunogenic. It expresses minor histocompatibility antigens and is rejected if transferred to an ectopic site in a presensitized host (Kirby et al. 1966). When the time of implantation nears, the antigens are not expressed on the outer surface of the 16 cell-stage blastocyst, but only on the inner cell mass (Håkansson et al. 1975; Searle et al. 1976), which leaves no possibility for a maternal immune response against tissue antigens at that time. At the time of implantation, lymphocytes infiltrate around the blastocyst in the endometrium in normal pregnancy.

The invading trophoblastic buds express HLA antigens of the class I type (Sunderland et al. 1981). During the development of the placenta, the trophoblast differentiates into the inner cytotrophoblast, which expresses class I HLA antigens, and the outer syncytiotrophoblast, which is in contact with the maternal circulation and expresses tissue-specific minor histocompatibility antigens. No trophoblast cells express class II antigens DR DQ, but DP antigens have been demonstrated on extravillous trophoblast (Sutton et al. 1986; Starkey 1987).

In a study of maternal–fetal histocompatibility for alleles at HLA class II loci, HLA-DQA1 and HLA-DQB1 were examined. Significantly more couples with recurrent spontaneous abortion were found to share two HLA-DQ as compared to normal fertile couples. The low number of HLA-DQA1-compatible fetuses found suggests that these fetuses are aborted early in pregnancy (Ober et al. 1993).

A new set of HLA antigens that differ from the other class I antigens A, B, and C and that have been designed HLA-G have been identified on trophoblast and the extraplacental fetal membranes (Ellis 1990). A failure of maternal immune cells to attack these membranes has been suggested to be due to the ability of chorion cells selectively to transcribe class I HLA genes and/or to process the products of these genes differently from other types of cells (Hunt and Fishback 1989).

Evidence has accumulated that in many species, including humans, natural killer (NK) cells tend to be cytolytic to target cells which are deficient in self human leukocyte antigen (HLA) class I molecules (Ljunggren and Kärre 1990). It has been proposed that HLA-G may protect trophoblast against maternal decidual NK cell attack by providing the necessary HLA class I profile, whereby trophoblast is disguised as "self" (King and Loke 1991). Recently, it has been found that trophoblast also expresses HLA-C on its cell surface (Loke and King 1996). These data have led to the hypothesis that co-expression of HLA-G and HLA-C provides trophoblast with a set of class I molecules for optimal NK recognition, although it is not clear at present how uterine NK cells interact with trophoblast HLA-G and HLA-C (LOKE and KING 1996).

NK-like large, granular lymphocytes have been detected in the human decidua during early pregnancy (BULMER et al. 1991). Decidual NK-like cells do not lyse trophoblast by themselves, but after stimulation with interleukin-2 (IL-2) they are converted to lymphokine-activated killer (LAK) cells that can kill human trophoblast cells (KING and LOKE 1991). NK -cell activity decreases significantly as pregnancy advances after the first trimester.

3.4 Helper/Suppressor Cells (CD4/CD8) and Cytokines

Pregnant females are biased towards humoral rather than cell-mediated immunity; T_H1 cytokines IL-2, Interferon gamma (IFN-γ), and tumor necrosis factor (TNF) compromise pregnancy, and T_H2 cytokines interleukins IL-4, IL-5, IL-6, and IL-10 are produced at the maternal–fetal interface. T_H2 cytokine IL-10 can downregulate the cytokine synthesis of T_H1 cells, and the T_H1 cytokine IFN-γ inhibits proliferation of T_H2 cells. Based on these facts, it is hypothesized that during pregnancy there is a balance between T_H1 and T_H2 activity and that fetal survival is improved when the T_H1 responses are downregulated by T_H2 cytokines (WEGMANN et al. 1993). There is substantial evidence to support this theory. One of the mechanisms of fetal damage in response to IL-2 and IFN-γ may be the induction of NK activity. In mice, activation of NK cells correlates with fetal resorption, which, however, can be prevented by anti-NK antibody treatment (WEGMANN et al. 1993).

This theory has gained support from later studies. In an abortion-prone mice model, IL-10, which may downregulate T_H1 response, prevents fetal loss. Alloimmunization reverses the fetal loss and is shown to enhance the placental production of T_H2 cytokines IL-4 and IL-10 (CHAOUAT et al. 1995). Accordingly, it has been found that a subset of women with recurrent abortion are deficient in transforming growth factor-β2-producing "suppressor cells" in uterine tissue near the placental attachment site (LEA et al. 1995).

T_H2-type immunity against trophoblast (IL-4, IL-5, IL-10) may be a natural response contributing to successful pregnancy, and T_H1 immunity (IL-2, TNF-β, IFN-γ) is associated with unexplained recurrent abortion and is thought to play a role in reproductive failure (HILL et al. 1995). Animal experiments supporting this theory have been reported (CHAOUAT et al. 1995). In an editorial comment (DUDLEY 1995), several questions were raised, e.g., what mechanisms regulate cytokine production by immune effector cells in the decidua, does HLA-G function to regulate cytokine responses through effector cells in the decidua, and can any simple, reproducible, and meaningful tests of maternal immune function be developed that have any predictable value for pregnancy outcome?

As examined using flow cytometry and an NK cytotoxicity assay, it has been shown that decidual NK cell responses in an embryonic pregnancies and in recurrent spontaneous abortions differ from those in normal pregnancies. However, it remains to be elucidated whether this difference is pathogenic or is a mere response to a dead embryo (CHAO et al. 1995).

The immunophenotypic characteristics of endometrial leukocytes from non-pregnant women with recurrent abortion have been determined by flow cytometric analysis. In the recurrent aborters, the percentage of endometrial $CD8^+$ T lymphocytes was significantly decreased, and the CD4 to CD8 ratio was increased. A normal proportion of $CD8^+$ and $CD20^+$ cells in the endometrium and a normal CD4 to CD8 ratio was a prognostic sign of successful subsequent pregnancy (LACHAPELLE et al. 1996).

Circulating lymphoid cells with cytotoxic activity against placental cells have been demonstrated by in vitro tests on blood lymphocytes from women with ongoing recurrent miscarriage (YOKOYAMA et al. 1994). A high preconceptional NK activity in women with recurrent miscarriages is found to predict subsequent pregnancy loss (AOKI et al. 1995). This is in accordance with the observation in mice that NK-type cells mediate early spontaneous abortion (CLARK et al. 1994). After allogeneic leukocyte immunotherapy, NK activity has been shown to decrease in women who maintained their next pregnancy. In contrast, the NK cell activity did not change in those women who aborted their next pregnancy. This effect on NK cell activity is monocyte dependent (HIGUCHI et al. 1995). It seems clear, however, that the antitrophoblast activity is also regulated systemically and is dependent upon $CD8^+$ cells (CLARK 1994).

In an abortion-prone mice model, abortions can be prevented by alloimmunization using paternal leukocytes and also by administration of granulocyte-macrophage colony-stimulating factor (GM-CSF). It was found that $CD8^+$ cells are essential for this protection (CLARK et al. 1994). Accordingly, miscarriages in women with recurrent abortion might be explained by the coexistence of a defective activation of $CD8^+$ suppressive mechanisms and circulating antiplacental cell cytotoxicity (CLARK 1994).

4 Possible Causes of Recurrent Pregnancy Loss

4.1 Antiphospholipid Antibody Syndrome and Other Autoimmune Aberrations

Autoantibodies against phospholipids, such as anticardiolipin and phosphatidylserine, react with vascular endothelium in the placenta, leading to intrauterine fetal death and pregnancy loss (BRANCH et al. 1985; LOCKSHIN et al. 1985; HUGHES et al. 1986). The antiphospholipid syndrome also includes a severe tendency towards developing thrombosis and thrombocytopenia.

Many, but not all women with systemic lupus erythematosus (SLE) have an increased tendency towards pregnancy loss. In a Swedish study of unselected patients with SLE, 54% had elevated serum concentrations of anticardiolipin antibodies, and in 10% of these women levels were very high (STURFELT et al. 1987). Among clinically healthy Swedish women with habitual abortion, anticardiolipin antibodies were demonstrated in nearly the same proportions: 42% had increased levels, and in 10% of the women very high levels of anticardiolipin antibodies were found concomitant with decreased levels of complement factor C4 (UNANDER et al. 1987, 1991). Several other autoantibodies may be demonstrated in women with recurrent abortion, which suggests that recurrent pregnancy loss may be a marker for subclinical autoimmune disease. Placental lesions have been studied in women with different autoimmune diseases such as SLE, autoimmune thyroid diseases, idiopathic thrombocytopenic purpura, systemic sclerosis, scleroderma, and multiple sclerosis. Placental vascular lesions were found to contain deposits of lgM and complement factors C3 and C1q (LABARRERE et al. 1986).

4.2 Immunization Treatment

Based on the clinical observations in transplantation patients and the theory based on the cross-reactions between antigens on trophoblast and on leukocytes, immunization treatment using leukocytes has been proposed to treat women with recurrent abortion (TAYLOR and FAULK 1981; BEER et al. 1981).

Several different protocols for immunization treatment have been developed (for a review, see UNANDER 1992). The criteria used for inclusion/exclusion of patients for treatment differ, as do the origins of the cells used for immunization, the numbers of immunizations, and the time relationships between immunizations and pregnancy. The leukocytes used for immunization are either from a third party or from the woman's own husband, and they are given to the women in transfusions of either pooled buffy coats or leukocyte-rich erythrocyte concentrates or in intravenous, intradermal, and intracutaneous injections of separated mononuclear leukocytes. A different protocol uses trophoblast membrane preparations.

When judging the outcome of pregnancies after immunotherapy for recurrent abortion, it should be remembered that untreated pregnancies after repeated miscarriages or intrauterine fetal deaths carry increased risks for intrauterine fetal death, intrauterine growth retardation, prematurity, and congenital malformations (FUNDERBURK et al. 1976; SCHOENBAUM et al. 1980; MCINTYRE et al. 1986).

4.3 HLA Compatibility

Many reports have been published showing diverse results of HLA sharing within couples with recurrent abortion or no such increased sharing. Since trophoblasts do not express classical HLA antigens and no allogeneic variation of trophoblast antigens has been found, the role of HLA compatibility has been questioned. Among the inbred Hutterite population, HLA compatibility is connected with lower fertility and increased miscarriage rates (OBER et al. 1988). Increased sharing of HLA antigens has been found among couples with three or more spontaneous abortions in a large, ethnically homogenous Chinese population in Taiwan (Ho et al. 1990). Extended MHC haplotypes, disadvantageous for reproduction, have also been found in an isolated Finnish population (Laitinen 1993). These studies support the hypothesis that recessive lethal genes linked to the HLA loci play a role in the pathogenesis of recurrent spontaneous abortions.

A possible explanation for success of leukocyte immunization in couples with increased HLA compatibility could therefore be that immunization may induce the production of antibodies directed against the products of lethal genes linked to the HLA loci. Such antibodies might be able to modulate antigens on the surface of the developing embryos carrying the lethal genes.

4.4 Antipaternal Cytotoxic Antibody

A lack of development of antipaternal cytotoxic (anti-HLA) antibody during pregnancy has been claimed to be a sign of an abnormal immunologic reaction to pregnancy, and the development of such cytotoxic antibody after immunization with paternal cells has been claimed to be correlated to successful outcome of subsequent pregnancy (Mowbray et al. 1985, 1987). However, only 25% of primigravida have cytotoxic antibodies at time of their first delivery. The incidence of such antibodies increases with increasing numbers of pregnancies, but the percentage of women who have delivered four times without any detectable antipaternal cytotoxic antibody is still 43%–63% (Terasaki et al. 1970; Tongio et al. 1972). No correlation has been shown between the course and result of pregnancy and the presence or lack of such antibodies. A prospective study of 226 normal pregnant women showed that 62% of women who had live births never developed any antipaternal cytotoxic antibody during pregnancy and that most women who developed antibody did so after 28 weeks of gestation (Regan and Braude 1987). Thus the low incidence of cytotoxic antibody among aborting women is probably explained by their gestations being insufficiently long to cause a response. Accordingly, the production of previously absent antipaternal cytotoxic anti-HLA antibody cannot explain the success of immunization treatment.

4.5 Blocking Antibodies

Blocking antibodies in pregnant sera detected by mixed lymphocyte reaction (MLR) blocking assay have been implicated as an essential factor in successful pregnancy. Factors that can block cellular immune responses can be demonstrated during and after pregnancy in the serum of females (Youtananukorn and Matangkasombut 1972). In mice, this blocking activity is an IgG_2 antibody, possibly complexed with embryonic antigens (Tamerius et al. 1975). Close correlation between the amount of serum-blocking antibodies and trophoblast survival has been observed, indicating immune dependency of trophoblast growth (TAKEUCHI 1980). There are several reports of lack of blocking factors in women with unexplained recurrent abortion (ROCKLIN et al. 1976; STIMSON et al. 1979; TAKEUCHI 1980; UNANDER and OLDING 1983). Blocking activity is unrelated to cytotoxic activity, although blocking activity is found more often in samples containing cytotoxic antibodies. Immunization treatment has been shown to induce previously absent blocking factor in habitually aborting women (UNANDER et al. 1985; TAKAKUWA et al. 1986; TAKEUCHI 1990), and data have shown a correlation between the development of blocking antibody after immunization treatment and a subsequent successful pregnancy (UNANDER and LINDHOLM 1986; TAKAKUWA et al. 1990).

The objection has been raised that blocking factors have not been shown to be antibodies and that their nature should be more precisely defined (SARGENT et al. 1988). We have tested different Ig fractions from sera with blocking capacity in one-way MLC and found that the blocking capacity resided in the IgG fraction. Accordingly, the blocking factor studied by us is either IgG or something that is separated with IgG (A.M. UNANDER, unpublished data). This is also true for the blocking effect studied by others (WERNET and KUNKEL 1973; GATTI et al. 1973; TAKEUCHI 1980; TAKAKUWA et al. 1986; CATTO et al. 1986). Serum samples tested by us for blocking capacity in one-way MLC were heat inactivated (UNANDER et al. 1985). Thus our results cannot be influenced by complement-activating antibodies such as the cytotoxic anti-HLA antibodies.

Objections have also been made that blocking capacity is not always demonstrable in a woman's serum during successful pregnancy (SARGENT and REDMAN 1985; SARGENT et al. 1988). However, vast amounts of antibodies able to block cell-mediated immune responses can be eluted from the placenta (REVILLARD et al. 1976). One explanation for the blocking antibody not being found in all successful pregnancies may be that the assays are too insensitive. Antibodies that are produced may be adsorbed to the placenta in an amount that leaves only a small proportion in the blood and makes determination of the remaining antibodies in the circulation difficult. A blocking effect of the woman's serum can be detected as early as the 12th week of gestation in most normal primigravid women (ROCKLIN et al. 1976; TAKAKUWA et al. 1986; CATTO et al. 1986). Blocking antibodies include auto-anti-idiotypic antibodies binding to maternal T cell receptors for paternal major histocompatability complex (MHC) types (SUCIO-FOCA et al. 1983). After development of a more sensitive assay, antibodies to anti-HLA-DR were detected in all early pregnancies studied (MARUHASHI et al. 1984). Nevertheless, since HLA-DR is not expressed on trophoblast, it remains unclear why antibodies against anti-HLA-DR should be relevant in successful pregnancy.

Spontaneous abortion in mice may be prevented by preimmunization with splenocytes that express the paternal haplotype (CHAOUAT et al. 1983). Based on data from this animal model, it has been proposed that successful vaccination against abortion may act primarily by augmenting suppressor cell activity in the decidua at the implantation site (CLARK et al. 1987). Further experiments show that spontaneous abortion in mice may also be prevented by preimmunization with anti-idiotypic antibodies to antipaternal antibody (CHAOUAT and LANKAR 1988). Accordingly, passive immunization with intravenous Ig that was thought to contain anti-idiotypic antibodies has been tried in humans (MÜLLER-ECKHARDT et al. 1989).

Blocking antibodies may affect the afferent and/or the efferent arm of cell-mediated immunity generated against fetal antigens (ROBERT et al. 1973; TAKEUCHI 1990). Human blocking factors are shown to be IgG, directed against HLA or closely related MHC antigens (GATTI et al. 1975). Blocking antibodies have been claimed to be directed against one of two cross-reactive trophoblast-lymphocyte antigens (MCINTYRE and FAULK 1982). Noncytotoxic Fc receptor-blocking antibodies detected by the EA rosette inhibition assay (EAI) have also been suggested to act as blocking antibodies in pregnancies (POWERS et al. 1983; CATTO et al. 1986). This EA inhibitory activity in maternal serum persisted in the IgG preparation, in the $F(ab)_2$ fragments, and also after platelet absorption (CATTO et al. 1986).

It has been shown that the blocking antibodies in a woman can be removed by absorption with syncytiotrophoblast plasma membrane prepared from her own placenta, whereas preparations from placentas from other women cannot absorb her blocking antibodies (GOTO et al. 1989). It is therefore speculated that blocking antibodies may be directed against alloantigenic antigens expressed on trophoblasts and closely associated with class II MHC antigens that are not expressed on trophoblast (GOTO et al. 1989). As mentioned above, class II antigens DP can be demonstrated on extravillous trophoblast, although all trophoblast is negative for HLA DR and DQ (SUTTON et al. 1986). The relevance of this is as yet unclear, since extravillous trophoblast is not in contact with the maternal circulation.

Flow cytometric methods have been used in further work on the antibody status of women with habitual abortion after leukocyte immunization. Flow cytometry has shown that, in most women who develop blocking antibodies after immunization with their husband's cells, antibodies directed against both T and B cells can be demonstrated by flow cytometry (GILMAN-SACHS et al. 1989). The same group earlier showed that immunization with paternal cells induces the formation of antibodies against the husband's B cells (BEER et al. 1985).

We have found that women with habitual abortion who had received repeated third-party leukocyte-rich erythrocyte concentrates and experienced live birth had developed antibody against their husband's $CD4^+$ lymphocytes parallel to the formation of blocking factors in one-way MLC against the husband's cells. Neither was true for those women who aborted again after immunization treatment (ENSKOG et al., to be published). Our hypothesis is that, in some aborting couples, the husband's alloantigens are too weak alone to induce alloreactivity in the woman. Immunization of the woman with third-party cells would induce processing and subsequent presentation of antigens from these foreign cells. Among these presented antigens might be alloantigens shared by the blood donor and the husband, and the allostimulation of the woman might also be directed against these shared epitopes. Subsequent exposure to the husband's cells might lead to further alloreactivity in the woman against the husband's minor antigens. An alternative explanation for our findings is that the third-party cells may activate the woman's allogeneic response, which may then be directed specifically against her own husband's antigens exposed to the woman's immune system as expressed on sperm, leukocytes in the ejaculate, and trophoblast (ENSKOG et al., to be published). This is in accordance with previous findings that reproductive success can be improved in allogeneic mice with increased pregnancy loss by nonspecific stimulation of the maternal immune system by complete Freund's adjuvant (TODER et al. 1989). Neither the formation of antibodies against B cells (BEER et al. 1985; GILMAN-SACHS et al. 1989) nor the formation of anti-idiotypic antibodies (SUCIO-FOCA et al. 1983; MARUHASHI et al. 1984) are excluded by our data.

An integrated model has been proposed for the immune response of the mother toward the fetus during pregnancy. This model includes blocking antibodies, growth factors, suppressor factors, and cytotoxic factors (TAKEUCHI 1990). Predominantly novel MHC antigens expressed on trophoblast might induce a protective immune reaction, such as production of blocking antibodies, growth factors for trophoblasts, and generation of suppressor cells. This protective immune reaction might block a cytotoxic immune reaction generated by the classical MHC antigens that are to some extent expressed on trophoblast. If novel MHC antigens are repressed and classical MHC antigens are inappropriately expressed, the cytotoxic immune reaction would not be blocked, this generating trophoblastic damage. As concluded by TAKEUCHI (1990), continued studies on MHC genes and products of trophoblasts and their immunobiological significance are important for elucidation of the immunoregulatory mechanisms in pregnancy.

5 Conclusion

In spite of many beautifully hypothesized roles of classical immunologic phenomena in reproduction (CLARK 1993), many contradictory data have been published. Thus the true immunopathologic events that are critical for the maintenance of pregnancy and for pregnancy loss are still unclear.

Acknowledgements. This work was supported by grants from the Medical Research Council of Sweden (Projects no. 7326 and 7942), the Expressen Prenatal Research Foundation, the Göteborg Medical Society, the Swedish Society of Medicine, the Åhlén Foundation, and the Åke Wiberg Research Foundation.

References

Aoki K, Kajiura S, Matsumoto Y, Ogasawara M, Okada S, Yagami Y, Gleicher N (1995) Preconceptional natural-killer-cell activity as a predictor of miscarriage. Lancet 345:1340–1342

Beer AE, Billingham RE (1974) The embryo as a transplant. Sci Am 230:36–46

Beer AE, Quebbeman JF, Ayers JWT, Haines RF (1981) Major histocompatibility complex antigens, maternal and paternal immune responses, and chronic habitual abortions in humans. Am J Obstet Gynecol 141:987–999

Beer AE, Semprini AE, Xiaoyu Z (1985) Pregnancy outcome in human couples with recurrent spontaneous abortions: HLA antigen sharing; female serum MLR blocking factors; and paternal leukocyte immunization. Clin Exp Immunogenet 2:137–153

Branch DW, Scott JR, Kochenour NK, Hershgold E (1985) Obstetric complications associated with the lupus anticoagulant. New Engl J Med 313:1322–1326

Bulmer JN, Morrison L, Longfellow M, Riston A, Pace D (1991) Granulated lymphocytes in human endometrium: histochemical and immunohistochemical studies. Hum Reprod 6:791–798

Burlingham WJ (1988) What is known about blocking factors in renal allograft recipients. Am J Reprod Immunol Microbiol 16:15–20

Catto GRD, Power DA, McLeod AM (1986) Blocking antibody in pregnancy. In: Clark Da, Croy BA (eds) Reproductive immunology. Elsevier, Amsterdam, pp 85–90

Chao KH, Yang YS, Ho HN, Chen SU, Chen HF, Dai HJ, Huang SC, Gill TJ 3rd (1995) Decidual natural killer cytotoxicity decreased in normal pregnancy but not in anembryonic pregnancy and recurrent spontaneous abortion. Am J Reprod Immunol 34:274–280

Chaouat G, Lankar D (1988) Vaccination against spontaneous abortion in mice with preimmunization with an anti-idiotypic antibody. Am J Reprod Immunol Microbiol 16:146–150

Chaouat G, Kiger N, Wegmann TG (1983) Vaccination against spontaneous abortion in mice. J Reprod Immunol 5:389–392

Chaouat G, Meliani AA, Martal J, Raghupathy R, Elliot J, Mosmann T, Wegmann TG (1995) IL-10 prevents naturally occuring fetal loss in the CBA x DBA/2 mating combination, and local defect in IL-10 production in this abortion-prone combination is corrected by in vivo injection of IFN-τ. J Immunol 154:4261–4268

Clark DA (1993) Paraimmunology and receptors on decidual T cells: conflict or confirmation? Am J Reprod Immunol 29:35–38

Clark DA (1994) Maternal aggression against placenta? Am J Reprod Immunol 31:205–207

Clark DA, Slapsys R, Croy BA, Krcek J, Rossant J (1984) Local active suppression by suppressor cells in the decidua: a review, Am J Reprod Immunol 5:78–83

Clark DA, Chaouat G, Guenet JL, Kiger N (1987) Local active suppression and successful vaccination against spontaneous abortion in CBA/J mice. J Reprod Immunol 10:79–85

Clark DA, Chaouat G, Mogil R, Wegmann TG (1994) Prevention of spontaneous abortion in DBA/2-mated CBA/J mice by GM-CSF involves CD8+ T cell dependent suppression of natural effector cell cytotoxicity against target cells. Cell Immunol 154:143–152

Clarke B, Kirby DRS (1966) Maintenance of histocompatibility polymorphisms. Nature 211:999–1000

Daya S, Gunby J (1994) The effectiveness of allogeneic leukocyte immunization in unexplained primary recurrent spontaneous abortion. Am J Reprod Immunol 32:294–302

Daya S, Johnson PM, Clark DA (1989) Trophoblast induction of suppressor-type cell activity in human endometrial tissue. Am J Reprod Immunol 19:65–72

Dudley DJ (1995) Recurrent pregnancy loss and cytokines not as simple as it seems. JAMA 273:1958–1959

Ellis S (1990) HLA G: at the interface. Am J Reprod Immunol 23:84–86

Enskog A, Robbins D, Kjellsson B, Unander AM, Söderström T. Anti-husband T-helper cell antibody formation predicts outcome of immunotherapy in women with habitual abortion and lack of MLC blocking antibodies (to be published)

Faulk WP, Mclntyre JA (1981) Trophoblast survival. Transplantation 32:1–5

Faulk WP, Temple A, Lovins RE, Smith N (1978) Antigens of human trophoblasts: a working hypothesis for their role in normal and abnormal pregnancies. Proc Natl Acad Sci USA 75:1947–51

Funderburk SJ, Guthrie D, Meldrum D (1976) Suboptimal pregnancy outcome among women with prior abortions and premature births. Am J Obstet Gynecol 126:55–60

Gatti RA, Yunis EJ, Good RA (1973) Characterization of a serum inhibitor of MLC reactions. Clin Exp Immunol 13:427–437

Gatti RA, Svedmyr EAJ, Leibold W, Wigzell H (1975) Characterization of a serum inhibitor of MLC reactions. III. Specificity. Cell Immunol 15:432–451

Gilman-Sachs A, Luo SP, Beer AE, Beaman KD (1989) Analysis of anti-lymphocyte antibodies by flow cytometry of microlymphocytotoxocity in women with recurrent spontaneous abortions immunized with paternal leukocytes. J Clin Lab Immunol 30:53–59

Goto S, Takakuwa K, Kanazawa K, Takeuchi S (1989) MLR-blocking antibodies are directed against alloantigens expressed on syncytiotrophoblasts. Am J Reprod Immunol 21:50–53

Håkansson S, Heyner S, Sundqvist KG, Bergström S (1975) The presence of paternal H-2 antigens on hybrid mouse blastocysts during experimental delay of implantation and the disappearance of these antigens after onset of implantation. Int J Fertil 20:137–140
Hamilton TA, Wada HG, Sussman HH (1980) Expression of human placental cell surface antigens on peripheral blood lymphocytes and lymphoblastoid cell lines. Scand J Immunol 11:195–201
Harrison RF (1992) Human chorionic gonadotrophin (hCG) in the management of recurrent abortion; results of a multi-centre placebo-controlled study. Eur J Obstet Gynaecol Reprod Biol 47:175–179
Higuchi K, Aoki K, Kombara T, Hosoi N, Yamamoto T, Okada H (1995) Suppression of natural killer cell activity by monocytes following immunotherapy for recurrent spontaneous abortions. Am J Reprod Immunol 33:221–227
Hill JA, Polgar K, Anderson DJ (1995) T-helper 1-type immunity to trophoblast in women with recurrent spontaneous abortion. JAMA 273:1933–1935
Ho HN, Gill TJ 3rd, Nsieh RP, Hsieh HJ, Lee TY (1990) Sharing of human leukocyte antigens in primary and secondary recurrent spontaneous abortions. Am J Obstet Gynecol 163:178–188
Hughes GRV, Harris NN, Gharavi AE (1986) The anticardiolipin syndrome. J Rheumatol 13:486–489
Hunt JS, Fishback JL (1989) Amniochorion: immunological aspects – a review. Am J Reprod Immunol 21:114–118
King A, Loke YW (1991) On the nature and function of human uterine granular lymphocytes. Immunol Today 12:432–435
Kirby DRS, Billington WD, James DA (1966) Transplantation of eggs to the kidney and uterus of immunized mice. Transplantation 4:713–718
Klopper A (1980) The new placenta proteins. Placenta: 1:77–89
Labarrere CA, Catoggio LJ, Mullen EG, Althabe OH (1986) Placental lesions in maternal autoimmune diseases. Am J Reprod Immunol 12:78–86
Lachapelle MH, Miron P, Hemmings R, Roy DC (1996) Endometrial T. B, and NK cells in patients with recurrent spontaneous abortion. Altered profile and pregnancy outcome. J Immunol 156(10):4027–4034
Laitinen T (1993) A set of MHC Haplotypes found among Finnish couples suffering from recurrent spontaneous abortions. Am J Reprod Immunol 29:148–154
Lea RG, Underwood J, Flanders KC, Hirte H, Banwatt D, Finotto S, Ohno I, Daya S, Harley C, Michel M, Mowbray JF, Clark DA (1995) A subset of patients with recurrent spontaneous abortion is deficient in transforming growth factor β-2-producing "suppressor cells" in uterine tissue near the placental attachment site. Am J Reprod Immunol 34:52–64
Ljunggren HG, Kärre K (1990) In search of the "missing self": MHC molecules and NK cell recognition. Immunol Today 11:237–244
Lockshin MD, Druzin ML, Goel S, Quamar T, Magid MS, Jovanovic L, Ferenc M (1985) Antibody to cardiolipin as a predictor of fetal distress or death in pregnant patients with systemic lupus erythematosus. New Engl J Med 313:152–156
Loke YW, King A (1996) Immunology of human implantation: an evolutionary perspective. Hum Reprod 11:283–286
Maruhashi T, Takakuwa K, Kajino T, Kanazawa K, Takeuchi S (1984) Characterization and detection of blocking antibodies in early pregnant sera. Am J Reprod Immunol 5:99–104
Mclntyre JA, Faulk WP (1982) Allotypic cross-reactive (TLX) surface antigens. Hum Immunol 4:27–35
Mclntyre JA, Fault WP, Nichols-Johnson VR et al (1986) Immunologic testing and immunotherapy in recurrent spontaneous abortion. Obstet Gynecol 67:169–175
Medawar PB (1953) Some immunological and endocrinological problems raised by the evolution of viviparity in vertebrates. Soc Exp Biol 7:320–338
Mowbray JF, Gibbings C, Liddell H, Reginald PW, Underwood JL, Beard RW (1985) Controlled trial of treatment of recurrent spontaneous abortion by immunisation with paternal cells. Lancet 1:941–943
Mowbray JF, Underwood JL, Michel M, Forbes PB, Beard RW (1987) Immunisation with paternal lymphocytes in women with recurrent miscarriage. Lancet 2:679–680
Müller-Eckhardt G, Heine O, Neppert J, Künzel W, Müller-Eckhardt C (1989) Prevention of recurrent spontaneous abortion by intravenous immunoglobulin. Vox Sang 56:151–154
Noonan FP, Halliday WJ, Morton H, Clunie GJA (1979) Early pregnancy factor is immunosuppressive. Nature 278:649–651
Ober C, Elias S, O'Brien E (1988) HLA sharing and fertility in Hutterite couples: evidence for prenatal selection against compatible fetuses. Am J Reprod Immunol 18:111–115

Ober C, Steck T, van der Ven K, Billstrand C, Messer L, Kwak J, Beaman K, Beer A (1993) MHC class II compatibility in aborted fetuses and term infants of couples with recurrent spontaneous abortion. J Reprod Immunol 25:195–207

Olding LB, Johnsen SA, Unander M, Westberg NG, Wilhelmsson L (1982) Strong suppression of maternal leukocytes by fetal T lymphocytes in human pregnancy – one of nature's ways of prohibiting rejection of the fetus? Transplant Proc 14:146–148

Olding LB, Oldstone MBA (1974) Lymphocytes from human newborns abrogate mitosis of their mothers' lymphocytes. Nature 249:161–162

Opelz G, Sengar GPS, Mickey MR, Terasaki PI (1973) Effect of blood transfusions on subsequent kidney transplants. Transplant Proc 4:253–257

Parazzini F, Acaia B, Ricciardiello O et al (1988) Short-term reproductive prognosis when no cause can be found for recurrent miscarriage B J Obstet Gynaecol 95:654–658

Power DA, Catto GRD, Mason RJ, McLeod AM, Stewart GM, Stewart KN, Shewan WG (1983) The fetus as an allograft: evidence for protective antibodies to HLA-linked paternal antigens. Lancet 2:701–704

Proud G, Shenton BK, Smith BM (1979) Blood transfusion and renal transplantation. Br J Surg 66:678–682

Regan L, Braude PR (1980) Is antipaternal cytotoxic antibody a valid marker in the management of recurrent abortion? Lancet 1987:2

Revillard JP, Brochier J, Robert M, Bonneau M, Traeger J (1976) Immunologic properties of placental eluates. Transplant Proc 8:275–279

Robert M, Betuel H, Revillard JP (1973) Inhibition of the mixed lymphocyte reaction by sera from multipara. Tissue Antigens 3:39–56

Rocklin RE, Kitzmiller JL, Carpenter CD, Garovoy MR, David JR (1976) Maternal-fetal relation. Absence of an immunologic blocking factor from the serum of women with chronic abortions. New Engl J Med 295:1209–1213

Rocklin RE, Kitzmiller JK; Kaye MD (1979) Immunobiology of the maternal-fetal relationship. Ann Rev Med 30:375–404

Sargent IL, Redman CWG (1985) Maternal cell-mediated immunity to the fetus in human pregnancy. J Reprod Immunol 7:95–104

Sargent IL, Wilkins T, Redman CWG (1988) Maternal immune responses to the fetus in early pregnancy and recurrent miscarriage. Lancet 2:1099-1104

Schoenbaum SC, Manson RR, Stubblefield PG, Domy PD, Ryan K (1980) Outcome of delivery following induced and spontaneous abortion. Am J Obstet Gynecol 136:19–24

Searle RF, Sellens MH, Elson J, Jenkinson EJ, Billington WD (1976) Detection of alloantigens during pre-implantation development and early trophoblast differentiation in the mouse by immunoperoxydase labelling. J Exp Med 143:348–359

Singal DP, Joseph S (1982) Role of blood transfusions on the induction of antibodies against recognition sites on T lymphocytes in renal transplant patients. Hum Immunol 4:93–108

Starkey PM (1987) Reactivity of human trophoblast with an antibody to the HLA class II antigen, HLA-DP. J Reprod Immunol 11:63–70

Stimson WH, Strachan AF, Shepherd A (1979) Studies on the maternal immune response to placental antigens: absence of a blocking factor from the blood of abortion-prone women. Br J Obstet Gynaecol 86:41–45

Sturfelt G, Nived O, Norberg R, Thorstensson R, Krook K (1987) Anticardiolipin antibodies in patients with systemic lupus erythematosus. Arthr Rheum 30:382–388

Sucio-Foca N, Reed E, Rohowsky C, Kung P, King DW (1983) Anti-idiotypic antibodies to anti-HLA receptors induced by pregnancy. Proc Natl Acad Sci USA 80:830–834

Sunderland CA, Naiem M, Mason DY (1981) The expression of major histocompatibility antigens by human chorionic villi. J. Reprod Immunol 3:323–331

Sutton L, Gadd M, Mason DY et al (1986) Cells bearing class II MHC antigens in the human placenta and amniochorion. Immunology 58:23–29

Takakuwa K, Goto S, Hasegawa I, Ueda H, Kanazawa K, Takeuchi S, Tanaka K (1990) Result in immunotherapy on patients with unexplained recurrent abortion: a beneficial treatment for patients with neative blocking antibodies. Am J Reprod Immunol 23:37–41

Takakuwa K, Kanazawa K, Takeuchi S (1986) Production of blocking antibodies by vaccination with husband's lymphocytes in unexplained recurrent aborters: the role in successful pregnancy. Am J Reprod Immunol Microbiol 10:1–9

Takeuchi S (1980) Immunology of spontaneous abortion and hydatidiform mole. Am J Reprod Immunol 1:23–28

Takeuchi S (1990) Is production of blocking antibodies in sucessful human pregnancy an epiphenomenon? Am J Reprod Immunol 24:108–119

Tamerius J, Hellström I, Hellström KE (1975) Evidence that blocking factors in the sera of multiparous mice are associated with immunoglobulins. Int J Cancer 16:456–464

Taylor CG, Faulk WP (1981) Prevention of recurrent abortion by leukocyte transfusions Lancet 2:68–70

Taylor PV, Gowland G, Hancock KW, Scott JS (1976) Effect of length of gestation on maternal cellular immunity to human trophoblast antigens. Am J Obstet Gynecol 125:528–531

Terasaki PM, Mickey MR, Yamazaki JN, Vredevoe D (1970) Maternal-fetal incompatibility. Transplantation 9:538–543

Toder V, Blank M, Drizlikh G, Nebel L (1982) Placental and embryo cells can induce the generation of cytotoxic lymphocytes in vitro. Transplanatation 33:196–198

Toder V, Strassburger D, Carp H, Irlin Y, Lurie S, Pecht M. Trainin N (1989) Immunopotentiation and pregnancy loss. J Reprod Fertil. Suppl 37:79–84

Tongio MM, Berrebi A, Mayer S (1972) A study of lymphocytotoxic antibodies in multiparous women having at least four pregnancies. Tissue Antigens 2:378–388

Unander AM (1992) Immunization treatment in habitual abortion using third party leukocytes. Transfusion Med Rev 4:1–16

Unander AM, Lindholm A (1986) Transfusions of leukocyte-rich erythrocyte concentrates: a successful treatment in selected cases of habitual abortion. Am J Obstet Gynecol 154:516–520

Unander AM, Olding LB (1981) Ontogeny and postnatal persistence of a strong suppressor activity in man. J Immunol 127:1182–1186

Unander AM, Olding LB (1983) Habitual abortion: parental sharing of HLA antigens, absence of maternal blocking antibody, and easily suppressed lymphocytes in the women. Am J Reprod Immunol 4:171–178

Unander AM, Lindholm A, Olding LB (1985) Blood transfusions generate/increase previously absent/weak blocking antibody in women with habitual abortion. Fertil Steril 44:766-771

Unander AM, Norberg R, Hahn L, Arfors L (1987) Anticardiolipin antibodies and complement in ninety-nine women with habitual abortion. Am J Obstet Gynecol 156:114–119

Unander AM, Norberg R, Arfors L, Enskog A, Haeger M, Lindholm A, Robbins D, Siösteen CC, Söderström T, Stigendal L, Wennerström H (1991) Opinions on treatment of women with habitual abortion based on investigations for blocking antibody and autoantibodies. Am J Reprod Immunol 26:32–37

Wegmann TG, Lin H, Guilbert L, Mosmann TR (1993) Bidirectional cytokine interactions in the maternal-fetal relationship: is successful pregnancy a TH2-phenomenon? Immunol Today 14:353–356

Wernet P, Kunkel HG (1973) Demonstration of specific T-lymphocyte membrane antigens associated with antibodies inhibiting the mixed leukocyte culture in man. Transplant Proc 5:1875–1881

Yamada H, Polgar K, Hill JA (1994) Cell mediated immunity to trophoblast antigens in women with recurrent spontaneous abortion. Am J Obstet Gynecol 170:1339–1344

Yokoyama M, Sano M, Sonoda K, Nozaki M, Nakamura G, Nakano H (1994) Cytotoxic cells directed against placental cells detected in human habitual abortion by an in vitro terminal labeling assay. Am J Reprod Immunol 1994 31 (4):197–204

Youtananukorn V, Matangkasombut P (1972) Human maternal cell mediated immune reaction to placental antigens. Clin Exp Immunol 11:549–556

Youtananukorn V, Matangkasombut P, Osathanondh V (1974) Onset of human maternal cell-mediated immune reaction to placental antigens during the first pregnancy. Clin Exp Immunol 16:593–598

Transfer of Maternal Leukocytes to the Infant by Human Milk

A.S. GOLDMAN and R.M. GOLDBLUM

1 Introduction

Human milk contains a complex immune system that consists not only of a host of soluble direct-acting antimicrobial agents (GOLDMAN and SMITH 1973), anti-inflammatory factors (GOLDMAN et al. 1986), and immunomodulating agents (GOLDMAN 1993) but also of living cells. The discovery of leukocytes in human milk began with microscopic examinations of human milk by the first microscopist, ANTHONY VAN LEEWENHOEK (1695). His observations lay fallow until ALFRED DONNÉ (1837) the French physician who first adapted plate photography to microscopy, reported the presence of globules and granular bodies in human milk. Most of the globules were probably milk fat globules, myriads of which are normally found in human milk. Many years later when staining techniques became available, some of the *corpuscles de Donné* were found to be cells.

The identity of these cells, however, remained unclear until more sophisticated microscopic and cytochemical staining methods were applied (SMITH and GOLDMAN 1968; CRAGO et al. 1979). Special stains were required because the morphology of most cells in human milk is obscured by large numbers of intracytoplasmic lipid vacuoles and membranes. These studies demonstrated that neutrophils, macrophages, and lymphocytes are present in human milk, and that the dominant cell

---

Department of Pediatrics, Immunology/Allergy Division, Children's Hospital, 301 University Boulevard, University of Texas Medical Branch, Galveston, TX 77555–0369, USA

populations in early human milk secretions are neutrophils and macrophages (Smith and Goldman 1968). Furthermore, many milk leukocytes were found to be living, motile, and interactive (Smith and Goldman 1968, 1970; Smith et al. 1971). It was also noted that other leukocytes commonly associated with inflammation, such as basophils, mast cells, eosinophils, and platelets, were excluded from human milk.

Succeeding experiments concerning leukocytes in human milk were hampered because their high lipid content made it difficult to isolate the major populations by buoyant density gradient techniques. However, more recently progress has been made in understanding their origins, numbers and phenotypic features, in vitro functions, and fate after transfer into experimental animals. This chapter reviews those investigations and analyzes the potential relationship between the cells and soluble defense agents in human milk.

2 Origins and General Features of Human Milk Leukocytes

It is likely that the leukocytes in human milk originate from blood. No leukocytes, other than a few macrophages, appear in the mammary gland until late pregnancy and throughout lactation. Based upon the specific pattern of leukocytes in human milk, oral immunization experiments in women (Goldblum et al. 1975) and observations in animal models concerning the origin of IgA-producing cells in the mammary gland (Roux et al. 1977; Weisz-Carrington et al. 1978), it seems likely that the homing of leukocytes to the mammary gland is controlled in part by hormones produced during late pregnancy and lactation.

The vast majority of B cells that home to the mammary gland transform into plasma cells that remain sessile in the mammary gland. In contrast, other leukocytes attracted to the site traverse the mammary epithelium and become part of the milk secretions. The highest concentrations of leukocytes in human milk occur in the first few days of lactation ($1–3 \times 10^6$/ml) (Smith and Goldman 1968; Tsuda et al. 1984). Earlier observations suggested that the relative frequencies of neutrophils, macrophages, and lymphocytes are 40%–65%, 35%–55%, and 5%–10%, respectively. More current estimates by flow cytometry suggest that the relative frequencies of neutrophils, macrophages, and lymphocytes in human milk are approximately 80%, 15%, and 4%, respectively (Bertotto et al. 1990; Wirt et al. 1992; Keeney et al. 1993).

3 Neutrophils in Human Milk

Because of the large number of intracytoplasmic inclusions, neutrophils and macrophages in human milk are difficult to identify by common staining methods. However, neutrophils can be identified by their high content of myeloperoxidase

(Crago et al. 1979; Tsuda et al. 1984), paucity of nonspecific esterase (Crago et al. 1979; Tsuda et al. 1984), poor adherence to collagen-fibronectin substrata (Tsuda et al. 1984), and low expression of CD14 (Keeney et al. 1993). The failure to distinguish between the two populations of phagocytes in human milk confounded previous investigations. For example, human milk neutrophils are phagocytic (Smith and Goldman 1968), but it remains uncertain whether the respiratory burst in stimulated, unfractionated milk leukocytes is due in part to neutrophils or derives solely from macrophages.

Human milk neutrophils do not respond well to chemoattractants by increasing their adherence, polarity, or directed migration in in vitro systems (Thorpe et al. 1986). In addition, they display a marked decrease in deformability (Buescher 1991). The decrease in neutrophil motility was not due solely to a diminished adherence to the test substrata, since a striking decrease in motility was observed in in vitro systems that are highly dependent on or relatively independent of adherence (Özkaragoz et al. 1988).

Although it was initially interpreted that the decrease in adherence (Thorpe et al. 1986), polarity (Thorpe et al. 1986), and motility (Hawes and Jones 1985; Thorpe et al. 1986) of neutrophils in human milk are due to inhibitors in human milk (Thorpe et al. 1986), further investigations suggested that a more reasonable interpretation is that milk neutrophils are activated. Indeed, the phenotypic features of human milk neutrophils are indistinguishable from activated blood neutrophils (Keeney et al. 1993; Table 1). In this respect the surface expression of CD11b, part of the integrin Mac-1 heterodimer, was found to be increased, whereas the expression of L-selectin is significantly decreased (Keeney et al. 1993). The phenotypic features have been reproduced by incubating blood neutrophils in human milk or a particulate fraction of milk rich in milk fat globules and other membranous materials. Further, activation of blood neutrophils by a particulate fraction of milk is abrogated by prior incubation with an inhibitor of phagocytosis, cytochalasin B.

Table 1. Phenotypic features of neutrophils and macrophages in human milk demonstrated by flow cytometry: the increased expression of CD11b and the decreased expression of L-selectin are consistent with cellular activation

Source of neutrophils	fMLP Stimulation	Fluorescence channel intensity	
		CD11b	L-selectin
Human blood			
	–	~ 300	~ 78
	+	~ 700	~ 19
Human milk	–	~ 500	~ 18

4 Macrophages in Human Milk

Macrophages in human milk display a high content of nonspecific esterase (CRAGO et al. 1979; TSUDA et al. 1984), adhere to collagen-fibronectin substrata (TSUDA et al. 1984), move spontaneously (SMITH and GOLDMAN 1968; ÖZKARAGOZ et al. 1988), phagocytize particles (SMITH and GOLDMAN 1968), mount a respiratory burst after in vitro stimulation (TSUDA et al. 1984; SPEER et al. 1985; 1986; CUMMINGS et al. 1985), and kill-ingested *Candida albicans* (CUMMINGS et al. 1985). It has been reported that the chemotactic response of human milk macrophages is lower than that of blood monocytes (CLEMENTE et al. 1986), but this may have been due to a confusion between neutrophils and macrophages in the tested specimens. In an in vitro model in which the movement of leukocytes into type I collagen gel was assayed cytochemically, the motility of macrophages in human milk was greater than that of blood monocytes (ÖZKARAGOZ et al. 1988; MUSHTAHA et al. 1989). Since their functional (ÖZKARAGOZ et al. 1988) and ultrastructural features (SMITH et al. 1971) are consistent with cellular activation, milk macrophages were examined for phenotypic markers of activation by flow cytometry (KEENEY et al. 1993). The expression of CD11b was increased, and expression of L-selectin was decreased, as found in activated mononuclear phagocytes (KEENEY et al. 1993; Table 1).

Milk macrophages also process and present antigens to T cells (OKSENBERG et al. 1985) and synthesize lysozyme and the third component of the complement system (C3) in rates that are similar to alveolar macrophages (COLE et al. 1982). The rate of synthesis of C2 by human milk macrophages is, however, less than that of the alveolar cells (COLE et al. 1982). In addition, human milk macrophages produce biologically significant quantities of prostaglandin E_2 (LE DEIST et al. 1986), plasminogin activator (LE DEIST et al. 1986), and platelet-activating factor-acetylhydrolase (FURUKAWA et al. 1993) and thus may be the source of much of these components in human milk. In contrast, there is virtually no evidence that human milk macrophages produce certain cytokines found in early human milk secretions, including tumor necrosis factor-α (MUSHTAHA et al. 1989; RUDLOFF et al. 1992), interleukin-1 (SUBIZIA et al. 1988; MUNOZ et al. 1990), interleukin-8 (PALKOWETZ et al. 1994), and interleukin-10 (GAROFALO et al. 1995). Human milk macrophages also contain IgA and IgM (CLEMENTE et al. 1986), but these immunoglobulins are not released from the cells in response to certain stimuli.

5 Lymphocytes in Human Milk

T cells and B cells comprise, respectively, about 83% and 4–6% of lymphocytes in early human milk secretions (BERTOTTO et al. 1990; WIRT et al. 1993; see above). The small number of natural killer cells in human milk as shown by flow cytometry

(WIRT et al. 1992) is in keeping with the low cellular cytotoxic activity of human milk leukocytes (KOHL et al. 1980), and the small number of B cells reflects the sessile nature of B cells that enter the lamina propria of the mammary gland to transform to plasma cells.

Both $CD4^+$ (helper) and $CD8^+$ (cytotoxic/suppressor) T cell subpopulations are present in human milk (BERTOTTO et al. 1990; WIRT et al. 1993), but the proportion of $CD8^+$ T cells in human milk is higher than that in human blood T cells (WIRT et al. 1993) as in other mucosal sites. Virtually all $CD4^+$ T and $CD8^+$ T cells in human milk bear the CD45 isoform CD45R0 that is associated with immunologic memory (BERTOTTO et al. 1990; WIRT et al. 1993; Table 2). In addition, the proportion of T cells in human milk that display other phenotypic markers of activation is much greater than those in blood (WIRT et al. 1993; EGLINTON et al. 1994; GIBSON et al. 1991). T cell receptors of the cells are primarily α/β, but the relative frequency of γ/δ_+ T cells is higher than that of blood T cells (BERTOTTO et al. 1990, 1991; GIBSON et al 1991).

T cells in human milk produce certain cytokines including interferon-γ (BEST-OTTO et al. 1990), macrophage migration inhibitor factor (KELLER et al. 1981), and monocyte chemotactic factor (KELLER et al. 1981). The production of interferon-γ is consistent with the CD45RO phenotype of T cells in human milk (BERTOTTO et al. 1990; WIRT et al. 1993) and the finding that $CD45RO^+$ T cells are the major source of that cytokine (DOHLSTEN et al. 1988). T cells may therefore be one of the sources of interferon-γ in human milk (BOCCI et al. 1993); EGLINTON et al. 1994). There is no evidence that other cytokines are spontaneously produced by leukocytes in human milk (GAROFALO et al. 1995; RUDLOFF et al. 1992; SKANSÉN-SAPHIR et al. 1993), although tumor necrosis factor-α (RUDLOFF et al. 1992), interleukin (IL) 1β (MUNOZ et al. 1990), IL-6 (SAITO et al. 1991; RUDLOFF et al. 1993), IL-8 (PALKOWETZ et al. 1994), IL-10 (GAROFALO et al. 1995), transforming growth factor (SAITO et al. 1993; PALKOWETZ et al. 1994), granulocyte colony-stimulating factor (GILMORE et al. 1994), and macrophage colony-stimulating factor (HARA et al. 1995) have been detected in human milk. It is unknown, however, whether some of these cytokines were produced by the leukocytes during their sojourn in the mammary gland.

Table 2. Phenotypic features of T cells in human milk and blood demonstrated by flow cytometry: the increased relative frequencies (percentages) of T cells positive for HLA-DR, CD25 (interleukin-2 receptor), and CD45RO are consistent with cellular activation

CD3+ T cells	$HLA-DR^+$	$CD25^+$
Human milk	87 ± 5	15 ± 6
Human blood	10 ± 4	6 ± 2
$CD4^+$ T cells	$CD45RA^+$	$CD45RO^+$
Human milk	3 ± 3	~ 100
Human blood	50 ± 14	75 ± 7
$CD8^+$ T cells	$CD45RA^+$	$CD45RO^+$
Human milk	24 ± 10	92 ± 5
Human blood	82 ± 3	58 ± 14

6 In Vivo Fate of Human Milk Leukocytes in the Recipient Infant

The in vivo fate and function of activated leukocytes from human milk in the recipient infant are undetermined. Mucous membrane sites in the upper alimentary/respiratory tract would seem to be potential sites for the entry and action of human milk leukocytes. There is some evidence from experimental animal models that milk lymphocytes enter tissues of the neonatal animal (Head et al. 1977; Hughes et al. 1988; Jain et al. 1989; Weiler et al. 1983). There has been considerable interest in the possibility that cellular immunity can also be transferred to the recipient human infant via sensitized T cells in human milk. Some observations suggest that cellular immunity to tuberculosis (Pabst et al. 1989) or to schistosomal antigens (Eissa et al. 1989) may be transferred to the infant by breastfeeding, but this remains controversial (Keller et al. 1987). In this regard, HLA types, the repertoire of T cell antigen receptors, and the special phenotypic features of T cells may be markers of maternal T cells transferred to the recipient infant through human milk. The rationale for possible example is as follows: Only small numbers of memory T cells are present in peripheral blood during the newborn period and early infancy (Hayward et al. 1989; Maccario et al. 1993; Chheda et al. 1996), but it is unclear whether the infants that were investigated were breastfed or not. Since T cells in milk are $CD45RO^+$, the occurrence of an increased number of $CD45RO^+$ T cells in human milk would suggest that some of the increment arises from a transfer of T cells from human milk.

7 Coda

The presence of living leukocytes suggests that human milk has certain characteristics of an immunologic tissue. These selected populations of leukocytes are induced to traffic and home to the mammary gland, exit through the parenchyma of the organ, and become activated. In contrast to elicited leukocytes at inflammatory sites, human milk leukocytes do not injure the mammary gland or the recipient infant.

If the results of cell transfer studies with human milk leukocytes in experimental animals are germane to humans, there is a strong prospect that these leukocytes aid in the defense of the recipient infant. Further characterization of the biology of the leukocytes in human milk is therefore desirable. Future studies may address (a) the ability of these maternal cells to resist the environmental conditions of the alimentary and respiratory tracts, their potential to interact and penetrate the epithelium of those sites, (b) the immunologic repertoire of $CD4^+$ and $CD8^+$ subpopulations of T cells in human milk, (c) ways in which these populations of milk leukocytes may influence and be influenced by the mucosal defense system of the developing recipient infant, and (d) whether these transferred cells have systemic effects. Such experiments may lead to a more profound understanding of the relationship between maternal leukocytes and the other elements of the complex defense system in human milk and the immune system of the developing infant.

References

Bertotto A, Castellucci G, Fabietti G, Scalise F, Vaccaro R (1990a) Lymphocytes bearing the T cell receptor gamma delta in human breast milk. Arch Dis Child 65:1274–1275

Bertotto A, Gerli R, Fabietti G, Crupi S, Arcangeli C, Scalise F, Vaccaro R (1990b) Human breast milk T cells display the phenotype and functional characteristics of memory T cells. Eur J Immunol 20:1877–1880

Bertotto A, Gerli R, Castellucci G, Scalise F, Vaccaro R (1991) Human milk lymphocytes bearing the gamma/delta T-cell receptor are mostly delta TCS1-positive cells. Immunology 74:360–361

Bocci V, von Bremen K, Corradeschi F, Luzzi E, Paulesu L (1993) Presence of interferon-γ and interleukin-6 in colostrum of normal women. Lymphokine Cytokine Res 12:21–24

Buescher ES (1991) The effects of colostrum on neutrophil function: decreased deformatbility with increased cytoskeletal-associated actin. In: Mestecky J, Blair C, Ogra P (eds) Immunology of milk and the neonate. Plenum, New York, pp 131–136

Chheda S, Palkowetz KH, Rassin DK, Schmalstieg FC, Goldman AS (1996) Deficient quantitative expression of CD45 Isoforms on $CD4^+$ and $CD8^+$ T-cell subpopulations and subsets of $CD45RA^{low}$ $CD45RA^{low}$ T cells in newborn blood. Biol Neonate 69:128–132

Clemente J, Leyva-Cobian F, Hernandez M, Garcia-Alonso A (1986) Intracellular immunoglobulins in human milk macrophages. Ultrastructural localization and factors affecting the kinetics of immunoglobulin release. Int Arch Allergy Appl Immunol 80:291–299

Cole F, Schneegener EE, Lichtenberg NA, Colten HR (1982) Complement biosynthesis in human breast milk macrophages and blood monocytes. Immunology 46:429–441

Crago SS, Prince SJ, Pretlow TG, McGhee JR, Mestecky J (1979) Human colostral cells. I. Separation and characterization. Clin Exp Immunol 38:585–597

Cummings NP, Neifert MR, Pabst MJ, Johnston RB Jr (1985) Oxidative metabolic response and microbicidal activity of human milk macrophages: effect of lipopolysaccharide and muramyl dipeptide. Infect Immun 49:435–439

Dohlsten M, Hedlung G, Sjogren H-O, Carlsson R (1988) Two subsets of $CD4^+$ T helper cells differing in kinetics and capacities to produce interleukin 2 and interferon-γ can be defined by the Leu-18 and UCHL1 monoclonal antibodies. Eur J Immunol 18:1173–1178

Donné A (1837) Du lait et en particulier de celui de nourrices, considéré sous le rapport de ses bonnes et de ses mavaises qualités nutritives et de ses altérations. Paris, Rue de Condé, no 15; Les Libraires de Médecine, Chevalier, Palais Royal, no 163

Eglinton B, Roberton DM, Cummins AG (1994) Phenotype of T cells, their soluble receptor levels, and cytokine profile of human breast milk. Immunol Cell Biol 72:306–313

Eissa AM, Saad MA, Ghaffar AK, el-Sharkaway IM, Kamal KA (1989) Transmission of lymphocyte responsiveness to schistosomal antigens by breast feeding. Trop Geogr Med 41:208–212

Furukawa M, Narahara H, Yasuda K, Johnston JM (1993) Presence of platelet-activating factor-acetylhydrolase in milk. J Lipid Res 34:1603–1609

Garofalo R, Chheda S, Mei F, Palkowetz KH, Rudloff HE, Schmalstieg FC Jr, Goldman AS (1995) Interleukin-10 in human milk. Pediatr Res 37:444–449

Gibson CE, Eglinton BA, Penttila IA, Cummins AG (1991) Phenotype and activation of milk-derived and peripheral blood lymphocytes from normal and coeliac subjects. Immunol Cell Biol 69:387–393

Gilmore WS, McKelvey-Martin VJ, Rutherford S, Strain JJ, Kell M, Miller S (1994) Human milk contains granulocyte-colony stimulating factor (G-CSF). Eur J Clin Nutr 48:222–224

Goldblum RM, Ahlstedt S, Carlsson B, Hanson LÅ, Jodal U, Lindin-Janson C, Sohl A (1975) Antibody forming cells in human colostrum after oral immunisation. Nature 257:797–798

Goldman AS, Smith CW (1973) Host resistance factors in human milk. J Pediatr 82:1082–1090

Goldman AS, Thorpe LW, Goldblum RM, Hanson LÅ (1986) Anti-inflammatory properties of human milk. Acta Paediatr Scand 75:689–695

Goldman AS (1993) The immune system of human milk. Antimicrobial, antiinflammatory, and immunomodulating properties, Pediatr Infect Dis J 12:664–672
Hara T, Irie K, Saito S, Tchijo M, Yamada M, Yanai N, Miyazaki S (1995) Identification of macrophage colony-stimulating factor in human milk and mammary epithelial cells, Pediatr Res 37:437–443
Hawes CS, Jones WR (1985) Human milk cell migration and production of moncyte chemotactic factor: lack of activity. Pediatr Res 19:996–999
Hayward AR, Lee J, Beverley PCL (1989) Ontogeny of expression of UCHL1 antigen on TcR-1$^+$ (CD4/8) and TcRδ^+ T cells. Eur J Immunol 19:771–773
Head JR, Beer AE, Billingham RE (1977) Significance of the cellular component of the maternal immunologic endowment in milk. Transplant Proc 9:1465–1471
Hughes A, Brock JH, Parrott DM, Cockburn F (1988) The interaction of infant formula with macrophages: effect on phagocytic activity, relationship to expression of class II MHC antigen and survival of orally administered macrophages in the neonatal gut. Immunology 64:213–218
Jain L, Vidyasagar D, Xanthou M, Ghai V, Shimada S, Blend M (1989) In vivo distribution of human milk leucocytes after ingestion by newborn baboons. Arch Dis Child 64:930–933
Keeney SE, Schmalstieg FC, Palkowetz KH, Rudloff HE, Schmalstieg FC Jr, Goldman AS (1993) Activated neutrophils and neutrophil activators in human milk. Increased expression of CD11b and decreased expression of L-selectin. J Leukoc Biol 54:97–104
Keller MA, Kidd RM, Bryson YJ, Turner JL, Carter J (1981) Lymphokine production by human milk lymphocytes. Infect Immun 32:632–636
Keller MA, Rodriguez AL, Alvarez S, Wheeler NC, Reisinger D (1987) Transfer of tuberculin immunity from mother to infant. In: Goldman AS, Atkinson SA, Hanson LÅ (eds) The effects of human milk on the recipient infant. Plenum, New York, pp 261–267 (Human lactation 3)
Kohl S, Pickering LK, Cleary TG, Steinmetz KD, Loo LS (1980) Human colostral cytotoxicity. II. Relative defects in colostral leukocyte cytotoxicity and inhibition of peripheral blood leukocyte cytoxicity by colostrum. J Infect Dis 142:884–891
Le Deist, de Saint-Basile G, Angeles-Cano E, Griscelli C (1986) Prostaglandin E2 and plasminogin activators in human milk and their secretion by milk macrophages. Am J Reprod Immunol Microbiol 11:6–10
Maccario R, Chirico G, Mingrat G, Aricò M, Lanfranchi A, Montagna D, Moretta A, Rondin G (1993) Expression of CD45R0 antigen on the surface of resting and activated neonatal T lymphocyte subsets. Biol Neonate 64:346–353
Munoz C, Endres S, van der Meer J, Schlesinger L, Arevalo M, Dinarello C (1990) Interleukin-1β in human colostrum. Res Immunol 141:501–513
Mushtaha AA, Schmalstieg FC, Hughes T Jr, Rajaraman S, Rudloff HE, Goldman AS (1989) Chemokinetic agents for monocytes in human milk: possible role of tumor necrosis factor-alpha. Pediatr Res 25:629–633
Oksenberg JR, Persitz E, Brautbar C (1985) Cellular immunity in human milk. Am J Reprod Immunol Microbiol 8:125–129
Özkaragoz F, Rudloff HE, Rajaraman S, Mushtaha AA, Schmalstieg FC, Goldman AS (1988) The motility of human milk macrophages in collagen gels. Pediatr Res 23:449–452
Pabst HF, Godel J, Grace M, Cho H, Spady DW (1989) Effect of breast-feeding on immune response to BCG vaccination. Lancet 1:295–297
Palkowetz KH, Royer CL, Garofalo R, Rudloff HE, Schmalstieg FC Jr, Goldman AS (1994) Production of interleukin-6 and interleukin-8 by human mammary gland epithelial cells. J Reprod Immunol 26:57–64
Roux ME, McWilliams M, Phillips-Quagliata JM, Weisz-Carrington P, Lamm ME (1977) Origin of IgA secretory plasma cells in the mammary gland. J Exp Med 146:1311–1322
Rudloff HE, Schmalstieg FC, Mushtaha AA, Palkowetz KH, Liu SK, Goldman AS (1992) Tumor necrosis factor-α in human milk. Pediatr Res 31:29–33
Rudloff HE, Schmalstieg FC, Palkowetz KH, Paszkiewicz EJ, Goldman AS (1993) Interleukin-6 in human milk. J Reprod Immunol 23:13–20
Saito S, Maruyama M, Kato Y, Moriyama I, Ichijo M (1991) Detection of Il-6 in human milk and its involvement in IgA production. J Reprod Immunol 20:267–276
Saito S, Yoshida M, Ichijo M, Ishizaka S, Tsujii T (1993) Transforming growth factor-beta (TGF-β) in human milk. Clin Exp Immunol 94:220–224
Schnorr KL, Pearson LD (1983) Intestinal absorption of maternal leukocytes by newborn lambs. J Reprod Immunol 6:329–337

Skansén-Saphir U, Linfors A, Andersson U (1993) Cytokine production in mononuclear cells of human milk studied at the single-cell level. Pediatr Res 34:213–216
Smith CW, Goldman AS (1968) The cells of human colostrum. I. In vitro studies of morphology and functions. Pediatr Res 2:103–109
Smith CW, Goldman As (1970) Interactions of lymphocytes and macrophages from human colostrum: characteristics of the interacting lymphocyte. J Reticuloendothel Soc 8:91–104
Smith CW, Goldman AS, Yates RD (1971) Interactions of lymphocytes and macrophages from human colostrum: electron microscopic studies of the interacting lymphocyte. Exp Cell Res 69:409–415
Speer CP, Schatz R, Gahr M (1985) Function of breast milk macrophages. Monatsschr Kinderheilkd 133:913–917
Speer CP, Gahr M, Pabst MJ (1986) Phagocytosis-associated oxidative metabolism in human milk macrophages. Acta Paediatr Scand 75:444–451
Subiza JL, Rodriguez C, Figueredo A, Mateos P, Alvarez R, de la Concha EG (1988) Impaired production and lack of secretion of interleukin 1 by human breast milk macrophages. Clin Exp Immunol 71:493–496
Thorpe LW, Rudloff HE, Powell LC, Goldman AS (1986) Decreased response of human milk leukocytes to chemoattractant peptides. Pediatr Res 20:373–377
Tsuda H, Dickey WD, Goldman AS (1984a) Separation of human colostral macrophages and neutrophils on gelatin and collagen-serum substrata. Cell Struct Funct 8:367–371
Tsuda H, Takeshige K, Shibata Y, Minakami S (1984b) Oxygen metabolism of human colostral macrophages. J Biochem 95:1237–1245
Van Leeuwenhoek A (1695) Epistola 106. Arcana naturae detecta delphis batavorum. Apud Henricum a Krooneveld
Weiler IL, Hickler W, Spenger R (1983) Demonstration that milk cells invade the neonatal mouse. Am J Reprod Immunol 4:95–98
Weisz-Carrington P, Roux ME, McWilliams M, Phillips-Quaglita JM, Lamm ME (1978) Hormonal induction of the secretory immune system in the mammary gland. Proc Natl Acad Sci USA 75:2928–2932
Wirt D, Adkins LT, Palkowetz KH, Schmalstieg FC, Goldman AS (1992) Activated-memory T cells in human milk. Cytometry 13:282–290

Subject Index

Current Topics in Microbiology and Immunology

Volumes published since 1989 (and still available)

Vol. 182: **Potter, Michael; Melchers, Fritz (Eds.):** Mechanisms in B-Cell Neoplasia. 1992. 188 figs. XX, 499 pp. ISBN 3-540-55658-3

Vol. 183: **Dimmock, Nigel J.:** Neutralization of Animal Viruses. 1993. 10 figs. VII, 149 pp. ISBN 3-540-56030-0

Vol. 184: **Dunon, Dominique; Mackay, Charles R.; Imhof, Beat A. (Eds.):** Adhesion in Leukocyte Homing and Differentiation. 1993. 37 figs. IX, 260 pp. ISBN 3-540-56756-9

Vol. 185: **Ramig, Robert F. (Ed.):** Rotaviruses. 1994. 37 figs. X, 380 pp. ISBN 3-540-56761-5

Vol. 186: **zur Hausen, Harald (Ed.):** Human Pathogenic Papillomaviruses. 1994. 37 figs. XIII, 274 pp. ISBN 3-540-57193-0

Vol. 187: **Rupprecht, Charles E.; Dietzschold, Bernhard; Koprowski, Hilary (Eds.):** Lyssaviruses. 1994. 50 figs. IX, 352 pp. ISBN 3-540-57194-9

Vol. 188: **Letvin, Norman L.; Desrosiers, Ronald C. (Eds.):** Simian Immunodeficiency Virus. 1994. 37 figs. X, 240 pp. ISBN 3-540-57274-0

Vol. 189: **Oldstone, Michael B. A. (Ed.):** Cytotoxic T-Lymphocytes in Human Viral and Malaria Infections. 1994. 37 figs. IX, 210 pp. ISBN 3-540-57259-7

Vol. 190: **Koprowski, Hilary; Lipkin, W. Ian (Eds.):** Borna Disease. 1995. 33 figs. IX, 134 pp. ISBN 3-540-57388-7

Vol. 191: **ter Meulen, Volker; Billeter, Martin A. (Eds.):** Measles Virus. 1995. 23 figs. IX, 196 pp. ISBN 3-540-57389-5

Vol. 192: **Dangl, Jeffrey L. (Ed.):** Bacterial Pathogenesis of Plants and Animals. 1994. 41 figs. IX, 343 pp. ISBN 3-540-57391-7

Vol. 193: **Chen, Irvin S. Y.; Koprowski, Hilary; Srinivasan, Alagarsamy; Vogt, Peter K. (Eds.):** Transacting Functions of Human Retroviruses. 1995. 49 figs. IX, 240 pp. ISBN 3-540-57901-X

Vol. 194: **Potter, Michael; Melchers, Fritz (Eds.):** Mechanisms in B-cell Neoplasia. 1995. 152 figs. XXV, 458 pp. ISBN 3-540-58447-1

Vol. 195: **Montecucco, Cesare (Ed.):** Clostridial Neurotoxins. 1995. 28 figs. XI., 278 pp. ISBN 3-540-58452-8

Vol. 196: **Koprowski, Hilary; Maeda, Hiroshi (Eds.):** The Role of Nitric Oxide in Physiology and Pathophysiology. 1995. 21 figs. IX, 90 pp. ISBN 3-540-58214-2

Vol. 197: **Meyer, Peter (Ed.):** Gene Silencing in Higher Plants and Related Phenomena in Other Eukaryotes. 1995. 17 figs. IX, 232 pp. ISBN 3-540-58236-3

Vol. 198: **Griffiths, Gillian M.; Tschopp, Jürg (Eds.):** Pathways for Cytolysis. 1995. 45 figs. IX, 224 pp. ISBN 3-540-58725-X

Vol. 199/I: **Doerfler, Walter; Böhm, Petra (Eds.):** The Molecular Repertoire of Adenoviruses I. 1995. 51 figs. XIII, 280 pp. ISBN 3-540-58828-0

Vol. 199/II: **Doerfler, Walter; Böhm, Petra (Eds.):** The Molecular Repertoire of Adenoviruses II. 1995. 36 figs. XIII, 278 pp. ISBN 3-540-58829-9

Vol. 199/III: **Doerfler, Walter; Böhm, Petra (Eds.):** The Molecular Repertoire of Adenoviruses III. 1995. 51 figs. XIII, 310 pp. ISBN 3-540-58987-2

Vol. 200: **Kroemer, Guido; Martinez-A., Carlos (Eds.):** Apoptosis in Immunology. 1995. 14 figs. XI, 242 pp. ISBN 3-540-58756-X

Vol. 201: **Kosco-Vilbois, Marie H. (Ed.):** An Antigen Depository of the Immune System: Follicular Dendritic Cells. 1995. 39 figs. IX, 209 pp. ISBN 3-540-59013-7

Vol. 202: **Oldstone, Michael B. A.; Vitković, Ljubiša (Eds.):** HIV and Dementia. 1995. 40 figs. XIII, 279 pp. ISBN 3-540-59117-6

Vol. 203: **Sarnow, Peter (Ed.):** Cap-Independent Translation. 1995. 31 figs. XI, 183 pp. ISBN 3-540-59121-4

Vol. 204: **Saedler, Heinz; Gierl, Alfons (Eds.):** Transposable Elements. 1995. 42 figs. IX, 234 pp. ISBN 3-540-59342-X

Vol. 205: **Littman, Dan R. (Ed.):** The CD4 Molecule. 1995. 29 figs. XIII, 182 pp. ISBN 3-540-59344-6

Vol. 206: **Chisari, Francis V.; Oldstone, Michael B. A. (Eds.):** Transgenic Models of Human Viral and Immunological Disease. 1995. 53 figs. XI, 345 pp. ISBN 3-540-59341-1

Vol. 207: **Prusiner, Stanley B. (Ed.):** Prions Prions Prions. 1995. 42 figs. VII, 163 pp. ISBN 3-540-59343-8

Vol. 208: **Farnham, Peggy J. (Ed.):** Transcriptional Control of Cell Growth. 1995. 17 figs. IX, 141 pp. ISBN 3-540-60113-9

Vol. 209: **Miller, Virginia L. (Ed.):** Bacterial Invasiveness. 1996. 16 figs. IX, 115 pp. ISBN 3-540-60065-5

Vol. 210: **Potter, Michael; Rose, Noel R. (Eds.):** Immunology of Silicones. 1996. 136 figs. XX, 430 pp. ISBN 3-540-60272-0

Vol. 211: **Wolff, Linda; Perkins, Archibald S. (Eds.):** Molecular Aspects of Myeloid Stem Cell Development. 1996. 98 figs. XIV, 298 pp. ISBN 3-540-60414-6

Vol. 212: **Vainio, Olli; Imhof, Beat A. (Eds.):** Immunology and Developmental Biology of the Chicken. 1996. 43 figs. IX, 281 pp. ISBN 3-540-60585-1

Vol. 213/I: **Günthert, Ursula; Birchmeier, Walter (Eds.):** Attempts to Understand Metastasis Formation I. 1996. 35 figs. XV, 293 pp. ISBN 3-540-60680-7

Vol. 213/II: **Günthert, Ursula; Birchmeier, Walter (Eds.):** Attempts to Understand Metastasis Formation II. 1996. 33 figs. XV, 288 pp. ISBN 3-540-60681-5

Vol. 213/III: **Günthert, Ursula; Schlag, Peter M.; Birchmeier, Walter (Eds.):** Attempts to Understand Metastasis Formation III. 1996. 14 figs. XV, 262 pp. ISBN 3-540-60682-3

Vol. 214: **Kräusslich, Hans-Georg (Ed.):** Morphogenesis and Maturation of Retroviruses. 1996. 34 figs. XI, 344 pp. ISBN 3-540-60928-8

Vol. 215: **Shinnick, Thomas M. (Ed.):** Tuberculosis. 1996. 46 figs. XI, 307 pp. ISBN 3-540-60985-7

Vol. 216: **Rietschel, Ernst Th.; Wagner, Hermann (Eds.):** Pathology of Septic Shock. 1996. 34 figs. X, 321 pp. ISBN 3-540-61026-X

Vol. 217: **Jessberger, Rolf; Lieber, Michael R. (Eds.):** Molecular Analysis of DNA Rearrangements in the Immune System. 1996. 43 figs. IX, 224 pp. ISBN 3-540-61037-5

Vol. 218: **Berns, Kenneth I.; Giraud, Catherine (Eds.):** Adeno-Associated Virus (AAV) Vectors in Gene Therapy. 1996. 38 figs. IX,173 pp. ISBN 3-540-61076-6

Vol. 219: **Gross, Uwe (Ed.):** Toxoplasma gondii. 1996. 31 figs. XI, 274 pp. ISBN 3-540-61300-5

Vol. 220: **Rauscher, Frank J. III; Vogt, Peter K. (Eds.):** Chromosomal Translocations and Oncogenic Transcription Factors. 1997. 28 figs. XI, 166 pp. ISBN 3-540-61402-8

Vol. 221: **Kastan, Michael B. (Ed.):** Genetic Instability and Tumorigenesis. 1997. 12 figs.VII, 180 pp. ISBN 3-540-61518-0

Springer and the environment

At Springer we firmly believe that an international science publisher has a special obligation to the environment, and our corporate policies consistently reflect this conviction.

We also expect our business partners – paper mills, printers, packaging manufacturers, etc. – to commit themselves to using materials and production processes that do not harm the environment. The paper in this book is made from low- or no-chlorine pulp and is acid free, in conformance with international standards for paper permanency.

Springer

FSC
www.fsc.org
MIX
Papier aus verantwortungsvollen Quellen
Paper from responsible sources
FSC® C105338

If you have any concerns about our products,
you can contact us on
ProductSafety@springernature.com

In case Publisher is established outside the EU,
the EU authorized representative is:
Springer Nature Customer Service Center GmbH
Europaplatz 3, 69115 Heidelberg, Germany

Printed by Libri Plureos GmbH
in Hamburg, Germany